W9-CAH-594

17 53

PRAISE FOR DREENA BURTON

"Combining a simple design with oodles of valuable veggie cooking info and mouth-watering recipes, Burton's latest cookbook features 'celebration' recipes and is every bit as good as her previous books, the now-classic *The Everyday Vegan* and the impressive follow-up *Vive le Vegan!*. . . . Vegan cooking is always a celebration when Burton's books are in the kitchen." —*Monday Magazine*

"You don't have to actually be a vegan to enjoy Dreena Burton's cookbooks and to make them a part of your usual kitchen library. This is healthy, nutritious cooking suitable for a family or anyone interested in eating for optimum health." —*January Magazine*

"Dreena has the know-how and a knack for whipping up inviting, festive dishes in minutes that anyone can enjoy as healthful weekday fare. . . . her Gimme Chimis is a mouth-watering creation that features nutritious ingredients in a south-of-the-border-style sauce with a touch of fire." —*Vegetarians in Paradise*

LET THEM EAT

Vegan!

ALSO BY DREENA BURTON

The Everyday Vegan

Vive le Vegan!

Eat, Drink & Be Vegan

LET THEM EAT
Vegan!

• • •

*200 Deliciously Satisfying Plant-Powered
Recipes for the Whole Family*

Dreena Burton

Da Capo
∞
LIFE
LONG

A MEMBER OF THE PERSEUS BOOKS GROUP

Newmarket Public Library

Copyright © 2012 by Dreena Burton
Photos by Hannah Kaminsky

All rights reserved. No part of this publication may be reproduced, stored in a retrieval
system, or transmitted, in any form or by any means, electronic, mechanical,
photocopying, recording, or otherwise, without the prior written permission of the
publisher. Printed in the United States of America. For information, address Da Capo
Press, 44 Farnsworth Street, 3rd Floor Boston, MA 02210.

Designed by Timm Bryson
Set in 10.5 point Warnock Pro by the Perseus Books Group

Cataloging-in-Publication data for this book is available from the Library of Congress.

First Da Capo Press edition 2012
ISBN: 978-0-7382-1561-7

Published by Da Capo Press
A Member of the Perseus Books Group
www.dacapopress.com

Note: The information in this book is true and complete to the best of our knowledge. This
book is intended only as an informative guide for those wishing to know more about
health issues. In no way is this book intended to replace, countermand, or conflict with the
advice given to you by your own physician. The ultimate decision concerning care should
be made between you and your doctor. We strongly recommend you follow his or her
advice. Information in this book is general and is offered with no guarantees on the part of
the authors or Da Capo Press. The authors and publisher disclaim all liability in
connection with the use of this book. The names and identifying details of people
associated with events described in this book have been changed. Any similarity to actual
persons is coincidental.

Da Capo Press books are available at special discounts for bulk purchases in the U.S. by
corporations, institutions, and other organizations. For more information, please contact
the Special Markets Department at the Perseus Books Group, 2300 Chestnut Street, Suite
200, Philadelphia, PA, 19103, or call (800) 810-4145, ext. 5000, or e-mail
special.markets@perseusbooks.com.

10 9 8 7 6 5 4 3 2

JUL 18 2012

With love to Charlotte, Bridget, and Hope.

Contents

11 *Dreena Dazs* 257

Plant Power: Your Time Has Come

When I started writing vegan cookbooks and later blogging about my journeys as a plant-powered mom and home cook, *vegan* was still kind of a dirty word—one synonymous with deprivation—and signaled an image of sprouts and a slab of wan tofu. Thankfully, in the past decade or so, veganism has come a long way. I've seen big changes in the food offerings and how we eat. When I first began eating vegan, there were very few substitutes for dairy products and meat and just a few nondairy milks. So we vegans had to be creative with the basics: beans, grains, nuts, seeds, vegetables, and fruit. I continued to create recipes in this framework while noticing more and more vegan convenience foods become available. The surge of animal-free packaged foods was accompanied by a swell of vegan support and excitement: We could have treats and substitutes that were as good as (or sometimes better than) their nonvegan equivalents. For a period of time, attention focused on these processed foods and recipes using refined ingredients and analogues, showing how exceptional or "sinful" animal-free foods could be.

But of course, there's always a rub: While these foods might qualify as vegan, they aren't always healthy. I'm not entirely against these foods. I understand that meat and dairy substitutes help people adapt their meals within their cooking comfort zones. Plus, we can all enjoy convenient treats when the bulk of our diet is wholesome. As you'll soon see, I shamelessly enjoy my ice cream! And, our girls enjoy an occasional veggie dog when we have burger night. But, we don't rely on vegan meats and other processed foods for our regular meals. My recipes won't have you veganizing a ground meat–based recipe with veggie ground round, or using vegan sour cream to make an artichoke dip. The tricky thing with processed foods is, because they are so convenient, they can comprise the bulk of the vegan diet, while the real (whole) foods are abandoned.

The reverse should be true. Whole foods, and lower-fat recipes based on plant power, should comprise 90 percent or more of our diet (optimally 100 percent, but I'm a realist and appreciate that most people need a little wiggle room). My own meals are filled with greens and beans, nuts and whole grains, and an abundance of veggies. When I create recipes, they unfold with health in mind and plant-powered foods in practice.

In recent years, I've seen the shift away from vegan junk foods back to the healthier basics. And, thanks to greater awareness of veganism in popular culture, we are now seeing folks who would never before have a plate without a piece of meat on it, coming to the table and leaving completely satisfied.

Eating vegan is about so much more than not eating animal foods. We know the importance of choosing whole plant foods, and largely organic and local foods, over highly processed foods. That's the health power of a plant-based diet. Eating a whole-foods vegan diet—with respect for lower-fat recipes featuring colorful, nutrient-dense vegetables and fruit, whole grains, beans, nuts, and seeds—is where it's at. These foods are the basis for delicious, nourishing, and, satisfying meals for everyone at the table—from the pickiest toddler (trust me on this one) to the green smoothie–drink-

ing spouse (trust me on this one, too). When we focus our diet on plant power, we feel better, look better, and want to do better. Before long, we find ourselves getting hooked on healthy foods. And why wouldn't we? When they taste delicious, make us feel good, improve our overall health, and are cruelty free—what's not to love?

Much like the recipes in my previous books, these recipes represent the nutritious (and delicious) snacks and meals our family eats. These recipes take it a step further, however. Unlike in my previous books, you won't find any white flour here—not even for cakes or cookies. And, while my cooking roots began with the beans, grains, nuts, and veggies basics, I provide more variety than ever before with this book. When I first started eating vegan, I, too, fell in the trap (albeit for a short while) of eating too many white-flour-based products such as pasta and bread. Now my recipes eschew white flour, and my cooking overall is more diverse, with a variety of vegetables and leafy greens, plenty of legumes, nuts and seeds, and whole grains. And, while some recipes are on the richer side, many more are lower in fat, so you can eat them every day.

These recipes are the kind of real-food nutritious recipes that everyone is looking for. Whether you are a busy single with a developing career and looking to recharge and renew your energy through a healthier diet, or need wholesome meals to nourish your active family, or have decided that dietary change is critical to sustain your vitality or change some developed health condition—this book will deliver the goods.

Preparing homemade food is also important. When you prepare your meals from whole, plant-based ingredients, you connect with your food. It is important to me that children see that dinner comes from washing, chopping, and cooking. It's equally important that we sit to dinner and take time to enjoy a home-cooked meal (even if it means much squirming, spilled drinks, and sister rivalry)! I see the energy and strength our good food gives our children. My children are plant powered—so much that I wouldn't mind a dimmer switch once in a while! And they have come to appreciate how real food tastes. Of course, they still enjoy treats—just like other children—but they have often discarded a lollipop because of its artificial flavorings, in lieu of something tastier and more wholesome.

Over the years, my recipes have highlighted unprocessed and whole-foods ingredients. This book will give you even more—more real-food recipes, plus plenty of allergen-free options specific to wheat, gluten, and soy. When I started baking with whole-grain flours, I branched out beyond wheat, and found I often enjoyed the results that alternative flours produced in baked goods. In this book, all of my recipes—sweet and savory—are either wheat free or have wheat-free substitutions (for some I offer an optional switch back to using wheat flour, for added convenience). Many are gluten free. I also have many soy-free and raw recipes. Although it's been said, "You can't please everyone," this book truly has a little something for everyone!

Beyond the recipes, this book gives you tips, techniques, notes, and lots of kitchen chatter—because, when I create a recipe I think of the people I can share it with. What might they need to know about the ingredients? Or specific techniques or substitutions? Since I enjoy providing oodles of notes for recipes (and my readers tell me they love them), you'll find lots of my "kitchen talk" through my recipes. From basic "Ingredients 411" to "Allergy-Free or Bust!" and "Savvy Subs and Adds" (see page xx for a full list), you'll find clear notes and suggestions that I learned while making these dishes time and again.

I also realize that some of you are looking for help with other aspects of food preparation, such as packed lunches and wheat-free baking tips. There are several informational sections at the front and back of the book: There is an in-depth pantry-meets-glossary—your "Plant-Powered Pantry" on page xxiii and "Plant-Powered Baking Notes" on page 170. When it comes to family matters, I discuss some of my experiences raising wee ones in "Powering the Vegan Family," page 269, and give you reams of ideas for packing lunches in "Plant-Powered Lunch Box," page 273. Finally, if you are trying to eat more nutrient-dense leafy greens, I give you two sections: "Let Them Eat Greens," page 279, with ideas on how to select, prep, and include more greens in your meals throughout the day . . . and "'Go Green' with Smoothies," page 26, to answer just about every question you might have on making delicious green smoothies to energize your day.

One final thing before you flip ahead: See the lists on xviii–xix for a quick-hit list of some specific examples of recipes that can cover your (wheat-free/gluten-free/oil-free/vegan sub-free/real-food-seeking/green-and-bean-loving/taste bud–pleasing) needs.

With all that, my wish is that these recipes entice your taste buds while nourishing your body and mind . . . that you find true favorites within these pages, and that maybe (hopefully) this book becomes well loved and covered with plant-powered splatters and stains! Let them eat vegan!

Before Strapping On That Apron
Read the Recipe First (Please!)

All too often, the excitement to dive into a new recipe turns into getting ahead of

So You Need . . .	I've Got You Covered With . . .
Everyday tips for eating more leafy greens?	"'Go Green' with Smoothies," page 26, and "Let Them Eat Greens," page 279
A salad with a creamy, rich, oil-free dressing that will convert even the most severe kale nay-sayers?	Kale-slaw with Curried Almond Dressing
Creamy dressings, sauces, and desserts that do not use vegan sour cream, cream cheese, or margarines?	Chapter 3
A tasty alternative to Parmesan that is soy free?	Brazil Nut Parmezan
A holiday main dish that is not a tofu turkey or any other shaped tofu loaf?	Winter Veg Chickpea Potpie and Festive Chickpea Tart
Creative, satisfying, bean recipes?	Jerk Chickpeas, Moroccan Bean Stew with Sweet Potatoes, Fragrant Kidney Bean Lentil Dal, Smoky Sweet Potato and Black Bean Salad, Thai Chickpea Almond Curry, Yellow Sweet Potato Chickpea Pie with Basil, and so on!
Veggie burgers that don't fall apart?	Nutty Veggie Burgers and Chickpea Pumpkin Seed Burgers . . . for starters!
Cookies that are healthier, with no white flours, and that are wheat free and gluten free?	Chapter 9

yourself and realizing you don't have an ingredient, have forgotten to include an ingredient, or have skipped a step. Not only does this make for (usually) a less than fab result, it is most irksome in the moment! Prevent the stress by reading through the recipe at least once before getting going. Seems obvious, but we've all been caught scoffing ourselves after realizing we've made a flub. Prevent the panic and read before you cook.

Readers of my previous books tell me they love the tips I give with every recipe; some say it's as if I'm in the kitchen with them, "talking them through the recipe." That's exactly what I've hoped to do with

So You Need . . .	**I've Got You Covered With . . .**
All right, really healthy cookies for your kids, with little or no sugar?	Wholesome Oat Snackles!, Cocoa Cookie Dough Balls, Pecan Date Nibblers, Breakfast Cookies . . . and more!
A gluten-free piecrust recipe that is dynamite enough to become your go-to pie crust recipe?	Gluten-Free Piecrust
Wheat-free cakes?	Chapter 10
Gluten-free cakes?	Chapter 10
Okay, well how about a sugar-free wheat-free cake?	Sugar-Free Chocolate Cake
Cake frostings that are soy free?	Chapter 10
Cake frostings that are margarine free?	Chapter 10
Luscious ice-cream recipes that are easy and soy free?	Chapter 11
Healthier and lower-fat versions of some of your favorite foods?	Panfried Falafel Patties, Three-Bean Salad, To-Live-For Pecan Pie, Award-Winning Frosted B-raw-nies, Artichoke and White Bean Dip, Classic Caesar Dressing, Whole-Grain Chia Pancakes . . . and more!

my recipes—welcome the reader, bring confidence to the process, and make it fun to create delicious vegan food. These recipes are no exception. They might be the most "note heavy" of the bunch!

To clarify some of these notes, I've done something new in this book. First, since some tips specific to ingredients apply to more than one recipe (e.g., how to remove vanilla seeds from a vanilla bean), rather than repeat them over and over in several recipes, I've added a "Kitchen Buzz" note to that ingredient in the upcoming section "Plant-Powered Pantry." Whenever there is some chit-chat from me about an ingredient, it will be denoted with "see 'Plant-Powered Pantry'" in the ingredient listing.

Next, I've categorized my recipe ramblings! When I test recipes, I play with scenarios that my readers might be faced with. For instance: if you don't have a barbecue grill, how can you adjust for oven-baking the eggplant for Creamy Grilled Eggplant Dip . . . or how might you make nut-free substitutions to dig into Mac-oh-geez! . . . or how can you make a recipe more kid-friendly—or alternatively—more suited to the grown-ups? I've done (most of!) the work for you, and share the fruits of my labor through the notes, which are categorized as:

Adult-Minded: I give you suggestions for ingredients and seasonings to use to kick up the flavor profile for mature palates.

Allergy-Free or Bust! Most of my recipes are either inherently wheat free or gluten free. But where substitutions can be made

for these food allergies—as well as for soy, tree nuts, and peanuts—they will be noted here (in addition to the ingredient listing).

If This Apron Could Talk: If my apron could speak, this is what it would tell you—all the extras I want to share from my own experiences with the recipe, be it a technique, something quirky about an ingredient, how to expedite for quicker fixes—this is my free pass to really get chatty with you!

Ingredients 411: Extra information about a particular ingredient in a recipe—when to use less/more, how to treat the ingredient, and any other specific ingredient tips that you might have a question about in that recipe.

Kid-Friendly: If you have kiddos, you know that some spices won't fly and some ingredients might bomb. In that case, tweak the recipe by changing one ingredient, or substitute a technique to change the consistency, and make it a hit. I give you plenty of kid-friendly advice along the way, as my own crew have given me ample experimentation!

Make It More-ish! Who doesn't want to make a recipe more indulgent or saucier once in a while? This will give you some ideas to do just that!

Protein Power: This tip explains when an ingredient such as hemp seeds or beans can enhance a recipe and boost the protein. Also handy for when you're asked, "But where do you get your protein?" for the umpteenth time!

Savvy Subs and Adds: When I experiment, I try variations on ingredients within food groups, so you have that flexibility with your own cooking. Sometimes adjustments are needed with these substitutions or additions (e.g., swapping acidic ingredients, flours, nut butters, or leafy greens,) and so I elaborate on these.

Serving Suggestions: Readers often want to know, "What sauce, salad, side, or other dish can I couple with this recipe?" Here I give you some of my favorite pairings.

Get Prepped

Don't scamper around the kitchen midrecipe, looking for that new bottle of vanilla or that seldom-used sifter (that you know is in the cupboard somewhere). I'm a hypocrite, because I do this far too often. Every time, it stresses me out! We all have good excuses, but let's face it: It's much easier to get your gear in front of you on the counter—not only the ingredients but your measuring cups, bowls, knives, and other equipment. The next section has a rundown of cooking equipment and other notes that might be handy to get you all set to go.

Make the Recipe As Is . . . and Then Play

It's usually best to get the sense of the original recipe before experimenting and tossing in another few herbs and veggies, or changing a variety of flour. Sometimes we experiment in the moment because we don't have the required ingredient (if so, please read previous suggestion). To get the idea of how the original recipe should taste, first try it as is. I give extra notes and tips throughout each recipe to help you customize for dietary needs or seasoning preferences. Once you've tried it as is, then play around, to see if you like the recipe better with more lemon juice, less nut butter, more nuts, and so forth.

Note for oil and salt restrictions: Although it is a good idea to first try the recipe as is, if you have personal restrictions for oil and salt intakes, obviously please adjust the recipes as you need to. Most of my savory recipes use minimal amounts of added oil and just enough salt to round out flavors. The salt and oil can always be further reduced, however, if needed. Similarly, I use reduced amounts of sugar and oils in most of my baked goods, particularly for items such as muffins and cereals. The sweeter goodies are meant to be just that—treats for special occasions. Still, I have tested my heart out to give you the most bang for your health buck, using healthier flours that are wheat and gluten free, and less-refined sweeteners (and less of them). My approach to an enjoyable and healthy plant-based diet is to eat a lot of the good stuff (85 to 90 percent whole grains, legumes, vegetables, fruits, nuts, and seeds), and then you have some wiggle room (pants size included) for healthier indulgences.

Tools to Get the Cooking Job Done

Okay, got a cute apron? No? Really, yours is stodgy? Come on, splurge on something fun and frilly already! Unless of course you're a guy. Sure, you may have the stodgy one.

Besides that apron, what do you really need to get cooking? Mostly just your gumption and the food, but there are definitely some appliances that make your job a lot easier. These are my "can't-live-without" tools:

Blender. When I say I can't do without a blender, mostly I mean my Rambo-meets-blender, the Blendtec. Before my Blendtec came along, I was doing fine with my regular standing blender and immersion blender. Then I was introduced to the Blendtec and my world of blending changed. No longer do I burn out motors on immersion and jug blenders. No longer do I curse in the kitchen (fine, that's a lie). But, this high-powered blender deserves a shrine on my countertop, I love it that much. It can take on any monster green smoothie with any combination of chunky (and frozen) fruits and greens, and whizzes up in minutes raw desserts and dressings with nuts. I have joked that it is my fourth child. Our girls know the difference, of course. But they also know not to get in the way of me and my Blendtec. When I'm with that machine, I mean business!

Food processor. As much as I worship the power of my blender, I still use and love my food processor. It's just essential for grating vegetables (in larger quantities) and making large batches of dips such as hummus. If you are in the market for a food processor, I recommend one with a bowl that holds at least 12 cups. That way you can manage large batches of food effortlessly.

Immersion blender. Before the Blendtec joined our family, I used my immersion blender for quite a lot, including smoothies, dressings, sauces, soups, and more. However, I did expect too much at times, and did burn out a motor or two trying to blend raw-food dips (with hard nuts). Still, immersion blenders are very handy for certain applications, most notably soups and dressings. When you need to puree a soup, it is much faster, easier, and cleaner to simply immerse the wand in the pot than to transfer your soup to a standing blender. It is also great for vinaigrettes: It fits perfectly inside a jar or deep cup, and will whiz up your dressings in just seconds, with very little cleanup. (Take-away from this: minimal cleanup!)

Kitchen rasp. An inexpensive kitchen tool, and one of my favorites. The concept for kitchen rasps grew from a similar tool used in woodworking. They are positively fabulous for grating nutmeg and zesting citrus, and can also be used for grating chocolate, garlic, and ginger.

Mixer (and ice-cream maker attachment). I'll confess: I resisted using a mixer for a long time, because I always strive to offer recipes that can be made without too much fancy equipment. But, truth is, for certain things, such as frostings and stiffer cookie doughs, a mixer is pretty much essential. Sure, you can work it out yourself with elbow grease, but it makes the process very arduous, time consuming, and probably so unenjoyable that you won't repeat it. That's not the idea! Cooking and baking should be at least partially fun. I have a KitchenAid mixer, and the neat thing about this appliance is that an ice-cream maker attachment can be used with the base. The ice-cream bowl attachment sits in your freezer until you're ready to make sweet, luscious ice cream! Then you simply attach the bowl to the base of the mixer, and pop on a paddle attachment, and you're ready to churn. It's a beautiful thing.

Some other necessary items for the kitchen include:

- good knives (chef's knife in particular, and also some smaller sharp and serrated knives)
- heat-resistant spatula(s)
- wire whisk
- measuring cups/spoons (more than one set is useful)
- salad spinner
- grater
- stainless-steel or other quality set of pots and pans
- nonstick frying pan (two are useful, one for savory items such as burgers and other for such things as pancakes; brands with nontoxic coatings are available)
- metal baking pans and dishes (muffin pans, two 8-inch round cake pans, an 8-inch square pan, rimmed baking sheets)
- ovenproof glass/Pyrex bakeware (a few pie plates, a loaf dish, an 8 by 12-inch rectangular baking dish, and larger casserole dishes, preferably with lids

- springform pan (for cheesecakes and other cakes or pies)
- cooling racks
- cutting boards
- colander and strainers (a fine one for rinsing small grains and sifting baking agents)
- cake and/or cupcake caddy (if needing to transport birthday goodies!)
- parchment paper

Plant-Powered Pantry and Kitchen Buzz

Transforming how you eat requires more than recipes; some organization and planning is needed. But once you get into the swing of using and buying some new ingredients, it all becomes second nature.

This section gives you a comprehensive rundown of specific ingredients used in these recipes, including explanations of these foods and techniques on how best to use them within my recipes. While not an exhaustive list of foods you might find in any given vegan pantry, most of the core foods are covered.

Readers of my previous books have really enjoyed all the tips I give throughout recipes. Because some tips are applicable to an ingredient and repeat through more than one recipe, I have highlighted tips ("Kitchen Buzz") within specific ingredients here, rather than clutter the recipes with repetitive tips. As you go along, you will find notes in those recipes, with a reminder to "see 'Plant-Powered Pantry.'" This is usually to draw attention to a technical tip or helpful note about an ingredient, such as how to remove vanilla seeds from the bean pod.

Adzuki beans: Small, reddish beans with a slightly sweet flavor that digest more easily than other beans. Adzuki beans cook rather quickly (see "Guide to Cooking Beans," page 285).

Agar powder: Also called agar-agar, this powder is derived from seaweed and is used in place of gelatin. It has no flavor, can be easily dissolved in liquid, and gels upon cooling. Agar comes in different forms, including flakes and strands; I use the powdered form. Available in whole foods stores, Asian supermarkets, and some grocery stores.

Agave nectar: Pronounced "uh-gah-vay," this is a liquid sweetener made from the juice of the agave cactus plant native to Mexico. It has a mild flavor, more neutral than honey and maple syrup. In general, I prefer pure maple syrup and consider it a healthier sweetener. However, when a more neutral flavor is needed for baking or cooking, I will opt for agave nectar. Available in whole foods stores and some groceries.

Almond meal: Sometimes referred to as ground almonds, because that's basically what almond meal is—almonds that have been processed into a fine meal, almost like flour. Most almond meal is made from blanched almonds, with a creamy white color. But some brands are ground from whole unblanched almonds, and so it is flecked with pieces of the tan-colored almond skins.

Kitchen Buzz: You can buy almond meal in your grocery or health food store, but you can also make your own. Place whole almonds in a food processor and pulse until very crumbly—not too long or it will begin to turn into a paste.

Annie's Naturals Goddess Dressing: A brand of thick, flavorful, all-natural dressing that is tahini based and does not have any added sweeteners.

Apple cider vinegar: This light brown vinegar is made from fermented apples, and has a mild fruity taste. Look for organic, unpasteurized apple cider vinegar that has some edible sediment (known as "the mother") floating at the bottom of the bottle.

Applesauce: I keep jars of organic unsweetened applesauce on hand for use in baking. It adds moisture and some sweetness to baked goods, and allows you to use less added fat through oils or otherwise. Our children also love applesauce on their toasted waffles, after a slather of almond butter!

Arrowroot powder: This tasteless thickener comes from the root of a tropical plant, and substitutes equally for cornstarch. Like cornstarch, it dissolves in liquid then must be brought to a boil to activate as a thickening agent. When dissolved it is cloudy, but turns clear once cooked.

Artichoke hearts: This vegetable is the un-opened flower and stem of a thistle—who knew?! Most of us are familiar with artichoke hearts, the edible portion at the center of the artichoke. If you are able to find frozen artichokes, they are far superior in flavor and texture to that of canned. Marinated artichokes can sometimes be substituted in recipes, though they absorb a briny flavor from the marinade that might be strong, depending on use (you can always rinse and pat dry marinated artichokes to help remove some of the marinade).

Balsamic vinegar: A popular Italian vinegar that has a wonderfully sweet robust flavor and relatively mild acidity. Look for organic varieties without sulfites.

Bananas (fresh and frozen): It's useful to buy more bananas than you will eat for snacking. Once overripe, they become sweeter and can be used in many desserts, including ice cream, muffins, cookies, and pies. Also, once frozen, they make green smoothies sing (see "'Go Green' with Smoothies," page 26).

Kitchen Buzz: Peel and slice overripe bananas in and store in resealable plastic bags or containers in your freezer. Much as you might store batches of seasonal berries for the winter, keep a couple of bags/containers of sliced bananas at the ready for smoothies.

Barley (pearl and pot): This is a grain that many of us grew up with, eaten in soups and stews. Most people are familiar with pearl barley, which is slightly chewy but also slightly creamy. It is a more processed (but not nonnutritious) form of barley whereby the grain has been hulled and polished. This yields an ivory-colored grain that cooks quicker and is also a little less chewy than its unprocessed form. Pot barley is less processed than pearl barley, and while still polished, more of the bran layer is retained. As such, it takes a little longer to cook.

Barley flakes: Much as how rolled oats are made from whole oats, barley flakes are made from the whole barley grain. Available in natural foods stores, though rolled oats can typically be substituted.

Barley flour: From the barley grain, this flour is light in color and mild in flavor and works well in baking and in combination with other flours. Available in whole foods stores and some grocery stores.

Beans: Beans probably need no definition; however, they do need more attention! Rich in protein and fiber, and vitamins and minerals, beans are one of the corner stones of a healthful vegan diet. Super versatile, they can be made into burgers and dips and sauces and put into stews and soups and casseroles and pastas. Beans are sometimes called legumes, which includes all varieties of peas, beans, and lentils: green peas, red lentils, yellow beans, kidney beans, adzuki beans, chickpeas, split peas, mung beans, and snow peas . . . and so many more! Although I would love to cook all my beans from scratch (see "Guide to Cooking Beans," page 285), time does not always permit with three kiddos and a busy schedule. So, I keep canned and dried beans on hand, in varieties that I use frequently (chickpeas, black beans, kidney beans, cannellini, and/or navy beans). Look for certified BPA-free canned beans—Eden Organic is one such brand. Because lentils cook quickly without needing presoaking, I generally cook these from scratch, and keep a variety on hand (green, French, red).

Blackstrap molasses: A syrup produced during the final stage of boiling sugar cane juice to make sugar. It is dark brown, thick, and has a strong, slightly bitter flavor. Regular molasses can be substituted and is less bitter, although it is not as nutritious. I often use blackstrap molasses in soups and savory dishes, as well as in baking.

Bouillon cubes: If you don't make your own or buy packaged stock, vegan cubes are the way to go. I prefer the bouillon cubes for a couple of reasons: (1) it takes up little cupboard space (unlike aseptic-packaged stocks), and has a longer shelf life; and (2) I typically prefer the flavor of these cubes to aseptic-packaged brands. I like the Harvest Sun brand of bouillon cubes, but there are other vegan bouillon cubes that will work well in these recipes.

Kitchen Buzz: For usage, one cube mixed with 2 cups of water equals 2 cups of stock, so you can halve cubes if needed and use with 1 cup of water to yield 1 cup of stock.

Brown basmati rice: Unhulled, thus retaining more fiber, brown basmati rice takes longer to cook than white basmati (see "Guide to Cooking Grains," page 283). Brown basmati is light and dry when cooked, not sticky like other varieties. The grain lengthens as it cooks and has a delicate nutty, buttery flavor and an aroma similar to popcorn. Available in health food stores and grocery stores.

Brown lentils: These are also called green lentils, and are the most common variety of lentils you see in stores. They are khaki in color, about the size of green peas, but shaped like flat disks. They have a pleasant earthy flavor and cook quickly (about 25 minutes). Like all varieties of lentils, they do not need to be soaked or precooked. Before using lentils, rinse to remove any small stones or particles.

Brown rice syrup: A thick, light brown sweetener made from rice; it sometimes also contains barley malt. It is less sweet than honey or sugar, and its sugars are absorbed more slowly in the bloodstream than other sweeteners. Because it is such a thick liquid, it does not always substitute well for maple syrup or agave nectar, but does work as a replacement for other thick sweeteners such as corn syrup and even honey.

Bulgur: Wheat kernels that have been first steamed and dried and then cut into smaller pieces for quicker cooking. Cracked wheat resembles bulgur but has not been precooked (steamed/dried), so it takes a little longer to cook. Bulgur is well known as the grain used in the popular tabbouleh salad.

Cannellini beans: The Italian name for white kidney beans; these are large, white, oval-shaped beans with a smooth, creamy texture and a nutty flavor. Other white beans such as navy often substitute well for cannellini beans.

Capers: The unripened buds of a Mediterranean plant that are pickled in a brine to give them a salty, pungent taste. They are dark olive green, have a small roundish shape, and come in different sizes; the smaller ones can be more expensive and are considered better quality. Rinse and drain capers before using. Widely available in grocery stores.

Cardamom (ground): A member of the ginger family, cardamom is ground from the seed that is encased in a cardamom pod. Wonderfully aromatic with a sweet flavor, this spice can be used in both sweet and savory dishes, and is a common ingredient in Indian cuisine. Although the ground form is less flavorful than grinding straight from the seed, it is more readily available.

Carob: Available in powder and chip form, carob comes from the pod of a legume-family tree native to the Mediterranean region. It is often used as a substitute for chocolate, although it really doesn't have the same flavor. Carob is sweet, whereas pure chocolate is bitter. But unlike chocolate, carob does not contain caffeine. Carob powder and chips are available in whole foods stores and some grocery stores.

Chia Seeds: This seed is a variety of the—you guessed it—"ch-ch-ch-chia" plant! This superseed is very tiny, smaller than a sesame seed, yet packed with a lot of nutritional power. Chia seeds have a very neutral flavor, which makes them very adaptable to baking and cooking. They are high in protein, containing all essential amino acids. They are also rich calcium and iron, vitamins A and C, and high in fiber and antioxidants. Chia seeds are a better source of omega-3 fatty acids than are flaxseeds. Also, unlike flaxseeds, chia seeds do not need to be ground for your body to absorb their nutritional value, though the ground form works well in many baking and cooking applications. They can be eaten whole, and can also be kept unrefrigerated. Chia seeds can also be purchased ground, which is handy for some cooking and baking purposes. Chia seeds are available in black and white seed colors; I prefer white chia seeds (and ground chia seeds).

Kitchen Buzz: I have found that you can typically use less ground chia as a substitute for ground flax meal. For instance if a recipe calls for 2 tablespoons of ground flax meal, 1 to 1½ tablespoons of ground chia will probably do just fine.

Chipotle hot sauce: Chipotle chile peppers are smoked and dried jalapeño chile peppers. They have a smoky, spicy flavor but are not as hot as other chile peppers. Look for chipotle hot sauces among other hot sauces in your grocery store. I use Tabasco brand.

Cocoa powder: Sometimes simply called cocoa, this is the dry powder that remains after pressing the cocoa butter out of chocolate liquor. When a recipe calls for unsweetened cocoa powder, use regular cocoa powder rather than Dutch-processed, as it is naturally acidic in nature, whereas Dutch-processed cocoa powder has been alkalized to reduce its acidity (for baked goods, this will impact the leavening reaction, as baking soda reacts well with regular cocoa powder's acidic nature and baking powder reacts with Dutch-processed cocoa). Cocoa powder is available in grocery stores, often in the hot beverages or baking aisles. See also Dutch-processed cocoa powder below.

Cocoa powder, Dutch-processed: Cocoa powder that has been processed with an alkali to neutralize its acidity. Dutch-processed cocoa powder has a richer, milder flavor than regular, but cannot always be substituted for standard cocoa powder in recipes (because of the difference in acidity). To be certain, use Dutch-processed cocoa powder only when specifically listed in recipes. Available in natural foods stores and some grocery stores.

Coconut butter: Made from the whole flesh or "meat" of the coconut, rather than just the oil (see below). It is thicker and drier than coconut oil, but also contains some fiber and protein, and other nutrients.

Some online sources may reference coconut butter as another name for coconut oil. Be certain that any reference to coconut butter in this book is specifically identifying the whole food of coconut butter. I use the Artisana brand; it is 100 percent coconut meat. There are other brands, too; if you cannot find it in your local store, it is worth ordering online.

Kitchen Buzz: Coconut butter does not need to be refrigerated. Keep it at room temperature for use in these recipes; it will be a little softer and far easier to measure.

Coconut milk (fresh and canned): Some of my recipes call for coconut milk. Where coconut milk is specified, I am referring to the canned variety—either regular or "lite." Regular coconut milk is quite thick and creamy, and will often separate with the liquids at the bottom and the thicker cream at the upper two-thirds of the can. In recent years, brands of refrigerated fresh coconut milk (sold in the dairy beverage section) have become available as substitutes for other nondairy milks such as almond, soy, and rice. These can usually be used where a nondairy milk is specified—but not when canned coconut milk is needed.

Kitchen Buzz: Some recipes call for separation of coconut milk liquid and cream; this can be made more efficient by refrigerating the can for a day or two. Don't shake the can before opening, otherwise you will begin to mix the solids and liquids again. The thick cream is easy to scoop out and skim from the separated liquid, and then used as a substitution to whipped cream. One of my favorite brands to use is Taste of Thai Organic. After refrigerating it, I am able to get up to about ¾ cup of cream with this brand. You will see this noted in some of the frosting recipes and also my Lemon-Scented Whipped Cream. These recipes specifically require the regular coconut milk rather than "lite." When a "lite" coconut milk can be used, it will be noted.

Coconut oil: Extracted from the flesh of coconut, this oil is used often in raw recipes, but also works well for frying and sautéing as it can be heated to higher temperatures before breaking down. It is sold in jars or plastic tubs; purchase the refrigerated brand of organic extra-virgin coconut oil. Available in whole foods stores or the natural foods section in grocery stores; look for organic extra-virgin coconut oil.

Kitchen Buzz: Coconut oil is solid when cold, but when kept at room temperature, is somewhat softened for easier measuring in these and any other recipes. I always keep mine at room temperature so it is softened and ready to use. If you find it is still hard and not easy to scoop at room temperature, try warming gently by placing the jar/tub in a hot water bath in a larger bowl or the sink.

Coconut sugar: Made from the nectar (or sap) of the coconut palm tree flower, this sugar has a beautiful, deep caramel color and similar flavor. It has a low glycemic index (35, with anything under 55 being considered low), which is significantly less than other granulated (and liquid) sweeteners, and is also high in some nutrients, including zinc, potassium, and iron. Nutritional nods aside, it is one of my favorite natural sweeteners just for flavor and color alone. Coconut sugar is available in many natural foods stores and online.

Kitchen Buzz: Sucanat is a reasonable substitute for coconut sugar.

Coriander seeds: This spice comes from the cilantro (coriander) plant, a leafy herb. It is commonly used in Indian cuisine, and has a very fragrant, lemony, and slightly floral flavor. The seeds can be found in grocery stores, in the spice or Indian food sections.

Corn flour: Flour that is made from finely ground cornmeal. It can come in fine and coarser consistencies. I use the Bob's Red Mill brand of corn flour, which is quite fine and powdery in consistency, with a pleasant yellow color. This brand is also stone ground, and so retains all parts of the corn kernel (some brands of corn flour do not, so check labels). In the United Kingdom and Australia, *corn flour* usually refers to what we know in North America as "cornstarch." When my recipes call for corn flour, do not substitute cornstarch.

Daiya cheese: While not an ingredient needed for my recipes, this tapioca-based cheese is widely recognized as the best vegan cheese.

Dried fruit: It's handy to have an assortment of dried fruit in your pantry for baking, but also for salads and some savory dishes. Look for unsulfured varieties (check that the ingredients do not include sulfites). Some brands are specifically labeled "unsulfured." You may notice some differences in the color and appearance of dried fruits that are unsulfured. For instance, dried apricots are brown rather than bright orange—but actually taste much better than does the bright orange fruit. Raisins, apricots, and cranberries are common dried fruits to keep stocked, but also consider goji berries, dried blueberries, dried apples, dried pineapple, and dried mangoes.

Earth Balance Buttery Spread: A brand of nonhydrogenated vegan tub margarine made from cold-pressed, non-genetically-modified oils, including soy (though a soy-free variety is also available), canola, and olive oils. While it is one of the best vegan dairy substitutes for both cooking and baking, these recipes do not rely on it. Available in whole foods stores and most grocery stores (either in the dairy case or in the natural foods refrigerated section).

Fennel: If you like the flavor of licorice or anise, you will love fennel. Eaten raw, its flavor is very pronounced, but the taste mellows greatly as you sauté, grill, roast, or otherwise cook it. Fennel looks somewhat like celery, with light green stalks and a white bulbous base. To use, trim the stalks to where they meet the bulb (fronds can be used as an herb similar to dill). Cut the bulb in half and remove the core, then slice or chop as needed. When shopping, look for firm, compact clean bulbs without any blemishes, and stalks that are fresh, green, and firm.

Fennel seeds: This spice adds a sweet licorice or anise flavor to dishes, and is often found in Italian cuisine. Available in grocery stores, either in the spice section or the ethnic foods section.

Flax meal: Flax meal is made from whole flaxseeds ground finely into a powdery or mealy form. Grinding enhances the nutritional absorption of flax seeds (which are high in omega-3 fatty acids). Flax meal also makes a wonderful egg substitute (see page 171), as it becomes quite gelatinous when combined with water or other liquid. You can grind your own flaxseeds, or buy ready-made flax meal (e.g., Bob's Red Mill) at whole foods stores or grocery stores. Flax meal has a high oil content and it can go rancid quickly; therefore, it's best to purchase it refrigerated or frozen (rather than at room temperature), and be sure to store in an airtight container in your freezer to retain its nutritional value and fresh flavor. You'll know if your flax has gone off with a quick sniff: fresh flax meal has a pleasant, sweet, nutty flavor and aroma, whereas old or rancid flax meal has a strong oily smell.

Flax oil: Derived from flaxseed, flax oil is rich in omega-3 fatty acids. It must be kept refrigerated, and cooking destroys its nutritional value, so use it cold, for instance in salad dressings or drizzled in a balsamic slurry on food. It doesn't have a long shelf life, so check the expiration date on labels when shopping and be sure to buy it refrigerated. A good-quality flax oil should not have much, if any, bitter aftertaste.

French (Le Puy) lentils: These lentils have a dark green/bluish hue, and compared to the brown/green variety of lentils, are slightly smaller and hold their shape better after cooking. I like how their texture is smooth rather than dry, and they have a slightly richer, less earthy flavor.

Goji berries: Touted as a superfood, these Himalayan berries deserve at least part of this hype, being rich in protein and antioxidants, having more vitamin C than oranges, and also being rich in vitamin A (which, among other things, is good for fighting viral infections). These berries resemble raisins in size, but with a flattened shape and dusty pink-red color. Their texture is chewy and slightly soft (though some brands may be softer and fresher than others). Goji berries are not inexpensive, and may be somewhat of an acquired taste. They aren't as sweet as other dried fruit such as raisins, or other dried berries such as blueberries.

Guar gum: A thickening and binding agent that is often used in gluten-free baking. Here, I also use it in my ice-cream recipes, as it adds a slight mallowy quality that gives it a textural edge. Guar gum comes from the seed of a beanlike plant. It is a powerful binder/thickener, similar to (but not always interchangeable with) xanthan gum. Available in natural foods stores and some grocery stores.

Hemp seeds: The hard outer shell of the hemp seed is removed to reveal the highly nutritious inner nut. Similar to sesame seeds in size, with a light yellow-green color, they have a light, soft texture with a little crunch. They can be sprinkled onto salads, sandwiches, or cereals, or used in baking and other recipes. Available in whole foods stores and some grocery stores.

Hemp seed nut butter: This highly nutritious butter is made from pureeing the shelled hemp seed nut. It can be used much like other nut butters in recipes. It has a greenish color and tastes somewhat like sunflower seeds. Roasted hemp nut seeds are also available in some areas, and they have a nuttier flavor that may be preferred by some. Available in whole foods stores and some grocery stores.

Hemp seed oil: Cold-pressing the hemp seed nut produces hemp seed oil. It has a green color and a mild, nutty taste. It works wonderfully in salad dressings and drizzled on meals, but like flax oil, it should not be used for cooking and requires refrigeration. Available in whole foods stores and some grocery stores.

Jicama: A tan-colored tuber that resembles a turnip, but is a little squatter. It has a pleasant, crunchy texture that is similar to that of water chestnuts, with a flavor like very mild green peas. When selecting a jicama, look for one that is firm with un-wrinkled skin and no blemishes.

Kamut flour: Made from the kamut grain, this wheat-free (but not gluten-free) flour has a slightly sweet and nutty flavor. It is a little coarser than other flours, and often works best when combined with other flours for baked goods such as muffins.

Kelp granules: A granulated form of kelp, that can be shaken much like salt but lower in sodium, and rich in such nutrients as iron and iodine. I like Maine Coast Sea Seasonings brand. I use these granules to give a subtle sealike flavor to certain recipes, but you can also sprinkle them on soups, salads, sandwiches, and other foods when you might reach for the salt shaker.

Lemongrass: Often used in Thai cooking, lemongrass slightly resembles a large scallion, having a slender stalk with a bulbous base. It is light green and yellow in color, with the outer leaves rather stiff and woody in texture. Lemongrass has a unique lemon flavor that is distinct from the lemon itself. Lemongrass is often added whole to soups and stews, to impart its marvelous taste. After trimming the stalk, the lower bulbous portion is then often bruised to help release its flavor, and added whole to simmer in recipes. Available in the produce section in most grocery stores.

Macadamia butter: A butter or paste much like almond or peanut butter, made from macadamia nuts. It is very light in color, with a beautifully mild nutty and but-tery taste. It makes a beautiful addition in many desserts. Available in many grocery stores and also health food stores.

Matcha green tea powder: A finely ground, high-quality powdered green tea unique to Japan. Made from stone-grinding the whole leaf, it has a beautiful vibrant green color and a slight bitter flavor. Matcha is high in antioxidants and also is also chlorophyll rich; and while it does contain caffeine, its caffeine is released more slowly and steadily than that from coffee beans.

Millet: A whole grain that is easy to cook (see "Guide to Cooking Grains," page 283), and also easy to digest. A nutritionally rich, gluten-free grain that is small and round with a light yellow color, millet can be used in place of brown rice or quinoa for meals. Its mild, mellow flavor is readily accepted by children and adults alike.

Millet flour: Made from whole millet, this gluten-free flour has a light creamy color, soft texture, and is fairly mellow in flavor compared to some other gluten-free flours.

Miso: A salty, thick paste made from fermented soybeans. Available in light and dark varieties, and also in combination with other grains like barley and brown rice. I use mostly brown rice and barley miso, since it has a mellow, mild flavor; however, sometimes I use red miso, which has a more robust flavor. Both are available in health food stores and grocery stores.

Mushrooms: Most of these recipes call for white button, cremini, or Portobello mushrooms for convenience. But, consider experimenting with varieties like shiitake, oyster, and chanterelles.

Neutral-flavored oil: Any oil that has a light or nondiscernible taste.

Kitchen Buzz: When my recipes specify a neutral-flavored oil, use one of these (or another with no noticeable flavor): avocado oil, almond oil, rice bran oil, grapeseed oil, or organic canola oil.

Nondairy milk: There are many choices for nondairy milks, including soy, rice, almond, oat, coconut (not canned but fresh, such as So Delicious), and hemp varieties. Many varieties work well in baking and cooking, including soy, almond, coconut, and also hemp and rice milk. Look for fortified varieties, and if using soy milk, be sure to buy those using organic, non-GMO soybeans. Experiment with different milks to find ones you like, depending on the use.

Kitchen Buzz: I personally prefer almond milk (especially unsweetened Blue Diamond Almond Breeze) for cooking and baking, followed by soy and coconut milks. Hemp milks have a more distinct flavor and rice milks can be sweet in flavor, which may be fine for baking (and drinking) but not always for cooking. With plain unsweetened almond milk, the flavor is clean and neutral, and the texture not too thin or thick, so it suits most recipes very well.

Nondairy yogurt: There are soy-, coconut-, and almond-based dairy-free yogurts. The coconut ones tend to be sweeter and less tangy than the soy, and so sometimes adjustments may be needed within a recipe to adjust for these flavor differences (e.g., adding some lemon juice to coconut yogurt). Where these adjustments are needed, it is specified within the recipe itself. Check the ingredients to make sure the brand you use is totally dairy free. If you don't care for store-bought yogurts, you can make my homemade cashew-based Vanilla Yogurt, page 235, in these recipes as well. While it doesn't contain the probiotics found in commercial yogurts, it is a quick scratch-made substitute to commercial yogurts that works well in the handful of recipes here that call for nondairy yogurt.

Nutritional yeast: Light, thin yellowish flakes (affectionately termed "nooch") that can be used as a nutritional supplement, but also have a cheesy, nutty flavor that works well in vegan foods. Nutritional yeast can be used in recipes or sprinkled directly on pasta, bread, and popcorn. It is rich in protein, minerals, and vitamins (especially B vitamins, including B_{12}), and is easy to digest. Nutritional yeast is grown on molasses, but is inactive (unlike baking yeast), and also differs from brewer's yeast and torula yeast. Look for the Red Star brand of nutritional yeast (sometimes called Red Star Vegetarian Support Formula or Red Star Yeast T6635+) to ensure it is fortified with vitamin B_{12}. Available in whole foods stores and bulk sections in grocery stores.

Nut butters: You will also need a variety of nut butters for these recipes, but the variety is more limited and includes almond, cashew, macadamia, and hazelnut butters. Most nut butters are ground from roasted nuts unless specified as "raw." You can keep both raw and roasted varieties on hand, or either/or, as you prefer.

Kitchen Buzz: Some of my recipes are raw and require both raw nuts and nut butters. But if you aren't adhering to a raw diet and are flexible with interchanging roasted nuts, then it's usually fine to do so unless the recipe specifies otherwise.

Nuts: From whole to butters, toasting and soaking, having a good variety of nuts in your pantry makes for more interesting vegan food! They can bring crunch and flavor, and also body and creaminess to dishes from dips, soups, and sauces to main dishes such as burgers, and finally to desserts. I store nuts in airtight containers, with backup stock in the freezer. If you don't use your stock of nuts very regularly, it's useful to keep them in the freezer so they don't go rancid, especially for oily nuts like walnuts and pecans—and also particularly in summer months. The majority of my recipes call for raw nuts: cashews, almonds, pecans, walnuts, pistachios, hazelnuts, pine nuts, and macadamia nuts (some are referenced individually here), but some call for toasted nuts such as almonds or pine nuts. You can toast nuts yourself, or keep some pre-roasted on hand. Some recipes (mostly raw) require nuts to be soaked in advance. There are reported digestive benefits for soaking nuts, but in my recipes the requirement is mostly for textural and technique benefits.

Kitchen Buzz: To toast nuts, place on a baking sheet lined with parchment paper. Place in oven preheated to 400°F, and bake for 7 to 12 minutes, tossing once or twice through the baking process to distribute even cooking, until golden and releasing a nutty aroma. Watch carefully as toasting times vary by nut, and they can turn from golden to burned in just seconds.

Soaking such nuts as almonds and cashews make them softer, which makes the puree creamier and the puree process easier and quicker. (Sometimes I don't opt to presoak the nuts in a raw recipe, and again, this is to achieve a certain consistency of the ingredients used in that recipe.) So, when you can, soak nuts where required for a recipe. To soak, place the nuts in a bowl of water and cover for several hours. Cashews will take 3 to 4 hours, almonds 6 to 8 hours. The nuts will become larger after soaking, as they swell from absorbing some of the water. Drain the soaking water, and rinse the nuts. Then store in the fridge for a couple of days until ready to use, or keep in the freezer for a few months. It is helpful to soak more than you will need for any given recipe. They can be frozen in batches, thaw well, and then are ready for use in recipes.

Oat bran: This is made from the outer layer, or husk, of the oat grain. It is high in dietary fiber and adds texture and heft to hearty baked goods such as muffins. Because it can go rancid more quickly than other flours and grains, it is best stored in a cool place, or even in the freezer. GF-certified oat bran exists, though it is not as readily available as other GF-certified oat products. It can be purchased online through Amazon.com or Onlyoats.ca.

Oat flour: One of my favorite alternative flours, oat flour is made from grinding oats, and has a slightly sweet flavor. It cannot always be substituted equally for wheat flour, but sometimes can, or can be combined with wheat or other nonwheat flour. Oats are wheat free, but may not always be gluten free (sometime cross-contamination occurs in processing). In gluten-free recipes, use GF-certified oat flour, such as Bob's Red Mill brand.

Kitchen Buzz: If you don't have oat flour, use rolled or quick oats and process them in a food processor or blender until very fine, like coarse flour. It is useful to grind a larger amount (a few cups), and then store in your pantry.

Olives: Move beyond canned black olives. Sure, they are fine for some recipes, but they actually have little to no flavor compared to other varieties. Kalamata olives have a strong, briny bite that is far more flavorful than common black olives. The pitted variety is great for convenience. Kalamata olives are widely available in stores, but specialty markets and natural foods stores will carry other varieties of pungent, dry-cured and briny olives that are worth sampling and trying in recipes. And mix up green and black olives in your

cooking from time to time. Green olives are unripened olives, whereas black/purple olives are fully ripe; after picking, the olives are cured or pickled.

Pasta (dried): Most dried pasta varieties are vegan, as they typically contain just flour (of some type) and water. Because traditional white pasta offers little nutritional value, I prefer to use kamut, brown rice, or whole wheat pastas. Other varieties of whole-grain pastas available include quinoa, wild rice (combined with brown rice), and corn. I like to stock a few different shapes of pasta, such as penne, rotini, spaghetti, linguine, macaroni, shells for stuffing with nut cheeses (e.g., Truffled Cashew Cheese), lasagna noodles, and alphabet shapes for the kids!

Kitchen Buzz: One thing to keep in mind is texture. Pasta aficionados are explicit about cooking pasta al dente, or with just a touch of firmness to the bite. This recommendation works for some varieties of pasta more than others (brown rice pasta doesn't really have an al dente point, in my opinion; it needs to be cooked through). Also, some of us like our pasta a little softer. So, follow the package directions for average cooking times, and then cook your pasta until done for you—whether that's with some firmness, or more fully cooked and softer.

Pine nuts: These seeds from the cones of several varieties of pine trees have a soft texture and earthy taste, and toasting enhances their nutty flavor. Keep them refrigerated or in the freezer, since they can go rancid quickly (like many nuts). When toasting/roasting, keep a sharp eye on pine nuts, as they turn from lightly golden to burned very quickly! Some stores carry pretoasted pine nuts, which are a handy pantry item. Available in refrigerated sections in grocery stores.

Pistachios: Green nuts with a delicate, slightly sweet taste and crunchy texture, pistachios work well in sweet and savory dishes. Stick with the brownish-green nuts; red pistachios have been dyed.

Plantains: A starchy fruit that closely resembles a banana, but larger in size and with a stubborn peel. Plantains are not eaten raw like bananas; rather, cooked, much like a starchy potato or sweet potato. They may be found at different stages of ripeness, from green to yellow and then blackened. When yellow-greenish, plantains are unripe and are quite starchy, firm, and not very sweet (much like a potato). They become sweeter as they turn more yellow, and once fully ripened (with a lot of blackened spots) they are quite sweet, fragrant, and softer in texture. Plantains are used in cooking at different stages of ripeness, depending on the sweetness and firmness desired for the recipe. If you buy plantains while yellow or green, they will ripen at room temperature within 4 to 7 days. To peel plantains, cut off the ends, slice the peel the length of the plantain, and then pull off the peel in one piece away from the plantain flesh. Available in most large grocery stores.

Poblano peppers: These "hot" peppers are actually mild on the heat register compared to other hot peppers (though they can vary in intensity from one pepper to another). They somewhat resemble a green pepper, but with a darker color and a more oblong, heart-shaped form. They can add mild heat to dishes, and most of this heat is found in the seeds and membranes. The skin is somewhat tough, and so they benefit from roasting or grilling to char and remove that outer layer before using in dishes. After roasting/grilling, they can be chopped and added to dishes, or cut in half and stuffed with fillings. Dried poblano chiles are called ancho chiles.

Portobello mushrooms: These mushrooms are known for their great flavor and "meaty" texture. They are large with a brown, round, flat cap, and a woody stem that is usually discarded or used in vegetable stocks. I typically remove the gills on the undersides of the mushrooms before using, because they leach a lot of black liquid when cooking. Available fresh in most grocery stores.

Potato starch: Sometimes referred to as potato starch flour, it is a gluten-free flour made from cooked potatoes. Do not confuse it with potato flour (which is heavy and has a distinct potato taste). Available in most grocery stores.

Powdered sugar: This may also be called confectioners' sugar or icing sugar, and is most often used in frostings and other specific dessert applications where a very fine, powdery form of sugar is needed.

Kitchen Buzz: I use Wholesome Sweeteners Organic Powdered Sugar, which is made from unrefined cane sugar (rather than icing sugar that is made from refined white sugar). You can easily make your own organic powdered sugar. To do so, use a blender and combine 1¼ to 1½ cups of unrefined sugar with 1 tablespoon of arrowroot powder or cornstarch. Blend on high speed until powdery, scraping down the jug once or twice. The arrowroot or cornstarch may not be needed with a very high-powered blender such as a Vitamix.

Pumpkin seeds: These shelled, flat, greenish seeds from our favorite autumnal vegetable are sometimes called pepitas. You can purchase them raw or lightly roasted, and I recommend having both on hand. Raw pumpkin seeds are terrific in dips and burgers, and even for snacking. Lightly roasted, they make great kid-friendly snacks and tasty toppers for salads and soups. Pumpkin seeds are rich in iron, and also good sources of protein and zinc.

Pure maple syrup: A natural sweetener from the sap of sugar maples, great in many desserts and baked goods. It's not to be mistaken for the cheaper "maple-flavored" syrup sold as pancake topping. Pure maple syrup is 100 percent maple syrup, with no artificial flavors, colors, or additives. Available in grocery stores; organic varieties are available in whole foods stores and some grocery stores.

Pure vanilla extract: Made from steeping pure vanilla beans in alcohol and water or a glycerin water base. Look for pure vanilla extract, checking the labels to ensure it's not artificial or imitation, which contains artificial colors and flavors, and does not have nearly the same flavor as pure vanilla. Available in grocery stores and organic varieties in whole foods stores.

Quick oats: These are rolled oats that are cut thinner for faster cooking. Not to be confused with "instant" oats, which are further processed and typically used in instant oatmeal breakfast pouches. GF-certified quick oats (e.g., Bob's Red Mill) are also available in stores and online.

Quinoa: Pronounced "keen-wa," this ancient grain is small in size but big in nutrition. Quinoa is a complete source of protein, and is high in calcium, iron, and phosphorous. Uncooked quinoa resembles flattened couscous, creamy beige in color (though there are other color varieties, including red and black) with a little ring around each grain that comes out like a tail when cooked. This ring holds the majority of quinoa's protein and gives it a slight crunch. Quinoa cooks quickly (see "Guide to Cooking Grains," page 283), has a light texture, and can be digested easily. It is best to rinse quinoa for a few minutes before cooking to remove the saponin, its natural pesticide, and to improve its flavor. Available in whole foods stores and some grocery stores.

Red curry paste: A key base for recipes in Thai cuisine, red curry paste can be made from scratch, with ingredients that include garlic, ginger, lemongrass, red chile peppers, and other seasonings such as cumin and coriander. Some recipes (and commercial brands) contain fish sauce, however. I use the Thai Kitchen brand, which does not contain fish sauce and can be combined with coconut milk, or in marinades, or other recipe applications.

Red lentils: These are small, pink-colored lentils that turn golden when cooked and have a mellow flavor. They cook very quickly (see "Guide to Cooking Beans," page 285), but do not hold their shape after cooking, so they are best in soups. Available in whole foods stores and grocery stores.

Rice flour: Flour made from finely milled rice. Rice flour is gluten free, and available in both brown and white flour forms. Because white rice flour is made from white rice rather than brown, it is not as nutritious as brown rice flour. It is sometimes preferable in baking or cooking, however, depending on the texture required for a recipe. You use brown or white rice flour in my recipes, as you prefer. Sweet rice flour is also available; it differs from white rice flour in that it is ground from sweet rice, and has a finer texture that is sometimes preferred in gluten-free baking. Available in whole foods stores and natural foods sections of grocery stores.

Roasted red peppers: Most grocers carry jars or bottles of roasted red peppers packed in oil, vinegar, or water. Look for varieties without chemicals or preservatives such as sulfites.

Kitchen Buzz: If you have extra time, try roasting red peppers yourself: Place lightly oiled peppers (whole or cut from the core) on a baking sheet and broil for 13 to 15 minutes, or until the skins are blistering and blackening in spots (whole peppers take a little longer than cut peppers). Transfer to a bowl and cover the bowl with plastic wrap to "sweat" for about 15 minutes. Then, once cool enough to handle, remove the skins from the peppers, and they're ready to use.

Rolled oats: When the whole oat groat grain is steamed, rolled, and flaked, you have rolled oats. Sometimes called old-fashioned oats, they work well in many savory and sweet recipes to add binding, density, and also chewiness. Sometimes quick oats can be substituted, as they are rolled oats that are flaked thinner for quicker cooking. GF-certified rolled oats (e.g., Bob's Red Mill) are also available in stores and online.

Sea salt: Sea salt is made from evaporated seawater. With little processing, trace minerals remain. Sea salt comes in a variety of colors, textures, and even flavors. Because sea salt varies from brand to brand, you may notice some taste "saltier" than others. The brand I have used is Bob's Red Mill, for consistency in testing. However, I sometimes use an iodized sea salt, and if you do the same, you may want to adjust salt measures slightly to taste.

Seeds: As with nuts, it is useful to have a variety of seeds (and some seed butters) in your pantry. Seeds that I use regularly include pumpkin, sunflower, hemp, and chia, and seed butters that I use often include tahini (sesame seed butter) and to a lesser extent sunflower seed butter. Seed butters are bitterer than nut butters, and are not always readily accepted by young palates. It is therefore useful to work them into recipes rather than eat straight. You can also try stirring pure maple syrup and cinnamon into something such as hemp seed butter or sunflower seed butter to make it more palatable.

Seitan: Although I do not call for seitan in any of my recipes specifically, I recognize that it is a beloved vegan staple and worth noting in this pantry list. Seitan, sometimes called wheat gluten, is a food made from the protein component of wheat flour—the gluten. That gluten component in the wheat flour is very elastic, and when combined with water and then seasoned and prepared (through simmering, steaming, baking, or other cooking methods), develops a texture resembling that of meat products. Seitan can be made from scratch or purchased premade in natural foods stores. Because it is made from wheat, it is obviously not suitable for those with a gluten or wheat intolerance. There are many recipes in this book in which seitan could be substituted (e.g., for the tofu in Tofu Baked in an Olive, Grape, and Herbed Marinade, or for part of the beans in Winter Veg Chickpea Potpie), and also sauces that would do flavor wonders for gluten dishes (e.g.,

Pumpkin Seed Chipotle Cream). If you are familiar with seitan, feel free to make such substitutions (optimally after trying the recipe first as is).

Shiitake mushrooms: These mushrooms have a brown, sometimes flat cap with a light underside, and a thin, stiff stalk. They have a distinct earthy flavor and a chewy, meaty texture. Available in most grocery stores.

Silken tofu: A smooth and silky variety of tofu sold in small, rectangular, aseptic boxes. An alternative processing of the soy milk creates a different texture than that of regular soft and firm tofu. Because silken tofu becomes so smooth and creamy when blended or pureed, it is often used to create smoothies, dips, and desserts. Its packaging allows for a long shelf life, even without refrigeration (although I prefer to refrigerate). Mori-Nu silken tofu (soft and firm varieties) can be found in most grocery stores, whole foods stores, and some Asian specialty stores.

Sorghum flour: A gluten-free flour that resembles whole wheat pastry flour in color and texture. It is made from a grain that originated from Africa, and has a rather nondistinct flavor (unlike some other gluten-free flours). It works well in combination with other flours for cookies, quick breads, cakes, and more.

Spelt flour (and sifted spelt flour): Available in whole foods stores and some grocery stores, this flour is made from spelt grain. It is a good substitute for common wheat flour, although typically not in direct 1:1 ratio; usually about 1¼ cups of spelt flour is needed to replace 1 cup of white wheat flour (and sometimes that measure varies).

Kitchen Buzz: If possible, buy a whole-grain spelt flour that has been sifted, to make your baked goods a little lighter in texture. If you cannot find a light or sifted spelt flour, you can sift the whole-grain flour yourself with a fine strainer to remove the coarse germ and make the flour lighter. Where my recipes call simply for "spelt flour," either whole-grain or light/sifted can be used. Otherwise, the recipe will specify "light or sifted spelt flour" for a lighter texture in the final product.

Steel-cut oats: Whole oat groat grains that have been cut into smaller pieces for quicker cooking, though they still take considerably longer to cook than do the more processed forms of oats (see "Guide to Cooking Grains," page 283). GF-certified steel-cut oats (e.g., Bob's Red Mill) are also available in stores and online.

Kitchen Buzz: Steel-cut oats can also be ground into a coarse flour for baking or other purposes by grinding in a blender until you reach a coarse, powdery texture.

Sucanat: A less-refined, granulated sweetener, standing for *Su*gar *ca*ne *na*tural. It has a caramel-brown color and a more rustic, coarser texture than do some other unrefined sugars. It also has a fairly prominent natural molasses flavor, which may or may not be desirable in a recipe.

Sweet potatoes (yellow and orange): Sweet potatoes may be termed yams in different areas. Most people know sweet potatoes to be the orange-fleshed tubers that find their way into a sugary sweet potato casserole. In Canada (and some other areas), orange sweet potatoes are classified as "yams" (both garnet yams and jewel yams). We also have yellow-fleshed sweet potatoes that are classified simply as "sweet potatoes." To hopefully clear any confusion, my recipes specify "orange-fleshed" and "yellow-fleshed" sweet potatoes (rather than use the term *yam*, which actually refers to a humongous starchy tuber with brownish barklike peel, which is unrelated to the sweet potato).

Tahini: Sometimes called sesame seed butter, this paste is made from pureeing white sesame seeds. It is often used in Middle Eastern recipes such as hummus and baba ghanouj. You may find raw tahini as well as regular tahini, which has been roasted. Raw tahini has a beautiful pale color and light, mellow flavor, though it can be about double the price of other kinds of tahini. As with all natural seed and nut butters, the oil in tahini rises to the top because there are no additives to suspend the oils, so stir the oil through the nut butter before using and then refrigerate. Available in whole foods stores and most grocery stores. Joyva brand of tahini is particularly nutty in flavor, far more than other brands that I have tried, and can almost pass as peanut butter.

Kitchen Buzz: Most often I use the Nuts to You brand of tahini in my recipes.

Tamari: A soy sauce made from fermented soybeans, without the colorings and additives found in many commercial brands. Tamari is also wheat free, unlike most soy sauces. Available at most grocery stores.

Tapioca starch flour: Sometimes simply referred to as tapioca flour, this is a gluten-free flour that is made from the cassava root. It works well in gluten-free baking to help sweeten flours such as rice, amaranth, and quinoa, but is also useful as a thickener (much like arrowroot or cornstarch) for sauces and pies. Tapioca flour is not the same as instant tapioca; it is finely ground into a flour that is easy to dissolve. Available in whole foods stores and natural foods sections of grocery stores.

Tempeh and marinated tempeh: A product that originated in Indonesia, tempeh is made from soybeans that have been cooked and combined with a culturing agent. The process turns the mixture into a solid cake form with the soybeans pressed together. Tempeh has more protein and vitamins than tofu does, and unlike tofu, is also high in fiber. The culturing process also makes tempeh a more digestible soy food. When buying tempeh, look for a firm cake that has a thin whitish bloom. It may have a few grayish or black spots, but should never have any pink, yellow, or blue coloration. Available frozen in grocery or whole foods stores, and in varieties that include grains, flax, and vegetables.

Kitchen Buzz: Tempeh should be steamed, sautéed, or otherwise cooked before eating. To reduce any bitterness, simmer it in vegetable broth for about 20 minutes before using. To enjoy it without much preparation, look for premarinated packages of tempeh. I really like Turtle Island Foods brand, whose flavors include coconut curry, sesame garlic, smoky maple, and lemon pepper. I simply bake the strips on a sheet lined with parchment until heated through and golden (panfrying would also work, but the toaster oven makes for quick time and easy cleanup), and then use in sandwiches, salads, and more.

Toasted sesame oil: Pressed from toasted sesame seeds, this oil has an intense sesame flavor and a dark golden color. Be sure to use it when recipes specifically call for it. The flavor is so strong, in fact, that you need just small amounts to season dressings, sauces, and other foods. (Lighter-colored sesame oil is not produced from toasted seeds and thus does not have the same rich flavor.) Available in whole foods stores, Asian markets, and grocery stores.

Tofu (firm and extra-firm; also see silken tofu): Made from soybeans, in a process not dissimilar from how cheese is made from milk. There are different textures of tofu, including soft, medium, firm, and extra-firm. Most of my savory recipes call for extra-firm tofu, which is available in most grocery stores as well as natural foods stores. When selecting tofu, be sure to buy an organic, non-genetically-modified brand.

Kitchen Buzz: I enjoy the texture of extra-firm tofu as is, but some prefer to make it denser, or "'meatier," if you will, by either pressing the tofu (with a tofu press or between weighted plates) or freezing and thawing. The freezing method is simple: Freeze the tofu (still in its package) and when read to use, thaw (you can quicken by placing the tofu package in a hot water bath). Both methods can help draw extra moisture out of the tofu and thereby make it denser and even firmer.

Unrefined sugar: Unlike common white and brown sugar, unrefined sugar retains some nutrients because it is partially refined or not refined at all. The term *unrefined sugar* can include such products as Sucanat, coconut sugar, and evaporated cane juice. Unrefined sugar has a golden color (light to dark beige), and some types (e.g., Demerara) have granules that are a little larger than that of standard white sugar. Be sure to check the label to ensure it is unrefined; organic sugar, for example, is now popular but is not necessarily unrefined. Finer granules are easier to bake with; Sucanat and most varieties labeled "unrefined sugar" work well.

Vanilla beans: These are the long, thin, leathery-looking beans of the vanilla orchid plant. Inside each bean are thousands of tiny vanilla seeds, which are used to make vanilla extract and other vanilla products.

When shopping for vanilla beans, check to see they are tender and pliable, rather than hard. They are fresher and easier to work with when slightly pliable.

Kitchen Buzz: To remove the vanilla seeds from the bean pod, slice the bean down the outer side, using a sharp-tipped knife, to open up lengthwise. Press open the sides, and using a blunt (butter) knife, scrape out all the tiny seeds from the bean on both sides. Add the seeds to your recipe as specified. The pod can be discarded or kept for other culinary uses; for instance, try inserting it into your jar of unrefined sugar, to impart a subtle vanilla essence.

Vegan mayonnaise: There are several varieties of vegan mayonnaise on the market; most people prefer the authentic taste of Vegenaise brand. I don't require use of vegan mayonnaises in my recipes, but offer it as an option to making your own. If you prefer to use a homemade mayonnaise to a store-bought version, try my "Almonnaise."

Vegan Worcestershire sauce: A Worcestershire sauce made without anchovies. I have found two brands available in whole foods stores: Annie's Naturals and The Wizard.

Vegetable stock: Widely available in grocery stores, natural foods markets, and online, vegetable stocks add depth of flavor to soups, stews, and other meals. If you don't make your own or buy packaged stock, you can also use bouillon cubes (see page xxvi).

Wild rice: Not actually a grain but a water-grown grass, wild rice has a purple-black color, a lovely nutty taste, and a chewy texture. It opens up and curls when fully cooked, exposing a white interior. Available in whole foods stores and most grocery stores.

Xanthan gum: A fine powder that is particularly useful in gluten-free baking to help bind ingredients and add stability and elasticity. Xanthan gum is also useful to thicken frostings and desserts, and is often found in store-bought salad dressings and sauces. Available in whole foods stores and some grocery stores.

1 Breakfast Bites and Smoothies

Breakfast is not always a sit-down meal. For many, it's a grab-and-go out the door kind of meal. Here, I'll give you recipes to meet both breakfast scenarios, with cereals, pancakes, muffins, healthy cookies, smoothies, and more. Muffins and other morning snacks are super versatile: not just to start the day, but to pack for lunches for yourself or the kids, or to satisfy late-night hunger pangs. If you love muffins, all of these contain whole-grain flours—no white flours, and no heavy amounts of sweeteners and oils. They are also all made with wheat-free alternative flours (see "Plant-Powered Baking Notes," page 170), from my new take on a bran muffin (Oat 'n' Applesauce Muffins), to my "sneaky" muffins—one with chia seeds (Chia Banana Muffins) and another with goji berries blended into the batter (Strawberry Goji Muffins).

If muffins aren't your cup of tea, check out my Breakfast Cookies, Wholesome Oat Snackles!, Monsta! Cookies, Cocoa Almond Jumbles, Proper Healthy Granola Bars, and a few more . . . perfect for lunches for you, the kids at school, or just after one of your nutrient-packed smoothies. Prefer a quick liquid? My morning starts with a green smoothie, and what follows is not just recipes for green (and other) smoothies, but also a full how-to guide to making green smoothies—from what greens to use, how to combine them properly with fruits, how to properly blend, other ingredients that can be added, and more. You'll be "going green" in no time!

When the weekend rolls around, take a morning and make it Pancake Day. These aren't the type of pancakes that sit like a brick in your stomach from heavy white flour, eggs, and butter; only whole-grain flours used here, and just a smidgen of oil, and most of my pancakes have no added sweeteners. So, make 'em often, and stack

1

'em high! Get some hemp or chia seeds in your cakes with Apple Spice Hemp Pancakes and Whole-Grain Chia Pancakes, or try something a little more decadent with Chocolate Drop Blueberry Pancakes. And if you'd prefer something savory, try out my "Momelet"—with two versions, one with soy but no nuts, and the other with nuts but no soy—I try to cover most of the allergy bases!

BF Blueberry Muffins

MAKES 10 TO 12 MUFFINS

wheat soy FREE

BF stands for "blueberry-free" (not "best friend" blueberry muffins, though that could work, too)! Confused? One of our daughters doesn't like blueberries, which baffles me. So when I make these muffins, I first fill a couple of muffin liners with the batter on its own, and then the remaining with the blueberries. I don't include this step in the directions below, but feel free to make a couple of BF Blueberry Muffins yourself, if needed! These muffins are delicious—tender, lightly sweet, and with a hint of lemon that accents the blueberries so nicely.

1¼ cups oat flour

¾ cup spelt flour

⅓ cup unrefined sugar (light-colored sugar is nicest for the final muffin color)

¼ teaspoon sea salt

1 teaspoon lemon zest

2 teaspoons baking powder

¼ teaspoon baking soda

2 tablespoons vanilla or plain nondairy yogurt (use soy-free yogurt or Vanilla Yogurt, page 235, for a soy-free option; see "Plant-Powered Pantry," page xxxiii)

2 tablespoons agave nectar or pure maple syrup

1 tablespoon freshly squeezed lemon juice

½ cup + 3 to 4 tablespoons plain nondairy milk

3 tablespoons neutral-flavored oil (see "Plant-Powered Pantry," page xxxii)

¾ cup frozen or fresh blueberries, tossed in 1 to 2 teaspoons of oat flour

Preheat the oven to 375°F. In a large bowl, combine the dry ingredients, sifting in the baking powder and baking soda. Stir until well mixed.

In another bowl, first combine the yogurt with the agave and lemon juice, stirring well, and then add the milk, starting with 3 tablespoons, and oil and stir until well mixed.

Add the wet ingredients to the dry, and mix just until well combined. If the batter is very thick, add the remaining tablespoon of milk. Otherwise, quickly but gently fold in the blueberries.

Pour the mixture into lined muffin pans (filling ten to twelve muffin cups). Bake for 18 to 22 minutes (longer for larger muffins, less time if all twelve muffin cups are filled), or until the muffins are set in the center (test by inserting a toothpick or skewer into the center of a muffin—it should come out clean).

Remove from the oven, let cool for a couple of minutes in the pan, and then transfer the muffins to cool on a cooling rack.

Ingredients 411: Add the blueberries at the very last moment, to limit the bleeding of the blueberries into the batter.

Make It More-ish! Chocolate chips are wickedly good with blueberries. Try adding a few tablespoons to the batter.

Coconut Banana Muffins

MAKES 11 SMALL TO MEDIUM
MUFFINS, OR 9 LARGER MUFFINS

wheat
soy **FREE**

During a grocery shopping one day, our daughter, then seven, asked for a coconut. She had somewhere heard or read about opening a coconut, and she pleaded with glee to try it ourselves. Well, we opened up that fruity beast, saved the coconut water, and peeled away the flesh. After all that work, our daughters didn't care for either the water or the coconut (figures)! I sweetened up the water with a touch of stevia and drank it myself. As for the coconut, I whipped up a few batches of muffins, which led me to testing this recipe. (Since then, I make these muffins with ready-made shredded coconut, thank you!)

TOPPING: (OPTIONAL)

1½ tablespoons unrefined sugar
½ teaspoon neutral-flavored oil (see "Plant-Powered Pantry," page xxxii)

1 cup whole-grain spelt flour
1 cup oat or barley flour
½ cup grated coconut (grate fresh coconut with the small-holed side of a grater, or simply used unsweetened dried coconut; see note)
¼ cup unrefined sugar
¼ to ½ teaspoon freshly grated nutmeg
¼ teaspoon (rounded) sea salt
2 teaspoons baking powder
½ teaspoon baking soda
¾ cup mashed overripe banana (1 to 1½ bananas)
¾ cup plain or vanilla nondairy milk
¼ cup pure maple syrup
2 teaspoons apple cider vinegar
1 teaspoon pure vanilla extract
3 tablespoons neutral-flavored oil (see "Plant-Powered Pantry," page xxxii)

Preheat the oven to 375°F.

In a small bowl, combine the topping ingredients, if using, and set aside until the muffin batter is ready.

In a large bowl, combine the dry ingredients, sifting in the baking powder and baking soda. Stir until well mixed.

In another bowl, combine the mashed bananas, milk, maple syrup, vinegar, vanilla, and oil. Add the wet mixture to the dry mixture, and gently fold and stir until well mixed.

Scoop the mixture into a lined muffin pan, filling nine muffin cups (for larger muffins) or eleven or twelve muffin cups (for smaller muffins). If using the topping, sprinkle a few pinches of it on top of each muffin.

Bake for 18 to 20 minutes (less time for smaller muffins, longer for larger), until a toothpick inserted into the center comes out clean.

Remove from the oven, let cool for a couple of minutes in the pan, and then transfer the muffins to cool on a cooling rack.

If This Apron Could Talk: If you have a mini-muffin pan, these make delightful mini-muffins, bake for less time, 14 to 15 minutes (for two dozen mini-muffins).

Ingredients 411: If using a finely shredded coconut, it will be more dense than a medium-shred. So, if you have a larger flaked coconut, you can use less milk, about ½ cup plus 1 to 2 tablespoons.

Pumpkin Oat Muffins

MAKES 12 MUFFINS

wheat *soy* FREE

Bring the enjoyment of pumpkin pie into delicious whole-grain, reduced-fat muffins (and, if you are whisked away by the pumpkin aroma, I think it's perfectly acceptable to top off your muffin with some nondairy whipped cream!).

TOPPING:

- 2 tablespoons unrefined sugar
- 1 teaspoon neutral-flavored oil (see "Plant-Powered Pantry," page xxxii)

- 1 cup spelt flour
- 1 cup oat flour
- ½ cup rolled or quick oats
- ¼ teaspoon sea salt
- ½ teaspoon ground cinnamon
- ¼ teaspoon freshly grated nutmeg
- ⅛ teaspoon ground allspice (optional)
- 2 teaspoons baking powder
- ½ teaspoon baking soda
- 3 tablespoons unrefined sugar
- 3 tablespoons pure maple syrup
- 1 tablespoon flax meal or ground white chia seeds
- ¾ cup plain nondairy milk
- 1 cup canned pumpkin pie mix (not pumpkin puree; I use Farmer's Market organic brand)
- 1 tablespoon freshly squeezed lemon juice
- 1½ teaspoon pure vanilla extract
- 3 tablespoons neutral-flavored oil (see "Plant-Powered Pantry," page xxxii)

Preheat the oven to 375°F.

In a small bowl, combine the topping ingredients and set aside until the batter is ready.

In a large bowl, combine the dry ingredients, sifting in the baking powder and baking soda. Stir until well mixed.

In another bowl, first combine the maple syrup with the flax meal, and then add the remaining wet ingredients and stir until well mixed.

Add the wet mixture to the dry mixture, and gently fold and mix until just combined (do not overmix). Spoon the mixture into a twelve-cup lined muffin pan. Sprinkle a little of the topping on each muffin.

Bake for 22 to 25 minutes, until a toothpick inserted into the center comes out clean.

Remove from the oven, let cool for a couple of minutes in the pan, and then transfer the muffins to cool on a cooling rack.

Adult-Minded: Bump up the allspice, add ⅛ to ¼ teaspoon of ground ginger for extra spice, and try adding ¼ to ½ cup of chopped walnuts or pecans.

Citrus-Scented Almond Muffins

MAKES 10 TO 12 MUFFINS

wheat *soy* **FREE**

This recipe I created after seeing an olive oil muffin recipe by Giada De Laurentiis from the Food Network. My version is quite different, including whole-grain flours and less oil, yet testers gave these muffins sparkling reviews!

1½ tablespoons ground flax meal, or 1 tablespoon (scant) ground chia seeds

1 cup plain or vanilla nondairy milk

¼ cup pure maple syrup

1 tablespoon apple cider vinegar

2½ to 3 tablespoons extra-virgin olive oil (see note)

1½ cups + 2 tablespoons barley flour

⅔ cup almond meal

⅓ to ½ cup unrefined sugar

¼ teaspoon (rounded) sea salt

1 teaspoon lemon zest (see note)

1 teaspoon orange zest (see note)

2 teaspoons baking powder

½ teaspoon baking soda

Preheat the oven to 375°F.

First prepare the wet mixture: Combine the flax meal with the nondairy milk and whisk well, and add maple syrup, vinegar, and olive oil. Set aside.

In a large bowl, combine the barley flour, almond meal, sugar, salt, and lemon and orange zest, and sift in the baking powder and baking soda. Stir until well mixed.

Add the wet mixture, and fold until well combined.

Scoop the mixture into lined muffin pans (filling ten to twelve muffin cups). Bake for 19 to 22 minutes, until the muffins are set in the center (test by inserting a toothpick into center of one of the muffins—it should come out clean).

Remove from the oven, let cool for a couple of minutes in the pan, and then transfer the muffins to cool on a cooling rack.

If This Apron Could Talk: Although olive oil isn't commonly used in baked goods, here it complements the fruity flavors of the citrus, and also the almond meal. So, definitely use it rather than substituting another oil.

Savvy Subs and Adds: If you don't have fresh citrus on hand, you can add a few drops of orange oil and lemon oil (about ¼ teaspoon each) if you keep those in your pantry.

Oat 'n' Applesauce Muffins

MAKES 12 MUFFINS

*wheat
(optionally) gluten
soy* **FREE**

This just might typify the crunchy-granola kind of muffin one would imagine vegans eat—full of wholesome goodness, with oats, oat bran, oat flour, and even ground white chia. Yep, this is a healthy muffin, just slightly sweet, but also tasty with warm spices of cinnamon, allspice, and a hint of ginger. It is especially nice warm, or gently reheated with a slather of nut butter.

¾ cup unsweetened applesauce
¾ cup vanilla nondairy milk
1½ tablespoons ground white chia seeds, or 2 tablespoons flax meal
¼ cup pure maple syrup
1 teaspoon lemon zest (optional)
½ tablespoon freshly squeezed lemon juice or apple cider vinegar
¼ cup neutral-flavored oil (see "Plant-Powered Pantry," page xxxii)
2 cups oat flour (see note for gluten-free)
½ cup oat bran (see note for gluten-free)
½ cup rolled or quick oats (see note for gluten-free)
⅓ cup unrefined sugar
¼ teaspoon (rounded) sea salt
1 teaspoon ground cinnamon
½ teaspoon ground allspice
¼ teaspoon ground ginger
2½ teaspoons baking powder
⅓ cup organic raisins, or a combination of raisins and cranberries

Preheat the oven to 375°F.

In a bowl, first combine the applesauce, milk, chia, maple syrup, lemon zest, lemon juice, and oil. Set aside.

In a separate, large bowl, combine the oat flour, oat bran, oats, unrefined sugar, salt, cinnamon, allspice, and ginger, sifting in the baking powder. Add the raisins. Stir to mix well.

Add the wet mixture to the dry ingredients. Mix just until well combined. Scoop the batter into a twelve-cup lined muffin pan.

Bake for 21 to 23 minutes, until the muffins are set in the center (test by inserting a toothpick or skewer into the center of a muffin—it should come out clean).

Remove from the oven, let cool for a couple of minutes in the pan, and then transfer the muffins to cool on a cooling rack.

Allergy-Free or Bust! For a gluten-free option, use GF-certified oat products. Gluten-free oat bran might be tricky to find but is available online (see "Plant-Powered Pantry," page xxxiv).

Chia Banana Muffins

MAKES 12 MUFFINS

wheat soy **FREE**

These whole-grain muffins are lower in fat than many muffin recipes, and also have the nutritional powerhouse of white chia seeds added to the mix. Plus, they're delish.

2¼ cups sifted or light spelt flour,
⅓ cup (scant) ground white chia seeds (see "Plant-Powered Pantry," page xxvi)
¼ cup unrefined sugar
¼ teaspoon sea salt
½ teaspoon freshly grated nutmeg
1 teaspoon ground cinnamon
2 teaspoons baking powder
½ teaspoon baking soda
1 cup pureed banana (see note)
1 cup vanilla or plain nondairy milk
⅓ cup pure maple syrup
1½ teaspoons pure vanilla extract
3 tablespoons neutral-flavored oil (see "Plant-Powered Pantry," page xxxii)

Preheat the oven to 375°F.

In a large bowl, combine the dry ingredients, sifting in the baking powder and baking soda. Stir until well mixed.

In another bowl, combine the pureed bananas, milk, maple syrup, vanilla, and oil.

Add the wet mixture to the dry mixture, and gently fold and stir until well mixed.

Scoop the mixture into eleven to twelve cups of a lined muffin pan.

Bake for 23 to 26 minutes, until a toothpick inserted into the center comes out clean.

Remove from the oven, let cool for a couple of minutes in the pan, and then transfer the muffins to cool on a cooling rack.

If This Apron Could Talk: Use an immersion blender to quickly puree overripe bananas. For the 1-cup yield, use about 2½ medium-size or 2 large bananas. Using a large cup and immersion blender, puree until smooth. You can also mash the bananas if you don't have an immersion blender, though the consistency will not be as smooth.

Make It More-ish! If you like, add about ⅓ cup of chopped nuts such as pecans or walnuts, or dark chocolate chips!

Savvy Subs and Adds: You can also use 2 cups of whole wheat pastry flour or 2⅓ cups of oat flour for a spelt flour substitute.

Strawberry Goji Muffins

MAKES 10 TO 12 MUFFINS

wheat soy FREE

The brilliant color of this strawberry-goji batter is incentive enough to whip up these muffins, though getting antioxidant- and vitamin-rich gojis and strawberries in a muffin is also pretty convincing!

1 cup oat flour
1 cup sifted or light spelt flour
⅓ cup unrefined sugar
¼ teaspoon (rounded) sea salt
¼ teaspoon ground cardamom or cinnamon
2 teaspoons baking powder
½ teaspoon baking soda
1 cup frozen strawberries
½ cup + 1 to 2 tablespoons plain or vanilla nondairy milk
¼ cup dried goji berries
¼ cup pure maple syrup
1 tablespoon freshly squeezed lemon juice
1 tablespoon arrowroot powder
2 tablespoons neutral-flavored oil (see "Plant-Powered Pantry," page xxxii)
1 to 2 teaspoons unrefined sugar, for topping (optional)

Preheat the oven to 375°F.

In a large bowl, combine the flours, sugar, salt, and cardamom, sifting in the baking powder and baking soda. Stir to mix well.

In a blender, combine the strawberries, milk, goji berries, maple syrup, lemon juice, and arrowroot powder (if you don't have a high-powered blender such as a Blendtec, you can place all these ingredients in the blender and let sit for a few minutes to help soften the gojis, while you prepare the dry mixture and your muffin pan). Puree until fully smooth; the goji berries should be pulverized.

Add the blended mixture, as well as the oil, to the dry ingredients. Mix until well combined.

Scoop the batter into lined muffin pans (filling ten to twelve muffin cups), and sprinkle with the optional sugar. Bake for 19 to 24 minutes, until the muffins are set in the center (they should look set on the surface, and you can test by inserting a toothpick or skewer into the center of a muffin—it should come out clean). (Alternatively, for smaller muffins, scoop about ¼ cup of batter into about fourteen lined muffin cups. Bake for 12 to 14 minutes, until they test for doneness as above.)

Remove from the oven, let cool for a couple of minutes in the pan, and then transfer the muffins to cool on a cooling rack.

Make It More-ish! If you'd like to add some whole goji berries to the muffins as well, go ahead and sprinkle a couple of tablespoons in with the dry ingredients. Also, a sprinkling of dark chocolate chips is always a welcome addition!

Steel-Cut Oats in an Instant!

MAKES 2 TO 3 SERVINGS

wheat
(optionally) gluten **FREE**
soy

Steel-cut oats are incredibly nutritious, and make the most satisfying cereal. But they take some time to cook, and we need quicker fixes in the morning. The trick to making these oats quickly is to first grind the oats in a blender. The oats then cook up more like a porridge, similar to the "cream of wheat" I remember from childhood, and cook in a mere five minutes! Now, you can have your morning steel-cut oats . . . in, well, almost an instant. Although children can sometimes be fussy about the texture of whole grains, you may find they love this oatmeal.

¾ cup ground steel-cut oats (see note) (use certified gluten-free oats for that option)
2 cups water (see note)
Pinch of salt
¼ to ½ teaspoon ground cinnamon
A few pinches of freshly grated nutmeg (optional)
4 to 6 tablespoons nondairy milk (plus more for serving, if desired; see note)
Optional toppings: chopped fresh fruit, nuts, dried fruit, and/or a sprinkle of unrefined sugar or a drizzle of maple syrup (also see note)

In a saucepan, combine the oats, water, salt, cinnamon, and nutmeg (if using) over medium heat. Whisk almost continuously while the mixture starts to come to a slow boil. Lower the heat to medium-low as the mixture thickens and starts to bubble. Once thickened, stir in the milk (use a large spoon at this stage as whisking will be difficult). The total cooking time should be just 4 to 5 minutes. Watch carefully and stir frequently, as once the mixture starts to thicken it can scorch at too high a heat setting.

Serve the oatmeal immediately, topping with another drizzle of nondairy milk (as oatmeal will thicken more as it sits), and adding the optional toppings if desired.

If This Apron Could Talk: Place steel-cut oats in a blender and pulse or puree until you have a flourlike consistency. I usually do this in batches of 2 to 3 cups, and store the extra "flour" in a container for quick use in cookies and this porridge. Measure out the ¾ cup needed for this recipe.

Protein Power: Stir in a few tablespoons of nut butter or peanut butter. It will melt and dissolve creamily with the oatmeal. Or sprinkle in ¼ cup of hemp seeds, or 2 to 3 tablespoons white chia seeds.

Savvy Subs and Adds:
- Try substituting organic apple cider (juice, that is; not vinegar!) for the water—a naturally sweet and delicious switch!
- If using a vanilla nondairy milk, it will add extra sweetness and a light vanilla flavor to this oatmeal. Feel free to sweeten more to taste with a sprinkling of unrefined sugar (coconut sugar is especially nice!), or a drizzle of pure maple syrup.
- If, like me, you have memories of oatmeal or cream of wheat topped with brown sugar, try coconut sugar. It has a caramel-like flavor and color, and while it's not in the oatmeal photo, it really is delicious sprinkled on top!

Apple Spice Hemp Pancakes

MAKES 10 TO 14 SMALL TO MEDIUM PANCAKES

wheat soy **FREE**

These wholesome pancakes have no added sugar, and yet borrow natural sweetness from the addition of cinnamon and apple. With pancakes this tasty and healthy, it's easy to oblige requests for seconds!

1¼ cups spelt flour (see note)
⅔ cup hemp seeds (see note)
2½ teaspoons baking powder
1 teaspoon ground cinnamon
¼ to ½ teaspoon freshly grated nutmeg
¼ teaspoon ground allspice
A few pinches of sea salt (a scant ⅛ teaspoon)
1½ cups + 2 to 3 tablespoons vanilla nondairy milk (see note)
1 tablespoon neutral-flavored oil (see "Plant-Powered Pantry," page xxxii)
¾ cup apple, peeled, cored, and diced

In a large bowl, combine the flour and hemp seeds, sifting in the baking powder. Add the cinnamon, nutmeg, allspice, and salt and stir well.

In a small bowl, combine the 1½ cups of milk, oil, and diced apple and stir well.

Add the wet mixture to the dry mixture and stir just until well combined.

Using the edge of a paper towel, lightly oil a nonstick skillet. On medium-high heat, heat the pan for a few minutes until hot, then lower the heat to medium or medium-low and let the pan rest there for a minute.

Using a ladle, scoop the batter into the pan to form pancakes. Cook for several minutes, until small bubbles form on the outer edge and into the center. Flip the pancakes to lightly brown the other side, 1 to 2 minutes. Repeat until all the batter is used, adding the remaining milk to thin the batter as needed (see note).

If This Apron Could Talk: If you are new to using hemp seeds, you can reduce the measurement to ½ cup and see how you like the pancakes with that amount added. Note that you may not need the extra 2 to 3 tablespoons of milk if you use fewer hemp seeds.

Savvy Subs and Adds:
- If you'd prefer to use whole wheat pastry flour, use just 1 cup, and you will need about 1½ cups of milk, plus another 1 to 3 tablespoons to thin the batter.
- Vanilla-flavored nondairy milk will add a touch of sweetness to this batter, and a little more flavor than will plain. Also, you will notice that the batter will thicken as it sits, so stir in another 2 to 3 tablespoons of milk as needed to thin out batter slightly while working in batches.

Chocolate Drop Blueberry Pancakes

MAKES 11 TO 14 MEDIUM TO LARGE PANCAKES

wheat *soy* **FREE**

There's something seriously addictive about blueberries and chocolate together. Just try and keep your fork away from these pancakes!

1½   cups + 2 tablespoons spelt flour
1   tablespoon baking powder
½   teaspoon ground cinnamon
⅛   teaspoon (rounded) sea salt
⅓   cup nondairy chocolate chips
1½   cups + 1 to 2 tablespoons vanilla nondairy milk (see note)
1 to 1½   tablespoons neutral-flavored oil (see "Plant-Powered Pantry," page xxxii) or organic extra-virgin coconut oil, melted
1   cup fresh or frozen blueberries (see note)

Place the flour in a large bowl and sift in the baking powder. Add the cinnamon, salt, and chips and stir well.

In a small bowl, combine 1½ cups of the milk with the oil and stir well.

Add the wet mixture to the dry mixture and stir just until well combined. Add the blueberries and gently mix (if using frozen, you can wait to add them just before you are ready to ladle).

Using the edge of a paper towel, lightly oil a nonstick skillet. On medium-high heat, heat the pan for a few minutes until hot, then lower the heat to medium or medium-low and let the pan rest there for a minute.

Using a ladle, scoop the batter into the pan to form pancakes. Cook for several minutes, until small bubbles form on the outer edge and into the center. Flip the pancakes to lightly brown the other side, 1 to 2 minutes. Repeat until all the batter is used, adding the remaining milk to thin the batter as needed (see note).

If This Apron Could Talk: Begin with 1½ cups of milk and whisk into the batter. At first the batter will be very thin, but give it a few minutes. Later, as you've worked through some of the batter, you'll notice that it might become too thick. So, add the remaining 1 to 2 tablespoons of milk, a little at a time, to thin the mixture if needed.

If using frozen blueberries, the pancakes will need a little longer to cook, as the batter needs to set up around the cold berries. If needed, lower the heat a little to allow the pancakes to set without overbrowning.

Protein Power: Slather your finished pancakes with a layer of cashew or almond butter—or even hemp nut butter. It will become melty with the warmth of the pancakes, and with a drizzle of pure maple syrup—just divine!

Whole-Grain Chia Pancakes

MAKES 12 TO 16 PANCAKES

 wheat soy **FREE**

Who says pancakes can't be healthy? These combine whole-grain flours with whole white chia seeds. They are fluffy, tender, delicious, and nutritious!

1¼ cups spelt flour
½ cup oat flour
¼ cup whole white chia seeds (not ground)
3½ teaspoons baking powder
½ to ¾ teaspoon ground cinnamon
¼ teaspoon freshly grated nutmeg
⅛ teaspoon sea salt
1¾ + 1 to 3 tablespoons plain or vanilla nondairy milk (see note)
½ teaspoon pure vanilla extract
1½ tablespoons neutral-flavored oil (see "Plant-Powered Pantry," page xxxii)

In a large bowl, combine the flours and chia seeds, sifting in the baking powder. Add the cinnamon, nutmeg, and salt and stir well.

In a small bowl, combine the 1¾ cups of milk, vanilla, and oil and stir well.

Add the wet mixture to the dry mixture and stir until combined. Let the batter sit for a couple of minutes while preparing the pan.

Using the edge of a paper towel, lightly oil a nonstick skillet. On medium-high heat, heat the pan for a few minutes until hot, then lower heat to medium or medium-low and let the pan rest there for a minute.

Using a ladle, scoop the batter into the pan to form pancakes (see note). Cook for several minutes, until small bubbles form on the outer edge and into the center and the pancakes are starting to look dry in spots on the top. Flip the pancakes to lightly cook other side, about a minute. Repeat until all the batter is used, adding the remaining milk to thin the batter as needed (see note).

If This Apron Could Talk: Begin with 1¾ cups of milk and whisk into the batter. At first the batter will be very thin, but give it a few minutes. The flour and chia seeds will quickly thicken the mixture. Later, as you've worked through some of the batter, you'll notice that it becomes much thicker. So, add an extra tablespoon of milk at a time, to thin the mixture if needed.

Ingredients 411: Be sure to buy whole white chia seeds (for optimal color in these pancakes), rather than the black chia seeds that you might find online or in stores.

Welsh Cakes

MAKES 20 TO 24 CAKES

wheat soy FREE

One day our daughter returned home from school and asked if I could make Welsh Cakes. Her class was doing medieval studies and was planning a feast, complete with Welsh Cakes. I modified the original recipe, removing white flour and also replacing the eggs and other ingredients. After testing this recipe several times, I decided that instead of panfrying the cakes (as is done traditionally), I would instead scoop the batter and bake the cakes much like cookies or small muffins. I prefer this baking method, as it is much easier—and I also like the results of puffier cakes! I have given directions for both cooking methods so you can do either.

1½ tablespoons flax meal, or 1 scant tablespoon of ground white chia seeds

3 tablespoons water

½ cup organic extra-virgin coconut oil (see note)

¼ cup fine-granule unrefined sugar

2¼ cups light or sifted spelt flour (see note)

1 tablespoon baking powder

½ teaspoon sea salt

¼ teaspoon freshly grated nutmeg

¼ teaspoon ground cinnamon

1 teaspoon lemon or orange zest (optional)

¼ to ⅓ cup raisins or currants

5 to 6½ tablespoons nondairy milk (as needed, a little less for whole wheat pastry substitution; see note)

Jam, for serving (optional)

Unrefined sugar, for coating or serving (optional, see page xlii)

Preheat the oven to 350°F (or see panfrying directions).

In a small bowl, first combine the flax meal with the water and set aside for it to become thick.

In a mixer fitted with the paddle attachment (see note), first combine the coconut oil and sugar and mix until creamy. Then add the flax mixture and mix again.

In a separate bowl, combine the flour, baking powder, salt, nutmeg, cinnamon, and zest. Stir well, then add about half of the dry mixture to the mixer. Mix on low speed for about 30 seconds, and then add the remaining dry ingredients and raisins.

Mix again, then begin to add the milk. Add a tablespoon at a time, until a dough forms (I typically use 5 or 5½ tablespoons, but you may need more, depending on the brand of flour and other variables). Try not to overmix; just stir until the dough comes together.

Scoop the mixture (using a cookie scoop is easiest), using 1 to 1½ tablespoons of batter per cake. If using the unrefined sugar, place in a small bowl. Take each scoop and lightly roll in the sugar to coat. Place on a baking sheet lined with parchment paper.

Bake for 19 to 20 minutes, then remove from the oven and let cool for a minute or two on the baking sheet. Then transfer to a cooling rack, or directly to a plate. For a more traditional type of serving, break open, spread on a little jam, and enjoy!

To panfry: Transfer the mixture to a lightly floured surface and roll out to a thickness of about ¼ inch. Using a cookie cutter (or the open side of a small cup), cut 2- to 3-inch rounds in the dough. Lightly oil a nonstick skillet, and heat on medium or medium-high heat. Add the cakes in batches and cook for 3 to 4 minutes on the first side and then 2 to 3 minutes on the second, until golden brown on the outside but soft inside (lower the heat if they are browning too much). Remove from the pan, lightly spread the top side with coconut oil or margarine, and sprinkle with unrefined sugar (if using).

If This Apron Could Talk: If you don't have a mixer, make this batter in a food processor: Briefly pulse the flour, sugar, baking powder, salt, nutmeg, and cinnamon to combine. Add the oil and pulse a few times, until the mixture is a coarse crumb (don't process fully or for too long). Next, pulse in the flax mixture and milk (I typically use 5 or 5½ tablespoons, but you may need more depending on the brand of flour and other variables) just until a dough begins to form. Remove the cover of the processor and check to see if the dough will hold when pressed together. If so, then pulse in the raisins and zest very briefly (just to combine, not to chop the raisins).

Savvy Subs and Adds: If you would like to make a wheat-based version, use whole wheat pastry flour. You will need 2 cups less 3 tablespoons of the flour, and between 4 and 5 tablespoons of nondairy milk.

Cocoa Goji Granola

MAKES 5½ TO 6 CUPS

*wheat
(optionally) gluten
soy*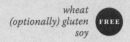

This granola is lightly sweetened, rather than sickly sweet as some commercial varieties of granola can be. Full of healthful ingredients, it makes a great snack to eat straight out of your hand!

2½ cups rolled oats (use certified gluten-free oats for that option)
½ cup millet
¾ cup hemp seeds
¼ cup unsweetened shredded coconut (see note)
3 to 4 tablespoons unrefined sugar (I use coconut sugar; Sucanat and date sugar are also good choices)
¼ cup sunflower seeds (see note)
¼ cup unsweetened cocoa powder
½ teaspoon ground cinnamon
⅛ teaspoon freshly grated nutmeg
¼ teaspoon (scant) sea salt
½ cup brown rice syrup
3 tablespoons organic extra-virgin coconut oil (at room temperature; see note)
1 teaspoon pure vanilla extract
⅓ to ½ cup goji berries (see note)
1 teaspoon orange zest

Preheat the oven to 300°F and line a large rimmed baking sheet with parchment paper.

In a bowl, combine the rolled oats, dry millet, hemp seeds, coconut, sugar, sunflower seeds, cocoa, cinnamon, nutmeg, and salt and stir until well mixed. Add the brown rice syrup, coconut oil, and vanilla and stir well (see note).

Transfer the mixture to the prepared baking sheet and spread out to distribute evenly. Bake for 28 to 30 minutes, stirring a couple of times throughout the baking process to ensure the mixture browns evenly.

Remove from oven, stir in the goji berries and orange zest, and let cool completely. Serve with cold nondairy milk, and store in an airtight container.

If This Apron Could Talk: If your coconut oil isn't warmed until liquefied, take a shortcut! Simply toss all ingredients as best you can and transfer to the prepared baking sheet. After 2 to 3 minutes of baking, the oil will have melted. Remove your baking sheet from the oven and now toss everything until well combined. Back into the oven it goes, but do remember to stir a couple of times again during the total baking time.

Savvy Subs and Adds: Chopped almonds are a natural complement to the orange and cocoa flavors in this granola, so feel free to replace the sunflower seeds (and/or the coconut) with some chopped almonds.

Not everyone is fond of goji berries. Feel free to substitute raisins or even cranberries (or combination of both) for the goji berries. Add them at the same time in the recipe, just after removing the granola from the oven.

Wholesome Oat Snackles!

MAKES 12 TO 14 SNACKLES

wheat
(optionally) gluten **FREE**
soy

Sometimes muffins and snacks can be a little on the sweet side for parents and adults who are looking to reduce the amount of added sweeteners in their diet. While most of my baked goods such as muffins are pretty healthful, these little snackles are particularly low in sweetener—and oil! They are great for packing in lunches, or to curb midmorning cravings. It's like having your oatmeal without the bowl!

1	cup rolled or quick oats (use certified gluten-free oats for that option)
1	cup oat flour (use certified gluten-free for that option)
⅓	cup raisins
¼	cup hemp seeds or unsweetened shredded coconut
1	teaspoon baking powder
1	teaspoon ground cinnamon
1	teaspoon lemon or orange zest (optional)
¼	teaspoon sea salt
	A few pinches of freshly grated nutmeg (optional, but nice flavor if not using zest)
½	cup unsweetened applesauce (see note)
¼	cup pure maple syrup (see note)
1	tablespoon neutral-flavored oil (see "Plant-Powered Pantry," page xxxii)
2 to 3	tablespoons nondairy chocolate chips (optional; you can omit if needing to reduce sugars)

Preheat the oven to 350°F. Line a baking sheet with parchment paper.

In a large bowl, combine the oats, oat flour, raisins, hemp seeds or coconut, baking powder, cinnamon, zest, salt and nutmeg, stirring to mix well. Add the applesauce, maple syrup, oil, and chocolate chips (if using). Stir until well incorporated

Use a cookie scoop (or take spoonfuls, about 1½ tablespoons in size) to transfer mounds of the batter to the baking sheet. Bake for 14 to 15 minutes, remove from the oven, and let cool on the pan for about a minute, then transfer to a cooling rack.

Savvy Subs and Adds: You can substitute ½ cup of pureed overripe banana for the applesauce. Since very ripened banana is typically sweeter than unsweetened applesauce (and also a little thicker), you can then reduce the maple syrup to 2 to 3 tablespoons and add 1 to 2 tablespoons of nondairy milk

To make these snackles slightly sweeter, add either extra raisins, or 1 to 2 tablespoons of an unrefined sugar such as Sucanat or coconut sugar. You can also add another 1 tablespoon of maple syrup (note that adding much more liquid sweetener will change the consistency of the batter).

Breakfast Cookies

MAKES 12 TO 14
AVERAGE-SIZE COOKIES

*wheat
(optionally) gluten
soy* **FREE**

These cookies are practically flour free—as well as sugar free, dairy free, *and* egg free! These gems are nutritious, using steel-cut oats, ground into a powdery flour substitute, combined with a healthy mix of natural sweeteners, dried fruit, and nut butter. Go ahead, indulge for breakfast . . . these are cookies you needn't feel guilty about eating first thing in the morning!

3 tablespoons pure maple syrup

2 tablespoons ground white chia seeds or flax meal

1 teaspoon pure vanilla extract

3 tablespoons brown rice syrup

2 tablespoons raw cashew butter (see note)

1½ tablespoons organic extra-virgin coconut oil (at room temperature) or organic neutral-flavored oil (see "Plant-Powered Pantry," page xxxii)

1 teaspoon orange or lemon zest (optional)

1¼ cups ground steel-cut oats (see page xl) (use certified gluten-free oats for that option)

½ teaspoon ground cinnamon

¼ teaspoon ground cardamom (or use freshly grated nutmeg or more cinnamon)

1 teaspoon xanthan gum

¼ teaspoon sea salt

1 teaspoon baking powder

3 to 4 tablespoons chopped unsulfured dried fruit (e.g., apricots, apples, cranberries, raisins, dates, goji berries)

2 tablespoons nondairy chocolate chips (try grain-sweetened chocolate chips, or omit for sugar-free version)

Preheat the oven to 350°F. Line a baking sheet with parchment paper.

In a mixer fitted with the paddle attachment, combine the maple syrup, chia, vanilla, brown rice syrup, cashew butter, oil, and zest. Blend for a minute or two until well mixed.

In a separate bowl, combine the dry ingredients, sifting in the baking powder, and stirring in the fruit and chips until well incorporated.

Add the dry mixture to the wet mixture. Churn with the mixer for a minute or so, until the mixture has come together.

Using a cookie scoop, transfer 1-tablespoon scoops of the batter to the prepared baking sheet. Bake for 11 to 12 minutes.

Remove from the oven, let cool for a minute or two on the pan, and then use a spatula to transfer to a cooling rack. The cookies will be soft, but will firm up while cooling. (Note: If using coconut oil, the cookies will be quite soft until they are completely cooled. Let them rest on the baking pan for an extra minute or two, and take care transferring to the cooling rack.)

If This Apron Could Talk: You can also make these cookies without a mixer. First combine the wet ingredients in a bowl (let the cashew butter and coconut oil come to room temperature first, to soften), and then the dry mixture in another bowl. Combine the two by hand, until well incorporated.

If you think about it ahead of time, remove your nut butter and brown rice syrup from the refrigerator and let sit at room temperature until softened or warmer. It will be easier to measure and mix with the wet ingredients.

Make It More-ish! These cookies are not meant to be a dessert cookie; rather, a healthy breakfast, snack, or "on-the-go" cookie. As such, they have a natural sweetness, but aren't nearly as sweet as dessert cookies. If you'd like them a little sweeter, try adding 2 tablespoons of unrefined sugar to the dry ingredients (or another couple of tablespoons of chocolate chips!).

Savvy Subs and Adds: While I love using raw cashew butter in these cookies, you can use other raw nut butters, such as almond butter, or also regular roasted nut butters (e.g., cashew or almond), or natural peanut butter. For a nut-free version, you can use seed butter such as tahini or pumpkin seed butter. For the best taste, use raw tahini instead of regular tahini (raw has a milder flavor than regular tahini). Because seed butters are not as naturally sweet as nut butters, you may want to add 1 to 2 tablespoons of unrefined sugar (or extra dried fruit) to the dry ingredients.

Cocoa Almond Jumbles

MAKES 13 TO 16 JUMBLES

wheat (optionally) gluten soy **FREE**

I designed these with my Banana Oat Bundles from *Vive le Vegan!* in mind. I wanted a variation that was nutty and chocolaty, and these baby jumbles were born! With rolled oats, ground almonds, almond butter, and applesauce—and no added oil—they are just the thing to satisfy that mid-morning hunger pang. Be sure to grab one still warm out of the oven.

1 cup	+ 2 tablespoons rolled or quick oats (see note) (use certified gluten-free oats for that option)
½	cup almond meal (see note for nut-free option)
¼	cup unrefined sugar (I like coconut sugar)
¼	teaspoon (scant) sea salt
¼	cup unsweetened cocoa powder
1	teaspoon baking powder
⅓	cup almond butter (see note for nut-free option)
¼	cup unsweetened applesauce
2½	tablespoons pure maple syrup or agave nectar
2	teaspoons pure vanilla extract
2 to 3	tablespoons nondairy chocolate chips (optional)

Preheat the oven to 350°F. Line a baking sheet with parchment paper.

In a large bowl, combine the oats, almond meal, sugar, and salt, and sift in the cocoa powder and baking powder.

In another smaller bowl, combine the almond butter with the applesauce, maple syrup, vanilla, and add the chocolate chips, if using. Stir to mix well.

Add the wet mixture to the dry mixture, and stir until well incorporated and the mixture is sticky and holding together when pressed.

Use a small cookie scoop (or take small spoonfuls and lightly roll in your hands) and transfer mounds of the batter to the prepared baking sheet. Bake for 12 to 13 minutes, remove from the oven, and let cool on the pan for about a minute, then transfer to a cooling rack.

Allergy-Free or Bust! To make these nut free, use these substitutions: Replace the almond butter with an equal amount of pumpkin seed butter, and replace the almond meal with ½ cup of oat flour. Also, increase the maple syrup to 3 tablespoons. I have noticed differences in the bitterness of pumpkin seed butters. In testing, my choice here is Nuts to You brand. Other brands will still work; you may just need to bump up the sweetener, using an extra sprinkle of unrefined sugar (rather than extra maple syrup so the batter doesn't become too loose).

If This Apron Could Talk: The batter will thicken more as the oats absorb the moisture of the wet ingredients, and the rolled oats will give a heartier type of snack cookie.

Ingredients 411: You can keep these healthier with less sugar added by leaving out the chocolate chips . . . but adding just a modest amount of chips doesn't hurt much!

Proper Healthy Granola Bars

MAKES 9 TO 16 BARS

wheat
(optionally) gluten **FREE**
soy

While some granola bars tout being "healthy," most really aren't, so I created these granola bars that are just right—not too sweet and that can be customized with some additions of spices or switches of dried fruit. I've been asked numerous times for a proper granola bar, and so here you have it!

½ cup brown rice syrup

1 tablespoon organic extra-virgin coconut oil, or 2 tablespoons nut butter (e.g., almond or cashew)

1 teaspoon pure vanilla extract

½ teaspoon agar powder (see note)

1½ cups rolled oats or barley flakes (use certified gluten-free oats for that option)

1 cup natural rice crisp cereal (not puffed rice, I use Natures Path brand)

½ cup raw sunflower seeds

¼ cup ground white chia seeds

¼ cup hemp seeds

½ cup raisins

3 tablespoons nondairy chocolate chips (optional)

¼ teaspoon sea salt

½ teaspoon ground cinnamon

Preheat the oven to 350°F. Line an 8-inch square cake pan with parchment paper.

In a small saucepan, combine the brown rice syrup with the oil, vanilla, and agar over medium-low heat. Stir and just gently heat through (do not boil, you are heating simply to melt the coconut oil and liquefy the brown rice syrup) and then remove from the heat. Set aside while preparing other ingredients.

Combine the oats, cereal, sunflower seeds, chia seeds, hemp seeds, raisins, chips, salt, and cinnamon in a mixing bowl and stir well.

Add the wet mixture to the dry mixture (scraping out all the sticky mixture from the saucepan) and stir very well, until the mixture will hold together somewhat when pressed with the back of your spoon.

Quickly transfer mixture to the prepared pan. Use a corner of parchment paper to press the mixture firmly and evenly into the pan. Bake for 17 to 20 minutes, until the bars are golden brown around the edges (but don't let burn), then remove from the oven and transfer to a cooling rack to begin to cool. Then, using a serrated knife, begin to score the bars while still hot/warm, marking out the bars as you'd like to cut them after cooling (They don't have to be cut all the way, just scored about halfway into the bars—this will make it easier to cut once chilled). Once cooled, transfer to the fridge until fully chilled.

After chilling, cut into bars along the scoring marks. Refrigerate in an airtight container, or in the freezer.

Ingredients 411: The agar helps give these bars a little extra firmness, but you can still make them without the agar if you don't have it on hand.

Monsta! Cookies

MAKES 12 TO 16
MONSTA! GOOD COOKIES!

wheat
soy **FREE**

Monsta, marvelous, magnificent, more-ish! These are jam-packed with healthful ingredients, and even though these are not your dessert kind of cookies, they will give that sweet tooth something to sing about!

⅓ cup organic extra-virgin coconut oil, or ⅓ cup (scant) neutral-flavored oil (see "Plant-Powered Pantry," page xxxii; also see note)

¼ cup pure maple syrup

¼ cup brown rice syrup (or more maple syrup)

2 tablespoons coconut or other unrefined sugar (optional; see note)

1 to 1½ teaspoons pure vanilla extract

1 cup light or sifted spelt flour

¾ cup oat flour

2 teaspoons baking powder

½ teaspoon ground cinnamon, or ¼ teaspoon freshly grated nutmeg

¼ teaspoon sea salt

½ cup unsweetened shredded coconut

2 tablespoons flax meal, or 1½ tablespoons ground white chia seeds

⅓ cup pecans or walnuts, lightly broken or chopped (for a nut-free version, use ¼ cup sunflower seeds)

¼ cup hemp seeds

¼ cup pumpkin seeds (or sunflower seeds if not substituting for walnuts, above)

Preheat the oven to 350°F. Line a baking sheet with parchment paper.

In a mixer fitted with the paddle attachment, combine the coconut oil, maple syrup, brown rice syrup, sugar (if using), and vanilla. Mix on low speed to incorporate for about a minute.

In a separate bowl, combine all the dry ingredients, except the nuts and seeds, and stir well.

Add about half of the dry mixture to the wet mixture. Churn with the mixer to start to incorporate, and then add the remaining dry mixture, as well as the nuts and seeds. Continue to stir on low speed, just until the mixture comes together and forms a dough on the paddle.

Scoop spoonfuls (1½ to 2 tablespoons in size; a cookie scoop works very well but isn't essential), and place on the prepared baking sheet. Bake for 14 minutes, then remove from the oven and let the cookies cool for about a minute on the baking sheet. Transfer to a cooling rack to cool completely.

If This Apron Could Talk: The unrefined sugar is optional—the cookies are still sweet and tasty without it, so if you don't want to use any granulated sugar of any sort, then omit it. But, for a slightly sweeter taste, you can include the 2 tablespoons of sugar.

Savvy Subs and Adds: If you prefer another oil to coconut, feel free to do so, just use a slightly scant measure.

Feel free to add ¼ cup of raisins, dried cranberries, or other dried fruit to the dry ingredients. You can include it as an addition, or as a replacement for some of the seeds or nuts.

Cocoa Cookie Dough Balls

MAKES 14 TO 16 DOUGH BALLS

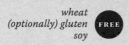

wheat
(optionally) gluten **FREE**
soy

Psst, these are really healthy. No need to tell the kids, or anyone else, for that matter; just eat them up knowing they are filled with almonds and oats, and sweetened only with dates and raisins.

½ cup raw almonds (see note for nut-free option)

½ cup + 2 tablespoons rolled oats (use certified gluten-free oats for that option)

A few pinches of sea salt (about a scant ⅛ teaspoon)

1 cup pitted dates

¼ cup raisins

¼ cup unsweetened cocoa powder

1 teaspoon pure vanilla extract

2 tablespoons nondairy chocolate chips or cocoa nibs (optional)

A few teaspoons of unsweetened cocoa powder, unrefined sugar, or a combination of both, for dusting/rolling (optional)

In a food processor, process the almonds until fine and crumbly. Then add remaining ingredients and (except the optional chocolate chips) pulse or process. Once the mixture starts to become crumbly, process fully for a minute or two. It will appear as if nothing is happening at first, that the mixture is just whirring around in crumbs, but soon it will start to become sticky. When you see it start to become a little sticky, add the chocolate chips and process again. Continue to process until it forms a ball on the blade. Stop the machine and remove the dough.

Take small scoops of the dough (1 to 1½ tablespoons in size) and roll in your hand. Repeat until you have rolled all of the dough. Toss or roll the balls in the coating, if using, and refrigerate. Eat and repeat often.

Allergy-Free or Bust! For a nut-free version, replace the almonds with just ¼ cup of raw pumpkin seeds, and add another ¼ cup of rolled oats.

If This Apron Could Talk: Make a double batch and freeze half. They thaw very well.

Kid-Friendly: These are excellent to pack in school lunches, with a nut-free option for you if nuts aren't permitted in your school.

Savvy Subs and Adds: Replace vanilla with ½ teaspoon almond extract or orange oil.

"Momelet"

MAKES 7 TO 9
SMALL "MOMELETS"

wheat
gluten
(optionally) soy 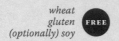 **FREE**

One of our daughters was curious about omelets and asked if we could eat them. I came up with these versions: one that's nut free and made with soy, and the other that's soy free and made with nuts! Of course, this does differ in some respects to an egg-based omelet; the soy version is slightly more "eggy" in texture, but not vastly so to detract from the soy-free version. Either way, it's a great, hearty breakfast or lunch dish for the whole gang.

SOY VERSION:

1 (12-ounce) package extra-firm silken tofu (see note)
½ cup corn flour or finely stone-ground cornmeal (see note)
2 teaspoons freshly squeezed lemon juice
¼ cup plain unsweetened nondairy milk (almond or soy preferred; see "Plant-Powered Pantry," page xxxiii)
1 tablespoon potato starch or arrowroot powder
1 teaspoon baking powder
½ teaspoon sea salt
¼ teaspoon onion powder
¼ teaspoon (rounded) turmeric
½ teaspoon yellow prepared mustard (usually gluten free, but check label)
½ teaspoon agave nectar
2 teaspoons olive oil
1 to 3 teaspoons olive oil, for oiling pan

In a blender, puree all the ingredients, except the oil for the pan, until very smooth, stopping to scrape down the sides as needed.

Heat a nonstick skillet over medium heat, and wipe the frying surface with a touch of oil.

Ladle ¼ to ⅓ cup of the mixture onto the skillet. Quickly use the base of the ladle to gently and gradually spread out the omelet (much like you would do to frost a cake; slowly bring the mixture from the center out to edges) to 5 to 5½ inches in diameter. Cook over medium heat for 3 to 4 minutes, or until you can see the surface area is setting up. Check the bottom of the omelet to see if it is golden brown in a few spots, and if so, flip over (if it is difficult to flip, it needs more time to set up).

If desired, sprinkle fillings over half of the omelet (to cover a half-moon), then after the second side has cooked for a couple of minutes, fold the unfilled side of the omelet over the filled side (see note for soy-free version). Let cook another minute or two to warm or melt the fillings, then serve. Repeat with remaining omelet mixture, reducing the heat a touch, if needed, as working through the batter.

Serve on their own, or sandwiched in bread, pitas, or tortillas with veggies, condiments (e.g., ketchup), or sauces (e.g., tahini sauce).

Ingredients 411: Opt for the standard extra-firm silken tofu, rather than the "lite" version. Also, in a pinch, soft tofu can be used in this recipe. One 10½-ounce package works fine.

¾ cup soaked raw cashews (will blend easier than unsoaked)

1 tablespoon ground white chia seeds

⅓ cup corn flour or finely stoneground cornmeal (see note)

1 tablespoon freshly squeezed lemon juice

1 cup + 3 tablespoons plain unsweetened nondairy milk (almond preferred; see "Plant-Powered Pantry," page xxxiii)

3 tablespoons potato starch or arrowroot powder

½ teaspoon sea salt

¼ teaspoon onion powder

¼ teaspoon (rounded) turmeric

½ teaspoon yellow prepared mustard (usually gluten free, but check label)

2 teaspoons olive oil

1 to 3 teaspoons olive oil, for oiling pan

SUGGESTED FILLINGS:

Cashew cheese or other nondairy cheese (e.g., Daiya)

Sliced green onions

Chopped fresh herbs

Chopped fresh tomatoes

Sautéed mushrooms

Chopped bell peppers

Fresh spinach leaves

Follow the previous directions. Note that the soy-free version doesn't need to be flipped before adding your optional fillings. It sets up a little differently, so once you see the surface area becoming a little firm, you can add the fillings, then fold over to finish cooking—or you can flip it if you prefer to brown both sides.

Adult-Minded: Sometimes I add ¼ cup of sun-dried tomatoes (packed in oil), drained, patted dry, and roughly chopped (optional) to the puree. They offer another flavor note to the omelet that adults especially might enjoy.

Ingredients 411: Very finely ground cornmeal is similar to corn flour in texture. However, if it is a medium grind, the cornmeal will be too granular. Look for an organic corn flour or fine stone-ground cornmeal. Bob's Red Mill brand is a good choice.

Let Them Drink Smoothies!

I'm not sure where I'd be without my morning smoothie. Usually it's a green smoothie—or purple, if blackberries or blueberries have their way! In winter months, I might opt for a creamy nut- and milk-based smoothie, but most often I feel very nourished and off to a good start when the greens get it on in my blender.

Don't keep your kale waiting! While I've included some recipes here, what's more important is the technique: Think of this as a basic instruction manual for any and all delicious smoothies. Ingredients can vary; the options truly are endless, from kale to spinach, nut butters, and frozen fruits. Go ahead, get your green on!

"Go Green" with Smoothies

The first time I heard about the idea of putting greens into a smoothie, I was turned off. I couldn't get past the idea of taking inherently bitter, sometimes fibrous, and stringy greens, and pureeing them into a drink. But what I soon discovered is, when you blend greens such as spinach, kale, or chard with sweet fruits such as bananas, apples, mangoes, oranges, and/or pineapples, you truly don't notice the taste of the greens. The sweetness of the fruit predominates.

Now, green smoothies rule our mornings. I make a large batch every morning that my husband and I share, and sometimes our kids do, too. When I first got started with green smoothies, I used a recipe. Now, I ad-lib our smoothies every day. Once you get started making green smoothies, you'll find yourself playing with your own combinations.

Here are some tips to get you drinking your greens:

Choose your greens. My favorite leafies to use are kale and collard greens. They are robust, store well in the fridge for a few days, and are very nutritious with more absorbable calcium and iron than greens such as spinach and Swiss chard. But, spinach and Swiss chard still offer many nutritional benefits, so definitely try them out. Also, as spinach and chard are milder in flavor than kale and collards, they are good "starter" greens for making smoothies. If you are new to the green smoothie business, start with something like spinach, and work your way into stronger-flavored greens such as kale. Try blending spinach with kale; once you get the knack of fruit-to-greens proportions, this will also help you determine how much sweet fruit (e.g., banana, mango, and pineapple) to combine with the greens for the best flavor. You can also experiment with other greens and lettuces, though I wouldn't recommend spicy greens such as arugula or mustard greens in a smoothie—they are just too strong and peppery. Save those for your sautés and salads!

Wash and stem greens. Some greens can hold more grit, so fully submerge the greens in a sinkful of water, then rinse and shake off the excess water. (Be sure to dry your extra greens before refrigerating. Use a salad spinner or shake to dry well. Once they are mostly dry, I store in the fridge by loosely wrapping in a dish towel, and then placing inside a large resealable plastic bag [leave unzipped]. I find the greens keep well for a couple of days, don't get soggy and rot, and stay nicely crisp.) With such greens as collards, chard, and kale, you'll want to separate the leaves from the thick stems. Holding the leaf in one hand, run your fingers of your other hand down the length of the stalk to strip the stalk (separating the leafy portion from the tough stem). The more tender parts of the stem (at the tops) will usually tear away with the leaves, and this is okay—they are tender enough.

Fruits to use—sweet and some frozen.
Bananas and mangoes: Adding these sweet fruits will balance the bitterness of the greens. Bananas are an obvious choice because most of us have them on hand, they ripen easily, and also they add creaminess to the drink. Greenish bananas, stay on the counter—you're not welcome to this smoothie party! Let your bananas over-ripen, and then peel, slice, and store them (in large resealable bags or in other airtight containers) in your freezer. If you aren't overly fond of bananas, try frozen mangoes. They are very sweet, and also lend a subtly creamy texture. I keep bananas in my freezer, and regularly buy bags of frozen mangoes. Either or both combine well with other fruits—and those not frozen—for a delicious smoothie. If using bananas or mangoes that are fresh and not frozen, you may want to add ice cubes in place of water for your blending, to chill your drink, as using all room-temperature fruits will give you a warmish smoothie (not the greatest).

Pears, grapes, melons—oh, my: Other fruits that work well in your smoothie include apples, pears, seedless grapes, pineapple, peaches, sweet apples and oranges, and honeydew melon or cantaloupe. These are usually kept refrigerated or at room temperature (though grapes are a great fruit to freeze, just not commonly kept frozen), and so combining with some frozen fruit is optimal. Including some frozen fruit of any kind nicely chills your green smoothie. Seasonal fruit are another consideration. During the fall and winter, I find myself making smoothies primarily with apples and oranges (along with frozen bananas and/or mangoes); and in the summer, I take advantage of local organic fruits such as peaches and berries.

Berry-licious: Can't leave the fruit topic without talking about berries: Fresh or frozen strawberries, blueberries, and raspberries are, of course, delicious in a green smoothie—and very nutritious. The only thing you need to know about using red or purple berries is that the color of the smoothie changes. No longer will it be a vibrant inviting green color; rather, a more swampy brownish color, particularly when using red berries. But if you can ignore the color aesthetic, by all means, include some berries! On the other hand, if you want to mask the green color (for children . . . or adults!), then blue or purple berries such as blueberries, blackberries, or açai pulp work magic.

Another green surprise: Another fruit that can be included is avocado. Technically it is a fruit, though not often thought of as a fruit because it isn't juicy or particularly sweet.

But it can add a luscious creaminess to your smoothie, so try adding half an avocado to your mixture and see how you like it.

Add-ins. Smoothies are the perfect place to get in nutritious bits and bobs that you might otherwise find tricky to include in your diet. Try seeds such as hemp, flax, or chia; nuts (or nut butters, such as like almond); or goji berries, spirulina, cocoa nibs, or a hit of fresh ginger. A high-powered blender (e.g., Blendtec) really does the best job with hard seeds and fruits. It will pulverize chia seeds and gojis to smithereens! Also consider adding a tablespoon or two of a smoothie infusion powder, to add extra flavor and also nutritional value. I really like Vega's Tropical Tango and Vanilla Almondilla Shake & Go, and typically add 1 to 2 tablespoons to my smoothie blend, choosing a flavor to complement the fruits used in the smoothie.

Don't Forget Other Veggies! Even though my focus is on getting the leafy greens into your smoothies, let's not forget that there are other veggies worthy of joining the smoothie club. And green smoothie veterans might appreciate lessening the fruit proportions to favor more vegetables, such as cucumber. Start with smallish measures (perhaps ¼ to ½ cup), as some vegetables impart strong and bitter flavor tones. Cucumber is rather mild, with a melonlike flavor, so you might try adding more. You can also try celery and carrots, used in combinations that complement those particular veggies (e.g., honeydew melon with cucumber; carrot with mango).

Blending. Blend the heck out of your smoothie! Make it smooth, not still grainy or chunky or with bits of leaves floating about. No, blend like mad! It can be thick, as you can always thin with water, but definitely needs to be smooth. If using a regular blender, you will need to blend for a couple of minutes. Blend until the greens are so pulverized that they are no longer visible, other than infusing your smoothie with a beautiful green color. If using a high-powered blender such as a Blendtec, simply run the whole juice cycle, and if needed, pulse again afterward if any chunks of frozen fruit remain. Kale leaves can take longer to fully blend than spinach or chard (especially depending on your blender). I find that frozen fruits, such as banana and mango, also help the blender cut through the greens. Add ½ to ¾ cup of water to get everything moving. (You can add more later to thin, if desired; the amount of water needed varies depending on the proportion of thick fruits, such as bananas, and the amount of very juicy fruit, such as melon or orange. Start with less, then add more if you need to. Better to have a thick smoothie that can be thinned rather than a watery smoothie.) You can use a regular blender or even an immersion blender; they simply take longer to fully smooth out, and require more patience and a little effort.

Taste. After blending, dip in a spoon to taste before serving up. If you need more fruit to balance the sweetness . . . or water to thin, add it now. You can also opt for nondairy milk if you like to replace part or all of the water, or even some nondairy yogurt. While I prefer plain ol' water in my morning monster smoothies, you may enjoy the creamier consistency that a nondairy milk adds to your concoction. Once you've made enough of these (again, whether with this recipe or just adding to your own smoothies), you'll probably skip this step, as you'll have a sense of proportions needed.

So, you've got the general idea, and here are some examples of smoothie combinations that I love. But, know that this list is by no means exhaustive! There are so many combinations, you just need to play around to find your favorites. I'm including kale and collards here as the base green, just because they are the ones I use most and they offer the most absorbable calcium and iron. Certainly chard or spinach can be substituted for kale and collards. I've also started with 1 to 1½ cups of greens, but by all means increase the ratio of greens to 2 cups or more as you become accustomed to the flavor. These suggestions should yield two pretty large smoothies, but measurements are quite approximate, so modify as you need.

Orange Juicius: 1 to 1½ cups of collard greens leaves, about 1½ cups of frozen banana chunks, one apple (core removed, skins intact), one orange (peeled), 1 to 2 tablespoons of hemp seeds, plus enough water to get it moving and thin out, if you like.

Tropical Twist: 1 to 1½ cups of kale leaves, about 1 cup of frozen banana chunks, ½ to 1 cup of frozen mango chunks, ½ cup of fresh pineapple (cubed), ½ cup of cucumber chunks (optional), 1 to 2 tablespoons of Vega Mango-Tango Smoothie Infusion, 1 tablespoon of salba seeds, plus enough water to get it moving and thin out, if you like.

Immunity Zinger: 1 to 1½ cups of kale leaves, 1 to 1¼ cups of frozen bananas chunks, one large or two small apples (core removed, skins intact), ½ to ¾ cup of frozen mango chunks, about ½ tablespoon of peeled ginger, ½ peeled lemon, plus enough water to get it all moving.

Berry Blaster: 1 to 1½ cups collard greens leaves, about 1½ cups of frozen banana chunks, about 1 cup of fresh or frozen strawberries, one apple, 1 to 2 tablespoons of Vega Vanilla Almondilla Smoothie Infusion (or ¼ teaspoon of almond extract [optional]), 2 tablespoons of goji berries, plus enough water to get it moving and thin out, if you like.

Purple People Feeder: 1 to 1½ cups of collard greens leaves, about 1½ cups of frozen banana chunks, about ½ cup of fresh or frozen blueberries, ½ cup of purple or red grapes or one red apple or pear, 1 to 2 tablespoons of flaxseeds, plus enough water to get it moving and thin out, if you like.

Smooth Talker: 1 to 1½ cups of kale leaves, 1 to 1½ cups of frozen banana chunks, about ½ cup of honeydew melon (cubed), ½ cup of cucumber, one orange or ½ cup of fresh pineapple (cubed), ½ avocado, plus enough water to get it moving and thin out, if you like.

Orange Blaster: 1 to 1½ cups of kale leaves; 1 cup of peach, nectarine, or mango chunks; two oranges (peeled); ⅓ cup of chopped carrot; ½ to ¾ cup of frozen banana; ½ cup of vanilla nondairy yogurt (optional); plus enough water to get it moving and thin out, if you like.

Get the idea? Start with your greens, add some frozen fruit and other sweet fruits, add a pop of flavor, if you want, occasionally sneak in some nutritional gangbusters such as white chia seeds, and throw in just enough water to make the whole thing sing. Easy-breezy, lemon-squeezy. And, you could add a squeeze of lemon, too, if you like.

Apple-a-Day Green Smoothie

MAKES 2 MEDIUM TO LARGE SMOOTHIES

wheat gluten soy **FREE**

Sure, an apple a day keeps the doctor away, but adding greens every day might just have your doctor asking *you* for health advice! While I'm pretty free-form with my smoothies these days, this recipe is a favorite combination. For more tips on making green smoothies, see page 26.

3 cups (packed) Swiss chard leaves, spinach, or kale (tough part of stalks removed and discarded) (see note and "'Go Green' with Smoothies," page 26)

1 to 2 small to medium-size apples (your fave; I like sweet Orin, Gala, Fuji)

1 to 1½ cups frozen sliced banana (fairly ripe/overripe is best)

½ to 1 cup frozen mango, or 1 fresh large orange (peel removed)

½ to ¾ cup cucumber, roughly cut in large chunks

1 to 1½ tablespoons whole flax or chia seeds, 2 to 3 tablespoons hemp seeds, or 1 to 2 tablespoons Vega Tropical Tango Shake & Go Smoothie (optional)

¾ to 1 cup water

Place all the ingredients in a blender and puree for a couple of minutes to ensure the flaxseeds are pulverized and well incorporated (if using a high-powered blender such as Blendtec, you won't need to puree as long; simply run on "whole juice" mode, and then pulse again afterward, if needed, if there are any remaining frozen bits of fruit to be incorporated).

Savvy Subs and Adds: Kale can easily be substituted, though the flavor of kale leaves is stronger than chard, so you might want to try 1½ to 2 cups of kale leaves and use the upper measurement of bananas for extra sweetness, and then adjust your smoothies after that.

Other fruits to switch to or add include fresh or frozen pineapple, fresh peeled orange, a handful of green grapes, and/or fresh or frozen berries (though the color will change from a vibrant green to a purplish or brown color when using berries).

Goji Strawberry Smoothie

MAKES 2 MEDIUM TO
LARGE SMOOTHIES

wheat
gluten **FREE**
soy

Goji berries are nutritional powerhouses, and easy to consume through this satisfying, tasty smoothie. The strawberries are a natural flavor pairing for goji berries, so use them if possible. If not, you can substitute another frozen berry such as blueberries. A high-powered blender (I use a Blendtec) is best for this smoothie, to fully pulverize the goji berries and tough flaxseeds. With a regular blender, you may have to puree longer or simply have a smoothie that's a little less, well, smooth . . . but still delicious!

1½ cups plain or vanilla nondairy milk
½ cup water (or more nondairy milk)
1½ cups frozen sliced banana (fairly ripe/overripe is best)
1 cup frozen or fresh strawberries
¼ cup goji berries
2 tablespoons flaxseeds
¼ teaspoon ground cinnamon (optional)

Place all the ingredients in a high-powered blender and puree for a few minutes to ensure the goji berries and flaxseeds are pulverized and well incorporated.

If This Apron Could Talk: Try these ideas to include goji berries in your daily diet: Add to cold and hot cereals; blend into smoothies; mix into vanilla nondairy yogurt; sprinkle in green salads (in place of dried cranberries); add to homemade jam and chutney recipes; use in place of raisins and dried cranberries in sweet recipes such as muffins, scones, quick breads, granola bars, and cookies; use in savory dishes such as pilafs and grain and bean salads; and add to your favorite trail mix (or buy trail mixes that include goji berries).

Ingredients 411: Goji berries are nutritional powerhouses. First, they are abundant in antioxidants. Antioxidants are measured by a scale called the ORAC test. The ORAC value for goji berries is between 20,200 and 30,000—compared to 2,400 for blueberries (which are well known for their high antioxidant level). Goji berries are also rich in protein, with eighteen amino acids, including the eight essential amino acids that make up a complete protein. To boot, gojis are rich in vitamin A—just 1 ounce of these berries (a mere 2½ to 3 tablespoons) will give you 140 percent of the RDA for vitamin A. Plus these tiny berries are also a better source of vitamin C than are oranges, and deliver trace minerals, including iron and zinc.

Hempanana Smoothie

MAKES 2 MEDIUM TO LARGE SMOOTHIES

wheat gluten soy **FREE**

This smoothie was a morning fix for me after I had our third baby. It satisfied my sweet tooth in a healthy way in the morning, and gave me essential fatty acids from the hemp seeds (as well as white chia seeds) that were beneficial for nursing.

½ cup hemp seeds

1 cup plain or vanilla nondairy milk

1 cup water (or more nondairy milk)

2 cups frozen sliced banana (fairly ripe/overripe is best)

½ cup or more frozen or fresh blueberries or strawberries (optional)

½ to 1 tablespoon whole white chia seeds, or 1 tablespoon ground white chia seeds (optional)

¼ to ½ teaspoon ground cinnamon

Place all the ingredients in a blender and puree for a few minutes to ensure the hemp and chia seeds are pulverized and well incorporated. If using frozen berries, you may need to add extra nondairy milk or water to help loosen the mixture, to puree it fully.

Ingredients 411: Hemp foods have become far more well known and popular since I first introduced them into my own recipes in *Vive le Vegan!* Is the hype deserved? You bet! Hemp seeds are a mighty little food, delivering complete protein, essential fatty acids, chlorophyll, antioxidants, and other vitamins and minerals. Hemp offers an almost perfect balance of the essential fatty acids, with a 3.75 to 1 (omega-6 to omega-3) ratio, compared to the recommended 4 to 1 ratio. Hemp seeds also offer complete protein, a mere 2 tablespoons dishing up 11 grams of protein! Hemp seeds resemble sesame seeds, but with a rounder shape, greenish tint, and much softer texture. They taste somewhat like sunflower seeds, but with a slight earthier and sweeter flavor. From hemp seeds, hemp nut butter can be made (just as almond butter is made from almonds). The nut butter has a distinctive greenish color (from the chlorophyll), and again, has a taste somewhat similar to sunflower seed butter.

2 Salads That Make a Meal

Salad is a funny term. The word implies "healthy," but how many macaroni, potato, and even marshmallow salads have you met that are anything but? On the other hand, usually salads are the side portion of greens and raw veg that some folks "have to get through" before going on to the best part of the meal (not naming any names here, but you know who you are, next to me at the table). But with hearty ingredients, flavorful herbs and seasonings, and plenty of substance from beans or grains, these recipes are both healthy and so delicious, you'll find yourself lingering over them. Here you'll find some classics with twists, such as Quinoa Niçoise and Three-Bean Salad. Try Smoky Sweet Potato and Black Bean Salad and you just might turn your back on your old black bean version. Know someone who needs help taking a leafy-greens plunge? The Kale-slaw with Curried Almond Dressing, with its julienned leaves of kale and other fresh vegetables mingled with a lightly spiced dressing, will have those salad haters thinking of kale as the new romaine, with my creamy nut-based dressings as your new Caesar.

Go ahead, serve up these salads as a meal—on their own, on top of greens, or add more greens and more veg for an even bigger salad! (Or, ahem, for those sitting next to me, tucked inside a pita with some green leafies snuck in.)

Three-Bean Salad

SERVES 6 AS A SIDE DISH

wheat
gluten **FREE**
soy

Does this recipe sound familiar? I remember a version of it that my mom served for potlucks and "cold-plate" dinners. Variations of this salad are also sometimes found at deli counters for take-out. What is fairly constant among the adaptations is the combination of chickpeas and kidney beans in a vinegar-prominent dressing. My version uses green onions in place of raw red or white onions, a touch of natural sweetener instead of white sugar, and the addition of raw apple to lighten up the flavors.

4 cups mixed chickpeas, kidney beans, and black beans (canned is okay; rinse and drain first)

½ cup seeded and chopped green or red bell pepper

¼ cup finely chopped celery

½ cup sliced green onions (mostly green portion)

3½ tablespoons apple cider vinegar

1 tablespoon extra-virgin olive oil (optional)

½ to 1 tablespoon pure maple syrup

½ teaspoon Dijon mustard

½ teaspoon + ⅛ teaspoon sea salt
Freshly ground black pepper

⅓ to ½ cup chopped apple (cored first, peeling optional), tossed in ½ teaspoon freshly squeezed lemon juice
Pinch or two of ground cloves

In a large bowl, combine all the ingredients (no need to mix the vinaigrette separately), tossing well to fully mix. Season to taste with extra salt and pepper if desired.

If This Apron Could Talk: This salad tastes best after it's had about a day to sit and the beans have absorbed some of the marinade. Be sure to toss again to redistribute any dressing lingering at the bottom of your container.

Kale-slaw with Curried Almond Dressing

MAKES 5½ TO 6½ CUPS

wheat gluten soy **FREE**

I've never cared much for traditional coleslaw, as I've never cared much for cabbage. But this slaw is a fresh take with nutrient-rich kale, along with crunchy carrots, fennel, and a touch of sweetness from apples and cranberries. The dressing really brings this slaw to life—don't skip it!

1 small to medium-size apple, cored and julienned (¾ to 1 cup), tossed in 1 teaspoon freshly squeezed lemon juice

2½ to 3 cups julienned kale (leaves cut/torn from stems and stems discarded) (see note)

1½ cups grated carrot

1 cup very thinly sliced or julienned fennel

¼ cup cranberries or raisins

⅔ to ¾ cup Creamy Curried Almond Dressing (or more, if desired; see note) (page 49)

2 to 4 tablespoons sliced or chopped raw almonds
Extra salt and pepper

Place the apple, vegetables, and cranberries in a bowl and toss. Add the dressing, starting with about ⅔ cup and adding more as desired, if you want a thicker coating of dressing. Toss to coat well, then let sit for 5 minutes or more to allow the kale leaves to soften slightly in the dressing. Serve, garnishing with a light sprinkling of almonds and extra salt and pepper, if desired.

If This Apron Could Talk: Kale salads can be quite versatile. Try another thick, creamy nut- or seed-based dressing, such as Citrus Tahini Dressing, Creamy Cumin-Spiced Dressing, or DJ's Hummus Salad Dressing. The key is to coat the leaves nicely, and let the salad sit for a few minutes before serving.

Savvy Subs and Adds: If fennel isn't your thing, substitute julienned jicama, thinly sliced celery (cut on a diagonal), or julienned red bell pepper, or some combination of these ingredients.

If you aren't sure if you'll like this much kale in the salad, try starting with 2 to 2½ cups, making up the difference with extra grated carrot or fennel.

Other veggies you can consider adding include chopped or finely sliced cucumber, red bell pepper, cherry tomatoes, grated beet ("pretty in pink" salad, anyone?). Or try some zucchini ribbons: Use a vegetable peeler to make thick ribbons—these can be the base of a salad all on their own! And other dried fruit, such as apricots, goji berries, and raisins, can be interchanged with the cranberries, if you prefer.

Quinoa Niçoise

SERVES 4 OR MORE

wheat gluten soy **FREE**

The best part of a salad Niçoise is everything but the fish and eggs! Here, quinoa mingles with some classic Niçoise ingredients, making this a flavorful and satisfying dish that can be eaten as a meal, or toted as a side dish for a picnic or party.

VINAIGRETTE:

- 3 tablespoons red wine vinegar (see note)
- 2 tablespoons apple cider vinegar (or more red wine vinegar)
- 1½ tablespoons pure maple syrup or agave nectar
- 1 tablespoon capers
- 1 tablespoon Dijon mustard
- ½ teaspoon sea salt
  Freshly ground black pepper
- 5 tablespoons extra-virgin olive oil (see note)
- 1½ tablespoons minced fresh tarragon

SALAD:

- ⅓ to ½ pound green beans, cut into bite-size pieces (1¾ to 2 cups; see note)
- 2 cups cooked Yukon Gold or red potatoes, cut into bite-size chunks (do not use russet potatoes; see note)
- 3 cups cooked quinoa, cooled (see note)
- ⅔ to ¾ cup kalamata or Niçoise olives, pitted, sliced or roughly chopped
- ¾ cup cherry tomatoes, halved
- 2 tablespoons sliced green onions or chopped chives (optional)
- 2 tablespoons chopped fresh flat-leaf parsley (optional)

To prepare the vinaigrette, combine all the ingredients, except the tarragon, in a deep cup or jar and blend with an immersion blender (or use a standing blender to puree everything). Once blended, stir in the tarragon, and set the dressing aside.

Prepare the salad: Cook the beans until just fork tender in small pot of simmering water. Drain, then rinse with very cold water (or submerge in a bowl of ice water) to stop the cooking process. Combine the beans and potatoes while they are still slightly warm (not hot), toss with the remaining ingredients in a large bowl, and stir in the vinaigrette. Season to taste with salt and pepper, if desired, and serve.

If This Apron Could Talk: I usually cook a large batch of quinoa when I'm making it for dinner, and then refrigerate the leftovers. But if you want to cook just enough quinoa for this recipe, you'll need roughly 1 cup of uncooked quinoa (to combine with 2 cups of water; see "Guide to Cooking Grains," page 283). You will probably have just a little more than 3 cups after cooking, so measure out the 3 cups after the quinoa is cooked and cooled.

Cook the potatoes ahead of time to make preparation of this salad easier. You can steam, boil, or bake the potatoes, or use leftover cooked potatoes. You will need about three small to medium potatoes.

Leftovers of this salad soak up all the seasoning in the vinaigrette. If you'd like additional moistness and also some vinaigrette "tang," toss another ½ tablespoon of red wine vinegar and olive oil into the salad.

Smoky Sweet Potato and Black Bean Salad

SERVES 3 TO 4

wheat gluten soy **FREE**

The sweet potatoes in this salad partially break down and help hold the other ingredients together. They offer sweetness and along with the beans a soft, toothsome texture, which is balanced by the crunchy, fresh red pepper and cucumber and the smoky essence in the spices added.

2	cups cooked sweet potato, cut into cubes (see note for baking tips)
2	(14-ounce) cans black beans, drained and rinsed
½ to ¾	cup seeded and diced red or yellow bell pepper
½	cup seeded and diced cucumber or peeled and diced jicama
2	tablespoons roughly chopped chives or sliced green onions (green portion)
2	tablespoons minced fresh flat-leaf parsley or cilantro
1 to 1½	teaspoons minced fresh oregano
4 to 5	tablespoons freshly squeezed lime juice (2 to 3 limes)
1 to 2	tablespoons olive, walnut, or avocado oil
1	teaspoon (touch scant) sea salt Freshly ground black pepper
½	teaspoon chipotle hot sauce (I use Tabasco brand; add another ½ teaspoon if you like it smokier/hotter)
1	teaspoon ground cumin
¼	teaspoon ground allspice
⅛ to ¼	teaspoon smoked paprika (start with ⅛ teaspoon, then adjust to taste)
¼	teaspoon pure maple syrup

Once the sweet potatoes are just warm or cool (see note), cut into cubes and place in a large bowl with the remaining ingredients (starting with 4 to 4½ tablespoons of the lime juice; I like to use close to 5 tablespoons). Toss well. Taste, and add additional lime juice, if desired, and season to taste with additional salt, pepper, paprika, or chipotle hot sauce, if desired. The salad is delicious at room temperature, but can be chilled for a picnic or to keep for lunches during the week.

If This Apron Could Talk: To bake the sweet potatoes, preheat the oven to 400°F and line a baking sheet with parchment paper. Bake the potatoes on the prepared pan for 40 to 60 minutes (baking time will depend on whether you are using smaller or larger sweet potatoes). Check the potatoes a few times in the last 10 to 15 minutes of baking. If you want a firmer bite to the sweet potatoes, bake for less time, until just al dente (cooked through, but with a slight give when pierced), which will help them hold more structure in the salad. I like the sweet potatoes cooked until mostly soft because I like how they meld into the salad and help it "hold" when serving/eating . . . but, it's up to you for your salad!

Make It More-ish! This would be delicious as a layered dip with guacamole. Distribute the salad over the bottom of a shallow casserole dish. Make a simple guacamole, and dollop or smooth over the top of the salad to distribute as evenly as possible. Scoop out portions to serve with tortilla or pita chips, or to wrap in lettuce leaves.

Quinoa Tabbouleh with Olives

SERVES 3 OR MORE
AS A SIDE DISH

*wheat
gluten* **FREE**
soy

Tabbouleh (sometimes spelled tabouli) is a popular Lebanese salad traditionally made with bulgur. My version is gluten free, using quinoa to replace the bulgur. I include olives in this version, as they really complement the flavors. Confused by the allspice? Don't skip it—it's authentic and delicious.

1½ to 1¾	cups cooked, cooled quinoa (see note)
2½ to 3	tablespoons freshly squeezed lemon juice
1½ to 2½	tablespoons extra-virgin olive oil
½	cup seeded and finely chopped cucumber
½	cup chopped tomatoes (juices gently squeezed out)
¼	cup chopped green onions (green part only)
1	cup minced fresh flat-leaf parsley
2 to 3	tablespoons minced fresh mint
¼ to ⅓	cup quartered pitted kalamata olives
1	teaspoon lemon zest
¼ + ⅛	teaspoon (or ½ teaspoon [scant]) sea salt
¼	teaspoon (rounded) ground allspice

In a large bowl, combine all the ingredients (starting with 2½ tablespoons of the lemon juice and 1½ tablespoons of the oil), mixing until well incorporated. Let sit for about 20 minutes, then taste. Add additional lemon juice and olive oil, if desired.

If This Apron Could Talk: If you've eaten or made tabbouleh before, you may notice that this recipe has less grain in proportion to the herbs and seasonings, even though I have used more quinoa than an authentic tabbouleh would bulgur! Authentic tabbouleh does not have a lot of bulgur, even though many deli varieties and recipes do. Instead, the salad is based more on the fresh herbs, with the bulgur used almost as you would a condiment. You can add less or more quinoa to your own preference, and adjust the salt and lemon juice accordingly to taste.

Ingredients 411: For best flavor and texture, use mostly the leafy portion of the parsley and the upper very tender stems, omitting the thicker lower stems. Mince the parsley with a chef's knife until very finely chopped. You will need one (or close to one) bunch of parsley to get this yield.

Savvy Subs and Adds: I like this salad without garlic, because it offers a cooling accompaniment to other more spicy dishes. But feel free to add a small or medium clove of garlic, grated or pressed, if you really love garlic flavor in tabbouleh.

3 Proud to Be Saucy and Dippy

I grew up in Newfoundland, and the term *saucy* is commonly used to refer to someone who is being a bit cheeky, sarcastic, just a bit of a smart aleck . . . yet with an affectionate ring. Yep, I was called saucy as a child more times than I've answered, "But where do you get your protein?" as an adult. I'm still saucy. Sometimes with words, but always with food.

Most of my meals have a saucy accompaniment of one kind or another. If it's not a salad dressing or "flax-y oil" (a slurry of flax oil and balsamic for drizzling on pizza, burritos, and more), then it's a creamy or slightly spicy sauce that accessorizes a meal just right, like an expensive pair of hoop earrings.

This chapter will give you all sorts of toppings for your salads, soups, pizza, pasta (though, be sure to check out Chapter 8, too), tofu, seitan, wraps, beans, tem-

pch, veggie burgers, potatoes, rice, quinoa . . . you getting the idea? Now picture your pastas and soups with nutty-cheesy Parmesan-like sprinkles, your veggie burger with "Almonnaise," that pizza with a fresh Basil Lemon Pistou, burritos with Chipotle Avocado Cream or Fresh Cream Sauce, potatoes with Raw Aioli, tempeh and tofu strips dipped into a Creamy Cumin-Spiced Dressing, rice and beans drizzled with Peanut Tahini Sauce, your holiday dinners with a savory Rosemary Gravy, a party plate of tortilla chips with "Vegveeta" Dip, and your salads with luscious but light Citrus Tahini Dressing or DJ's Hummus Salad Dressing.

When I'm not saucy, I'm a little dippy. Before you judge, try out the nutrient-rich dips made with beans and vegetables, such as Artichoke and White Bean Dip, Truffled Cashew Cheese, Creamy Grilled Eggplant

Dip (my eggplant-taming twist on baba ghanouj), or Grilled Onion Hummus with Hemp Seeds. Then, there are some nut-based spreads and cheeses. Not only delicious on their own with breads and raw crackers, you'll find yourself using Truffled Cashew Cheese paired with elegant soups and layered in lasagne, or switched with suggested fresh herbs for using in more sophisticated-tasting sandwiches and wraps. Spinach Cashew Pizza Cheese Spread, along with some piquant olives and juicy sliced tomatoes, will make an ordinary store-bought whole wheat pizza shell extraordinary. Go on, spread, scoop, and dip with gusto—just don't double-dip, please.

Yes, I'm proud to be saucy and dippy. Mind you, my family might have a different opinion.

DJ's Hummus Salad Dressing

MAKES ABOUT ¾ CUP

wheat gluten **FREE**

When I saw online that Trader Joe's had a bottled hummus salad dressing, I thought, "That's a great idea and I bet I can make it healthier"! Admittedly, I hadn't seen or tasted TJ's version, but took a gamble that my (DJ's) version would be healthier—and tastier.

¼ cup cooked or canned chickpeas (drain and rinse if canned)
¼ cup water
2½ tablespoons tahini
1 tablespoon freshly squeezed lemon juice
1 tablespoon red wine vinegar
1 teaspoon tamari
½ teaspoon Dijon mustard
2 to 3 teaspoons fresh oregano leaves (see note)
1 very small clove garlic, or ½ small to medium clove
1 to 1½ teaspoons agave nectar, or more to taste
¼ teaspoon sea salt
Freshly ground black pepper
1 to 2 tablespoons extra-virgin olive oil (optional)

Using a standing blender or an immersion blender and deep cup or jar, puree all the ingredients until smooth. Season to taste with additional salt or pepper, if desired, and using extra garlic to taste.

Kid-Friendly: Our kids love this dressing as is, but you might want to try omitting the oregano and using the nooch sub mentioned above—try 1 tablespoon to start, and then add more if you like.

Savvy Subs and Adds: If you don't have fresh oregano, don't use dried. Keep the flavor more vibrant and fresher by adding a tablespoon or so of chopped fresh parsley, or a lesser amount (1 to 2 teaspoons) of other fresh herbs such as thyme or rosemary. Fresh herbs can be omitted, however, and this will still have good flavor.

Other seasoning options include adding 1 tablespoon of nutritional yeast, or 1 to 2 tablespoons of chopped sun-dried tomatoes, 1 to 2 tablespoons of green onions, or 1 teaspoon of toasted sesame oil.

Serving Suggestions: Not just for drizzling on a common green salad, try tossing through julienned leafy greens like kale and chard. The dressing softens the greens and you'll find it's somewhat addictive to eat your beans 'n' greens!

Classic Caesar Dressing

MAKES 6 TO 8 SERVINGS
(ABOUT 1 CUP)

(optionally) wheat
(optionally) gluten **FREE**

This is a piquant Caesar dressing that is made without eggs or dairy. An alternative to my Raw Caesar Dressing from *Eat, Drink & Be Vegan*, it is very popular, but may not be an option for those with nut or seed allergies. It can be made in minutes and then tossed into a large bowl of romaine lettuce and croutons. This recipe yields a fairly substantial batch; you will likely have enough to refrigerate some for at least another meal or two.

½ cup firm silken tofu
1½ tablespoons extra-virgin olive oil (optional; see note)
1 tablespoon neutral-flavored oil (optional; see "Plant-Powered Pantry," page xxxii)
1 tablespoon freshly squeezed lemon juice
1 tablespoon apple cider vinegar
1 tablespoon mild miso (e.g., Genmai brown rice miso)
1 small to medium clove garlic (or larger clove, if you love raw garlic)
1 teaspoon Dijon mustard
1 teaspoon capers
½ teaspoon vegan Worcestershire sauce (omit or use gluten-free brand, for a wheat- or gluten-free option)
¼ teaspoon sea salt
Freshly ground black pepper (somewhat generous is good)
½ teaspoon agave nectar (plus more to taste, if desired)
1 tablespoon nutritional yeast (see note)
2 to 4 tablespoons plain unsweetened nondairy milk (almond or soy preferred; see "Plant-Powered Pantry," page xxxiii)

Using a standing blender or an immersion blender and deep cup or jar, puree all the ingredients (starting with 2 tablespoons of the oil) until very smooth. Add the additional oil and more agave nectar to taste, and season with extra salt and pepper as desired. This dressing is fairly dense and will thicken after refrigeration. Thin as desired while blending, adding about 2 tablespoons of milk, and then again after chilling, stirring in another tablespoon or more to your preferred consistency.

Ingredients 411: Using all extra-virgin olive oil as the oil in this dressing may give too pronounced an olive flavor for your liking, so I have opted to use 1½ tablespoons of olive oil plus 1 tablespoon of a neutral-flavored oil. The oil adds body and boosts the flavor profile, but you can reduce or omit the oil for a low-fat dressing if needed.

Kid-Friendly: If you love nutritional yeast, go ahead and add it into this dressing. It will give just a slight cheesy flavor that is enjoyable especially to kids. Be conservative with the garlic for the little ones.

Serving Suggestions: Try sprinkled with Cheesy Sprinkle or Brazil Nut Parmezan.

Creamy Cumin-Spiced Dressing

MAKES ABOUT 1¾ CUPS

wheat gluten soy **FREE**

This thick, creamy dressing can make a meal out of a salad. It offers the enchanting combination of cumin and cloves, flirting with some fresh herbs, a kick of lime juice, and a creamy base made with raw almonds. With its Southwest influence, this dressing can double as a sauce for burritos, enchiladas, or fajitas.

½ cup raw almonds
2 tablespoons freshly squeezed lime juice (see note)
1 tablespoon red wine vinegar
1 tablespoon olive oil (optional)
1 very small clove garlic (¼ average clove)
⅔ cup water or nondairy milk (plus 1 to 3 tablespoons more to thin as needed)
½ teaspoon sea salt
½ teaspoon pure maple syrup
¼ teaspoon ground cumin
Pinch of ground cloves
¼ cup fresh cilantro, or 2 tablespoon roughly chopped or torn fresh basil (see note)

Using a standing blender or an immersion blender and deep cup or jar, puree all the ingredients until very smooth, starting with ⅔ cup of water or milk and adding more to thin as needed. (A high-powered blender such as a Blendtec works best to smooth out the dressing; using an immersion blender or regular blender will leave a little more consistency and take a little longer.) This dressing thickens considerably after refrigerating, so add more water while blending or whisk into the dressing after chilling.

Savvy Subs and Adds: If you don't have limes, you can substitute 2 tablespoons of lemon juice, or 1 tablespoon of lemon juice plus another tablespoon of red wine vinegar.

Serving Suggestions: Try with Black Bean, Quinoa, and Sweet Potato Spicy Croquettes in place of the Pumpkin Seed Chipotle Cream, or with a salad to pair with Mexican Bean Soup.

Walnut Mustard Vinaigrette

MAKES ROUGHLY 1 CUP

wheat gluten soy **FREE**

This vinaigrette is tangy, but also thick and creamy with the addition of whole raw walnuts that are pureed right into the dressing. The walnuts and walnut oil also add healthy omega-3 fatty acids to this delicious vinaigrette, which can double as a veggie dip.

¼ cup balsamic or red wine vinegar

3½ tablespoons pure maple syrup

1 to 1½ tablespoons stone-ground prepared mustard

½ teaspoon (rounded) sea salt
Freshly ground black pepper

⅓ cup raw walnuts or pecans (see note)

2 tablespoons walnut oil

2 tablespoons extra-virgin olive oil

⅛ cup water (see note)

Using a standing blender or an immersion blender and deep cup or jar, puree all the ingredients until smooth. If you'd like to thin the dressing more, add a teaspoon or two of water at a time and puree, until thinned as desired. Alternatively, if you'd like to use this dressing as a veggie dip, add just 1 to 1½ tablespoons of water rather than the full ⅛ cup.

Savvy Subs and Adds: Try this with raw pecans instead of walnuts. They are a little sweeter and more buttery in flavor.

Raw-nch Dressing!

MAKES ABOUT 1¼ CUPS

wheat gluten soy **FREE**

This dressing is creamy and rich, and uses cashews instead of silken tofu or soy milk, for a creamy base. It is also very close to being a "'raw" recipe... to make it entirely raw, omit the Dijon mustard and replace the red wine vinegar with lemon juice or apple cider vinegar.

½ cup raw cashews

2 tablespoons freshly squeezed lemon juice

1½ teaspoons red wine vinegar (gives more flavor; see headnote for a raw version)

1 tablespoon extra-virgin olive oil (optional)

1 tablespoon raw tahini

¼ cup roughly chopped fresh flat-leaf parsley

2 teaspoons chopped fresh chives (optional; you can use more onion powder instead)

⅛ teaspoon garlic powder (see note)

⅛ teaspoon onion powder (see note)

¼ teaspoon Dijon mustard (omit for raw version)

½ teaspoon (scant) sea salt

⅛ teaspoon freshly ground black pepper

1 teaspoon raw agave nectar (or more to taste)

½ cup water or nondairy milk (or more to thin, as desired)

Using a standing blender or an immersion blender and deep cup or jar, puree all the ingredients until very smooth (it will take a couple of minutes). If you want to thin the dressing more, add water to your preferred consistency. This dressing will thicken some after refrigeration. You can thin it out by stirring in a few teaspoons of water, or keep it thick and use it as a dip for raw veggies.

Ingredients 411: I prefer a faint seasoning of garlic and onion in this dressing. I use just ⅛ teaspoon of the onion and garlic powders to lend a hint of flavor but not overwhelm the dressing. If you like more seasoning, feel free to use more onion powder (or extra chives), and more garlic powder (or even a tiny clove of garlic). Alternatively, you can omit both powders, if you prefer.

Savvy Subs and Adds: Try 2 tablespoons of fresh dill to replace some or all of the parsley.

Serving Suggestions: Not just for salad, this livens up tofu and tempeh dishes, and is magical with roasted baby potatoes.

Fresh Raspberry Vinaigrette

MAKES 1 TO 1¼ CUPS

wheat gluten soy **FREE**

When plump, fragrant raspberries are plentiful, use some in this vibrant dressing. It is best dressed on a simple salad of mixed greens with cucumber and avocado, with maybe a few basil leaves thrown in for good measure.

1¼ cup fresh raspberries
½ to 1 tablespoon red wine vinegar (see note)
½ teaspoon Dijon mustard
½ teaspoon sea salt
2½ to 3 tablespoons pure maple syrup or agave nectar
Freshly ground black pepper
3 tablespoons walnut oil or other oil of choice (see note)
½ cup toasted pecans (optional; see note)
1 tablespoon water (optional)

Using a standing blender or an immersion blender and deep cup or jar, puree all the ingredients, except the optional pecans and water, and blend until fully smooth and creamy. If straining (see note), strain and then return the vinaigrette to the blender. Add the pecans, if using, and pulse until well incorporated but still maintaining some texture. Add water to thin, if desired.

If This Apron Could Talk: If you are a stickler for not having seeds in the vinaigrette, strain through a fine sieve after blending. If using a high-powered blender, it pulverizes the seeds quite well, leaving not too many nibbly seeds noticeable. But straining is still an option. Simply strain the vinaigrette, return to it blender, and then pulse the pecans into the mixture, if using.

Ingredients 411: Depending on the sweetness of your berries and how much tang you enjoy in a vinaigrette, you can adjust the amount of red wine vinegar. Start with ½ tablespoon, then add the extra ½ tablespoon if you think you'd like the extra acidity.

The flavor of extra-virgin olive oil can be a little strong in this vinaigrette, competing with the flavor of the raspberries. But if you wish, use part walnut oil plus part extra-virgin olive oil, for a total of 3 tablespoons.

I quite like the nutty, sweet flavor of the pecans in this dressing. It's not essential, but consider trying it; it adds another dimension that is very pleasant.

Creamy Curried Almond Dressing (or Dip)

MAKES ABOUT 1 GENEROUS CUP

*wheat
gluten* **FREE**
soy

This dressing will definitely cling to your greens, and can easily be used as a dip as well. It is one of my favorites, with a very subtle curry flavor in a creamy, slightly sweet base. This is also the dressing for Kale-slaw with Curried Almond Dressing, a modern makeover of traditional coleslaw.

½   cup raw almonds
2½ tablespoons apple cider vinegar
2   tablespoons pure maple syrup or agave nectar
⅔   cup water (or more to thin as needed; see note)
1   very small clove garlic
1   teaspoon freshly grated ginger
½   teaspoon Dijon mustard
¼   teaspoon sea salt
    Freshly ground black pepper (optional)
⅛   teaspoon curry powder, or more to taste (see note)

Using a standing blender or an immersion blender and deep cup or jar, puree all the ingredients (starting with ½ cup of the water) until very smooth. (A high-powered blender such as a Blendtec works best to smooth out the dressing; using an immersion blender or regular blender will leave a little more texture and take a little longer.) Add additional curry to taste, and additional water to thin as desired (see note).

Adult-Minded: I like using about ⅛ rounded teaspoon of curry powder in this dressing, for a very muted flavor. But if you love curry, feel free to use more than this, adjusting to your own taste.

Serving Suggestions: I first tinkered with this recipe for a salad dressing. After making it, I realized it would work equally well as a dip. If using as a dip, use just ⅓ to ½ cup of water to puree and then refrigerate it, adding extra water later, if desired, to thin (it will thicken considerably after chilling). If using as a salad dressing, you can keep it thick, or thin it more as you prefer. I like it with about ⅔ cup of water as a salad dressing, which keeps it fairly thick, almost like a Caesar dressing consistency.

Creamy Carrot Miso Dip

MAKES ABOUT 1¼ CUPS

wheat gluten **FREE**

This dip is a refreshing departure from a bean-based dip, and nicely transforms hard, raw carrots into a creamy, light dip. Serve with vegetables, breads, or chips, or use in salads or dollop on soups, or whatever you fancy!

1 cup carrot that has been cut in disks or small chunks (roughly 4 to 4½ ounces)
⅓ cup raw cashews
2 to 2½ teaspoons apple cider vinegar
1 tablespoon red miso
1 small clove garlic (or ½ medium clove)
¾ teaspoon ground coriander
½ teaspoon Dijon mustard
¼ teaspoon sea salt
Freshly ground black pepper (use conservatively)
½ cup water (or more to thin as needed; see note)
1 tablespoon extra-virgin olive oil (optional, but adds nice flavor)

Using a standing blender (high-powered works best to smooth), puree all the ingredients (starting with 2 teaspoons of the vinegar) until very smooth. Taste and add extra vinegar if you wish, and season with additional salt and pepper, if desired. For a thinner dip, add more water (plus another 2 to 3 tablespoons more, if desired, to thin out a little more for use as a salad dressing).

If This Apron Could Talk: A high-powered blender can smooth out this dip with just ⅓ cup of water. You will need ½ cup for a regular blender, possibly more. Add just as much extra water as needed so as not to dilute the mixture. It will be thick with ½ cup of water, and will thicken more as it stands or chills.

Moroccan Carrot Dip

MAKES ABOUT 1¼ CUPS

wheat
gluten **FREE**
soy

Now give that carrot dip a sprightly, spicy twist with some Moroccan seasonings.

1 cup carrot that has been cut in disks or small chunks (roughly 4 to 4½ ounces)

⅓ cup raw cashews

2 to 2½ teaspoons apple cider vinegar

1 small clove garlic (or ⅓ medium clove)

½ to 1 teaspoon peeled and roughly chopped fresh ginger

⅛ teaspoon (scant) ground cinnamon

½ teaspoon ground cumin

½ teaspoon ground coriander

¼ teaspoon ground fennel

¼ teaspoon (rounded) sea salt (plus more, if needed)
Freshly ground black pepper (use conservatively)

½ cup water (or more to thin as needed; see note)

1 tablespoon olive oil (optional, but adds nice flavor)

Follow same directions as for the previous recipe, and season with additional vinegar and/or salt to taste.

Serving Suggestions: Surprise your guests with this uniquely flavored and colored dip—try serving as a centerpiece dip for crudités or with dipping breads. Also try tossing it into a salad, for a more substantial lunch salad.

Citrus Tahini Dressing

MAKES ABOUT ⅔ CUP

This dressing is slightly thick, thanks to the inclusion of tahini. There is very little added oil, and yet the dressing tastes full bodied and flavorful. The flavors are kid friendly, and so it makes eating salad a little more interesting for the little ones!

3 tablespoons freshly squeezed orange juice

1 tablespoon freshly squeezed lemon juice

2 tablespoons tahini

1 tablespoon red wine vinegar or apple cider vinegar

2 to 2½ tablespoons pure maple syrup (adjust to the tartness of the orange juice)

1½ to 2 teaspoons Dijon mustard

½ to 1 teaspoon roughly chopped fresh ginger

1 very small clove garlic (optional)

½ teaspoon sea salt

1 tablespoon hemp, walnut, or extra-virgin olive oil (optional)
Freshly ground black pepper

Using a standing blender or an immersion blender and deep cup or jar, puree all the ingredients (starting with 2 tablespoons of the maple syrup, until fully smooth and creamy. Add additional maple syrup to taste, if desired.

Kid-Friendly: When I omit the garlic and use the lesser amount of ginger, my kids really like this dressing.

Serving Suggestions: Try this on finely julienned greens. It is especially great with kale, as it helps mellow the flavor of the leaves. Chop your kale, then toss the dressing onto the leaves. Let sit for 10 or more minutes to allow the dressing to soften the greens. Add other salad fixings you might like, such as cherry tomatoes, grated carrot, chopped apple, or dried cranberries. As good as this dressing is on salads, don't limit it to just your greens. Try it on steamed broccoli or cooked quinoa, or mashed into chickpeas for a sandwich filling.

Peanut Tahini Sauce

MAKES JUST OVER 1 CUP

wheat gluten soy **FREE**

Peanut sauces are very popular, and most of us whip up tahini sauce from time to time (in my household, it's about every few days). This sauce isn't complicated or revolutionary, but it combines the best of both worlds, peanut sauce and tahini sauce, with seasonings to complement both nutty flavors.

¼ cup natural peanut butter (see note)

¼ cup tahini

1½ to 2 tablespoons freshly squeezed lemon juice or apple cider vinegar (adjust to taste)

⅓ to ⅔ cup water (or more as needed, if heating the sauce; see note)

1 very small clove garlic (or medium to large, if heating the sauce; see note)

1 teaspoon freshly grated ginger, or 2 teaspoons roughly chopped

¼ teaspoon (rounded) sea salt

1 teaspoon pure maple syrup or agave nectar

½ teaspoon toasted sesame oil

Using a standing blender or an immersion blender and deep cup or jar, puree all the ingredients (starting with 1½ tablespoons of the lemon juice and ½ cup of the water) until smooth. Add additional lemon juice and extra salt to taste. Also add the additional water to thin, as desired. Serve as is or serve warm, if desired. To heat the sauce, place in a saucepan over medium-low heat and whisk until it just starts to come to a low bubble. The sauce will thicken as it heats and cools, so you will want to whisk in an additional ¼ cup or more of water to thin it out. Also, because the cooking will mellow out the garlic flavor slightly, you can add more garlic, if you wish.

Allergy-Free or Bust: If you have a peanut allergy and want to replace the peanut butter, try pumpkin seed butter (Nuts to You is my favorite brand). Pumpkin butter is a little more bitter than peanut butter, so you may want to add another ½ to 1 teaspoon of sweetener.

Serving Suggestions: I sometimes heat this sauce to serve over a whole grain such as quinoa, brown rice, or millet. Alongside a salad or other veggies, and maybe some tofu or baked spuds, this makes quite a complete and delicious meal. Try with Tempeh Tickle, atop a whole grain such as millet or brown rice, drizzled over Gingered Broccolini, or over gently cooked (steamed or sautéed) bok choy.

Smoky Spiked Tahini Sauce

MAKES JUST OVER 1 CUP

wheat gluten soy **FREE**

Once smoked paprika entered my ingredients "hit list," I had to try it out in tahini sauce. It did not disappoint!

½	cup tahini
2	tablespoons freshly squeezed lemon juice
½ to ⅔	cup water (or more for a thinner sauce, if desired)
¼	teaspoon (rounded) smoked paprika (see note)
¼	teaspoon (rounded) sea salt (about ¼ + ⅛ teaspoon)
¾ to 1¼	teaspoons pure maple syrup or agave nectar (or more to taste)

Using a standing blender or an immersion blender and deep cup or jar, puree all the ingredients (starting with ½ cup of the water, ¼ teaspoon of the paprika, and ¾ teaspoon of the agave) until smooth. Add additional paprika and salt to taste; maple syrup to balance any bitterness, if needed; and water to thin, as desired.

Ingredients 411: I like the amount of smoked paprika at just a lightly rounded ¼ teaspoon, but you can try adding more if you love the flavor. Try ½ teaspoon and see how it works for you.

I always like a touch of sweetener in tahini sauce to offset the slight bitterness of the tahini. The amount you use depends on personal preference and also the brand of tahini used. Start with ½ to ¾ teaspoon, and add more if needed.

Serving Suggestions: This sauce is an absolute must as part of a falafel dinner platter. Serve alongside Panfried Falafel Patties, Quinoa Tabbouleh with Olives, and whole-grain pita bread. So satisfying and delicious! This sauce will also add a punch of flavor to wrap sandwiches and roasted vegetables.

"Almonnaise"

MAKES ABOUT 1 CUP

wheat gluten soy **FREE**

This thick, rich sauce can easily take the place of mayo for your favorite burgers or in sandwiches. You might just find yourself topping it on just about everything, from baked spuds to pasta, beans and rice, or just a big ol' dollop on a raw salad. Make a double batch (see note); it is that good.

¾ cup soaked raw almonds, drained (see notes)
1 tablespoon red wine vinegar or lemon juice
¼ teaspoon dill seeds, or ¼ teaspoon (scant) celery seeds (or omit both; see note)
¼ teaspoon dry mustard
¼ teaspoon (rounded) sea salt (about ¼ + ⅛ teaspoon)
½ cup water
2 tablespoons neutral-flavored oil (optional, can substitute 1 tablespoon water) (see "Plant-Powered Pantry," page xxxii)

Using a standing blender or an immersion blender and deep cup or jar, puree all the ingredients (starting with ½ cup of the water) until very, very smooth, scraping down sides as needed. (A high-powered blender works best to achieve a smooth consistency, but a regular blender or immersion blender can step in; just takes longer.) If the consistency is so thick that it isn't smoothing out, add another 1 to 2 tablespoons of water as needed.

If This Apron Could Talk: Soaking almonds makes them softer for pureeing, and will give a little creamier consistency and make the blending easier. See "Plant-Powered Pantry," page xxxiv. If you don't have time to soak the almonds, go ahead and still use ¾ cup of raw almonds—and just add more water, a tablespoon at a time, to get the mixture blended and thinned out.

The blender has an easier time working through this mixture if you double the batch. It's not essential, but if you think you will use it up within 4 to 5 days, consider a double whammy!

If you want to thin this puree more for a dressing or sauce, go ahead and add more water and maybe a touch more vinegar, until you have your desired taste and consistency.

Ingredients 411: I use raw almonds that have the skins intact, so this 'naise has some flecks of color from the almond skins. If you don't want this color, feel free to use blanched almonds.

Kid-Friendly: I love this 'naise best with the dill seed and also the dry mustard, but our kids like it without the dill (or celery seeds). Also, our children like the addition of just 1 tablespoon of nutritional yeast to this mixture—give it a try!

Raw Aioli

MAKES ABOUT 1 CUP

wheat
gluten **FREE**
soy

This rich aioli is entirely raw and unbelievably tasty! Try it with raw veggies, spread on sandwiches, or as a topping for baked potatoes, grains, or steamed veggies. It is thick enough to be used as a dip, but can be thinned as desired (see note).

⅓ cup raw cashews
⅓ cup raw Brazil nuts (or use more cashews)
2 teaspoons raw pine nuts
1½ to 2 tablespoons freshly squeezed lemon juice
1 small to medium clove garlic, quartered (or larger, to taste)
¼ teaspoon (rounded) sea salt
Freshly ground black pepper
½ cup + 1 to 2 tablespoons water (see note)
1 to 2 tablespoons walnut or olive oil (can omit, see note)
1 teaspoon lemon zest

Using a standing blender or an immersion blender and deep cup or jar, puree all the ingredients except the lemon zest (start with 1½ tablespoons of the lemon juice and ½ cup of the water). Start on low speed (if possible), and then work up to a high speed to finish blending. Puree until very, very smooth, adding more water to smooth out and thin, as desired. Add additional salt, pepper, and lemon juice to taste, and stir in the lemon zest. This sauce is fairly thick while pureeing and will thicken with refrigeration. To use as a dip, simply make ahead and refrigerate for an hour or more before serving. If you prefer a thinner consistency, add more water, ½ tablespoon at a time, as needed.

If This Apron Could Talk: Be sure to blend this sauce long enough to become creamy smooth. An immersion or regular blender will take several minutes of high blending to achieve a smooth consistency.

Ingredients 411: You can use a fruity extra-virgin olive oil here, or a more neutral, nutty oil (e.g., walnut). If you want a richer sauce, use the full 2 tablespoons, but certainly this can be made with 1 tablespoon of oil, or omitted altogether if you'd prefer no oil.

Serving Suggestions: This aioli is divine on just about any sandwich, and is also especially good on baked yellow- or orange-fleshed sweet potatoes. Also try a dollop in soups, such as Tomato Lentil Soup with Cumin and Fresh Dill.

Fresh Cream Sauce

MAKES ¾ TO 1 CUP

wheat gluten soy **FREE**

Sometimes you want a sauce that is creamy and smooth, but without any pronounced flavors such as garlic or spices. This sauce is it. It is creamy and cooling, and great for pairing with spicy dishes—but also many other things!

1 cup soaked raw cashews, drained (see "Plant-Powered Pantry," page xxxiv)

½ cup + 2 to 3 tablespoons water

¼ teaspoon (rounded) sea salt (about ¼ + ⅛ teaspoon)

2½ to 3 teaspoons freshly squeezed lemon juice

1 to 2 teaspoons extra-virgin olive oil (optional, but nice)

⅛ teaspoon agave nectar

Using a standing blender or an immersion blender and deep cup or jar, puree all the ingredients (starting with ½ cup + 2 tablespoons of the water) until very, very smooth. (A high-powered blender works best to give a very silky consistency.) Add extra water, if needed, to thin the sauce, and season to taste with additional salt, if desired. Serve swirled over spicy stews or burritos, or drizzled on pizza; or use as a salad dressing or as a condiment for sandwiches, baked spuds, sautéed greens . . . so many options.

Serving Suggestions: This sauce is one of my favorites, and I love it with spicy soups and bean dishes, burritos, and quesadillas. Make a quick-fix quesadilla by smashing some black beans with store-bought (or homemade) salsa and ground cumin. Layer on a whole wheat tortilla with chopped, grilled onions (grill thick rings of onion on a barbecue grill until caramelized and softened, or chop and caramelize in a non-stick skillet) and Daiya cheese. Top with another tortilla, then heat in a nonstick skillet until a little crispy on each side and the filling is hot with the cheese melted.

Chipotle Avocado Cream

MAKES ABOUT 1¾ CUPS

wheat gluten soy **FREE**

This sauce adds lusciousness to any Mexican-inspired meal, and is a must for Mexican Bean Soup.

1 cup (fairly packed) ripe avocado, cut into chunks (about 1½ medium-size to large avocados)

⅓ cup raw cashews (soaking beforehand is preferable but not essential; see "Plant-Powered Pantry," page xxxiv)

1½ to 2 tablespoons freshly squeezed lemon or lime juice

½ to ⅔ cup water

½ teaspoon sea salt

¼ teaspoon agave nectar or pure maple syrup (optional, or to taste; see note)

¼ teaspoon chipotle hot sauce (e.g., Tabasco brand), or more to taste, or omit (see note)

Using a standing blender or an immersion blender and deep cup or jar, puree all the ingredients (starting with ½ cup of the water). Start on a slow speed to incorporate the cashews, then increase speed to high until very smooth and creamy. Add additional water to thin, as desired, and salt, agave, and chipotle sauce to taste. Dollop on soup, or use as a dip with tortilla chips.

Adult-Minded: I like this sauce with a modest amount of chipotle hot sauce to give a hint of flavor but no added heat. If you like the heat, though, add more hot sauce to taste!

Kid-Friendly: Omit the chipotle hot sauce altogether, add another ¼ teaspoon of agave nectar, and use this sauce to top your kiddos' burritos, tacos, or even pasta or simple beans and rice.

Serving Suggestions: This sauce has star power beyond pairings with Mexican-inspired dishes. By merely omitting the chipotle seasoning, this sauce transforms into a creamy, sumptuous topping for just about anything, such as baked beans, rice and grain dishes, pasta casseroles, pizza, baked potatoes, salads, and stews.

Pumpkin Seed Chipotle Cream

MAKES ABOUT 1¼ CUPS

This cream has a smoky essence with an acidic hit from fresh lime juice.

wheat gluten soy **FREE**

3 tablespoons raw cashews
½ cup raw pumpkin seeds
2 tablespoons freshly squeezed lime or lemon juice
 A smidgen of fresh garlic (¼ to ½ small clove)
¼ teaspoon (rounded) sea salt (about ¼ + ⅛ teaspoon)
¾ cup plain unsweetened nondairy milk (almond or soy preferred; see "Plant-Powered Pantry," page xxxiii)
½ to 1 teaspoon Dijon mustard
½ to 1 teaspoon chipotle hot sauce (e.g., Tabasco brand; adjust to taste; I like ½ teaspoon)
1 tablespoon extra-virgin olive oil (optional, or use extra milk)

Using a standing blender or an immersion blender and deep cup or jar, puree all the ingredients. If using a immersion blender, start on low speed and then work up to a high speed to finish blending (it will take several minutes of high blending to achieve a smooth consistency). Puree until very, very smooth, adding more milk or water to smooth out and thin, as desired. Be sure to blend this sauce long enough for it to become creamy smooth. Add additional Dijon and/or chipotle hot sauce to taste. This sauce is fairly thick while pureeing and will thicken with refrigeration. To use as a dip, simply make ahead and refrigerate for an hour or more before serving. If you prefer a thinner consistency, stir in extra milk or a touch of water.

Serving Suggestions: This is an absolute must to spoon over Black Bean, Quinoa, and Sweet Potato Spicy Croquettes. It is also scrumptious with fried plantains. Peel and slice ripe (blackened) plantains on the diagonal and panfry in a smidgen of coconut oil over high or medium-high heat, seasoning with coarse sea salt, until browned and crispy, flipping as needed.

Basil Lemon Pistou

MAKES ½ CUP

wheat gluten soy **FREE**

Pistou is the French term for a sauce made with fresh herbs, garlic, and olive oil . . . much like a pesto but without the addition of nuts (or cheese). My version adds a fresh burst of lemon to brighten and lighten the flavors. If using the garlic, use a smallish clove (unless you are dearly committed to garlic)! Otherwise, the more subtle flavors of the lemon, basil, and olive oil will be overwhelmed.

3 cups (lightly packed) fresh basil (about 2½ ounces)
5 to 6 tablespoons extra-virgin olive oil
¼ teaspoon (scant) sea salt
1 to 1½ tablespoons freshly squeezed lemon juice (zest the lemon first, then collect the juices; see note)
1 small clove garlic (optional)
Freshly ground black pepper
½ teaspoon lemon zest

Using a standing blender or an immersion blender and deep cup or jar, combine all the ingredients (starting with 1 tablespoon of the lemon juice and 5 tablespoons of the oil) except the lemon zest. Puree until very, very smooth. Stir in the zest, and additional lemon juice and extra oil to taste, if desired (see note).

Ingredients 411:

• Start with 1 tablespoon of the lemon juice. Depending on how loose or tight your measure of basil leaves, you may want to add the remaining ½ tablespoon. Taste after the first 1 tablespoon measurement.

• If you find the mixture too tart after blending, add ¼ to ½ teaspoon of agave nectar.

Savvy Subs and Adds: You can try replacing 1 to 2 tablespoons of the oil with water. The final product won't be quite as rich and luscious, but it will still be full of flavor.

Serving suggestions: Serve, drizzled on cooked grains, pizzas, pastas, soups, steamed or grilled veggies, or over baked potatoes or yams. It is particularly delicious on Chickpea and Artichoke "Bliss in a Dish." Refrigerate in a glass bowl or jar with a tight-fitting lid. This *pistou* does not have a long shelf life, even with refrigeration, so try to use within a day or two at most.

Rosemary Gravy

MAKES 1½ TO 1¾ CUPS

wheat gluten **FREE**

Fresh rosemary really brings this gravy to life. It is made with gluten-free millet flour, which is very forgiving to work with, not forming clumps with whisking. Easy to make yet full-bodied in flavor, this gravy can be used for everyday meals or special holiday dinners.

3	tablespoons olive oil (or another oil, such as avocado)
3½	tablespoons millet flour
1¼ to 1½	cups water (see note)
1½ to 2	tablespoons tamari
1	small to medium clove garlic, grated (see note)
1 to 1½	teaspoons agave nectar or pure maple syrup
½	teaspoon dry mustard
	Freshly ground black pepper
1 to 1½	teaspoons fresh rosemary, chopped roughly

In a saucepan, combine the oil and flour and whisk together over medium heat. Whisk for a couple of minutes, then slowly add the water (starting with 1¼ cups) while continuing to whisk. Add the remaining ingredients (starting with 1½ tablespoons of the tamari and 1 teaspoon of the agave) and bring the mixture to a boil. Once at a boil and thickened, turn off heat or simmer over low heat until serving. Add the remaining water (or more) to thin, as desired; and add more tamari to season and darken in color, as desired, and additional agave to sweeten to taste.

Adult-Minded: Try adding a splash of red or white wine for added depth of flavor.

Ingredients 411:
- I like the level of saltiness using about 1½ tablespoons of tamari, but you can use more to taste, as noted in the directions.
- I use a kitchen grater to grate the garlic directly into the pot before heating. You can also sub ¼ to ½ teaspoon of garlic powder, to taste.
- When you first make this gravy, using about 1¼ cups of water seems about right. But it thickens even more after standing, and you may want even more than the full 1½ cups if the gravy has sat for a little while and needing reheating.

Kid-Friendly: Try adding 1 to 2 tablespoons of nutritional yeast to the gravy. Not too much, just a little, to contribute another flavor note that may be enjoyable for you (or children).

Serving Suggestions: Pair with "No-Fu Love Loaf," Smashing Sweet Spuds, White Bean Mashed Potatoes, Festive Chickpea Tart, baked white and sweet potatoes, and other veggie burgers or loaves.

Brazil Nut Parmezan

MAKES ABOUT 2 CUPS

wheat gluten soy **FREE**

There are many versions of vegan Parmesans available, and in fairness, none of them are really like dairy Parmesan. But, we don't need them to be! What we want is a tangy, salty, rich-tasting sprinkle that we can use for topping salads, pastas, pizza, and more. This topping delivers—yep, I'd say (borrowing Larry David's words), this sprinkle is prettay, prettay, prettay good!

1½ cups raw Brazil nuts (see note)
½ teaspoon (scant) sea salt
1½ tablespoons nutritional yeast
1 tablespoon freshly squeezed lemon juice

Preheat the oven to 275°F and line a baking sheet with parchment paper.

Process the Brazil nuts in a food processor or blender until fine and crumbly. Don't overprocess, or they will begin to heat and become pasty. Just pulse until finely crumbled.

Spread on the prepared pan. Toss in the salt, nutritional yeast, and lemon juice. Use your fingers to work these ingredients through the crumbled nuts.

Place in the oven and bake for 35 to 40 minutes, being sure to toss three or four times through the baking process (and check during last minutes of baking; the mixture should become dry and maybe a touch golden around the edges, but should not brown). Remove from the oven, let cool, and transfer to a container to refrigerate.

If This Apron Could Talk: After trying this for the first time, you might want to double your batch the next time round. It can disappear quickly! It's one of my husband's favorites; in fact, he keeps saying, "You should bottle this up and sell it"!

Kid-Friendly: Your little ones might love this just the way it is, but you can try bumping up the nooch another tablespoon to make it a little more cheesy. Also see Cheesy Sprinkle (recipe follows) for a cheesier-tasting topping.

Serving Suggestions: Any tomato-based pasta sauce will welcome this seasoning, as will a very modestly dressed pasta, such as one with olive oil and lemon juice. This topping works wonders on salads, and adds crunch and depth to cooked rice and other grains, as well as simple bean preparations.

Cheesy Sprinkle

MAKES ABOUT 1 SCANT CUP

wheat gluten soy **FREE**

This topping, affectionately called Cheesy Sprinkle in our house, will be a favorite for kids big and small. Try it on salads, tossed into pasta, sprinkled on rice and beans, worked into sandwich mixtures, as a pizza topping, or eaten off a spoon (yeah, I've done it before)!

½ cup nutritional yeast
¼ cup raw almonds (see note)
¼ cup raw cashews (or more raw almonds)
¼ teaspoon (rounded) sea salt (about ¼ + ⅛ teaspoon)
¼ teaspoon lemon zest (optional)

Put all the ingredients into a standing blender and pulse until very fine and crumbly. Don't overprocess, just pulse several times. That's it! Store in the refrigerator until ready to use.

Adult-Minded: Try adding ⅛ teaspoon of onion or garlic powder.

Kid-Friendly: I make this often for our kiddos, and make it quick and simple using just the nooch, nuts, and salt. You may enjoy added flavor depth from the zest, but it's not essential.

Savvy Subs and Adds: If you are inclined to use hemp seeds, you can them to replace ⅛ cup of the almonds, though for best flavor, don't substitute more than ⅛ cup.

Truffled Cashew Cheese

MAKES ABOUT 1½
(GENEROUS) CUPS

*wheat
gluten* **FREE**
soy

Cashew cheese is a favorite for eating on its own with veggies or crackers, or using in entrées to substitute for dairy cheese. The addition of truffle oil adds a particular sophistication to the flavor of the cheese. However, don't shy away from making this recipe if you don't have the truffle oil—see the note for other ideas.

2½ cups soaked raw cashews, drained (1¾ to 2 cups unsoaked; see "Plant-Powered Pantry, page xxxiv)
¼ cup freshly squeezed lemon juice (see note)
1 small to medium clove garlic
3 to 5 tablespoons water (as needed, to thin or smooth the cheese)
½ teaspoon sea salt
Freshly ground black pepper
1 to 2 teaspoons truffle oil (optional, see note)

In a food processor, blend all the ingredients until smooth (starting with 1 teaspoon of the truffle oil and adding 3 to 5 tablespoons of water or more, until creamy, thick, and smooth. Stop to scrape down sides of processor as needed. Add ½ to 1 teaspoon of the remaining truffle oil, to taste. Refrigerate in airtight containers, or freeze for later use.

If This Apron Could Talk: This cheese freezes very well. I typically make a double-batch, and freeze smaller portions that can be thawed for using within 3 to 4 days.

Kid-Friendly: Children may reject the essence of the truffle oil. This cheese is delicious without it, all on its own, or with some of the other seasonings mentioned above. If you kids love nooch, add that. Or, if they like olives, throw a few of those in, or pickles! This cheese is easy to customize and suit the taste buds of any picky eater.

Savvy Subs and Adds:
- After pureeing this mixture, taste, and if you'd like a zingier flavor, add another 1 to 2 teaspoons of lemon juice.
- I've also made this cheese with a combination of soaked Brazil nuts and cashews, a delicious variation.
- If you don't have truffle oil, simply make this cheese without it, and consider adding other flavor enhancers, such as fresh herbs (a handful of basil leaves, a few teaspoons of fresh thyme, or a couple of tablespoons of chopped chives), chipotle hot sauce, smoked paprika, kalamata olives, or an olive tapenade.

Cashew Chive Spread

MAKES 1¾ CUPS

wheat gluten soy **FREE**

This spread is a raw food recipe, and is similar to a cream cheese in consistency. It has a delicate herb and chive flavor, though you can always add additional herbs and chives for a stronger flavor, if desired. This mixture is terrific as a spread or dip for raw veggies or breads and crackers. Also think of using it in other ways, such as for a thin base layer on a pizza crust, or to layer in lasagna noodles or pasta shells in place of cheese.

1¾ cups raw cashews (see note)
3–3½ tablespoons freshly squeezed lemon juice
1 small to medium clove garlic
⅛ cup roughly chopped chives or green onions (green portion only)
1 tablespoon fresh dill, or ⅛ cup (packed) roughly chopped fresh basil
½ teaspoon sea salt
Freshly ground black pepper
½ cup water (plus more to thin the mixture, if needed)
2 to 3 teaspoons extra-virgin olive oil (optional)

In a food processor, combine all the ingredients (starting with 3 tablespoons of the lemon juice). Process and scrape down the bowl several times, and continue until the spread is very creamy, smooth, and thick. Taste, and if you'd like more lemony flavor, add the remaining ½ tablespoon of lemon juice. If too thick, add another few teaspoons of water, one at a time. This mixture will thicken and become denser after it has refrigerated for a day or two, so you may want to consider that when adding water to thin. Spread on bagels, toasted breads, crackers, or flatbreads, or use as a dip for veggies.

Savvy Subs and Adds: Brazil nuts are a nice substitute for some of the cashews. Try replacing ½ to ¾ cup of the raw cashews with raw Brazil nuts.

Spinach Cashew Pizza Cheese Spread

MAKES ABOUT 1½ CUPS

wheat gluten soy **FREE**

This spread is not unlike a pesto, but has a little more punch so it can hold its own on a pizza crust along with bold toppings. It's versatile enough to adapt to a pesto, however, or to use as a dip or spread for other snacks and meals. I like an extra dollop alongside my serving of pizza!

1¼ cup soaked raw cashews, drained (about 1 cup unsoaked; see "Plant-Powered Pantry," page xxxiv)
2 tablespoons freshly squeezed lemon juice (see note)
1 medium to large clove garlic
½ teaspoon (scant) sea salt
2 cups (packed) spinach leaves
2 tablespoons extra-virgin olive oil
1 to 1½ teaspoons roughly chopped fresh oregano (not dried)
⅛ teaspoon onion powder
Freshly ground black pepper (generous is good)

In a food processor, blend all the ingredients until very smooth. This will take a minute or two of processing, stopping to scrape down the sides of the processor a few times throughout. Once smooth, use immediately or refrigerate in an airtight container for 3 to 5 days. Use a spread as a base on pizzas, or bake portions in small ovenproof dishes until heated through and serve as a dip or spread. Can also be used cold as a dip or spread for sandwiches and wraps.

Ingredients 411: If you haven't soaked the cashews in advance, use 1 cup of raw cashews as is, adding a teaspoon or two of water, if needed, while pureeing.

Kid-Friendly: If you like nutritional yeast, add 1 to 2 tablespoons while pureeing. It will also make the spread more kid-pleasing!

"Vegveeta" Dip

MAKES ABOUT 1½ CUPS

wheat gluten soy **FREE**

This warm cheesy dip has a mild flavor that can be used to accompany many foods . . . and also combines very well with salsa to mimic the Velveeta salsa dip from years ago. I make this without nutritional yeast and it tastes fabulous, but if you love the nooch, feel free to add some!

½ cup raw cashews
1 tablespoon tahini, or ⅛ cup pine nuts
1½ tablespoons freshly squeezed lemon juice
½ tablespoons apple cider vinegar
1 cup plain unsweetened nondairy milk (almond or soy preferred; see "Plant-Powered Pantry," page xxxiii)
¼ cup water, or more milk
½ teaspoon sea salt
¼ teaspoon prepared yellow (check for wheat) or Dijon mustard
½ tablespoons arrowroot powder
½ teaspoon (scant) paprika
⅛ to ¼ teaspoon turmeric (for color)
1 tablespoon light-flavored olive oil (not extra-virgin) or other neutral-flavored oil (optional; see "Plant-Powered Pantry," page xxxii)
1½ to 2 tablespoons nutritional yeast (totally optional!)

Combine all the ingredients in a blender and puree until very, very smooth. Transfer the mixture to a small saucepan and heat over low or medium-low heat for 5 to 8 minutes, stirring frequently, until the mixture starts to bubble and thicken. To thin the sauce slightly, stir in another 1 to 2 tablespoons of milk. Avoid thickening the sauce over high heat or increasing the heat too fast, as this mixture can scorch quickly. Once the sauce has thickened, add your desired extras (see note), season with extra salt to taste, transfer to a serving dish . . . and dip!

Adult-Minded: For a nacho "Vegveeta"-style dip, try stirring in ⅓ to ½ cup of your fave salsa—this is a hit at our table! Other add-ins to consider include a handful of sliced green onions, chopped sun-dried tomatoes (oil-packed, drained) or chopped fresh tomatoes, sliced olives, chopped fresh flat-leaf parsley or cilantro, or for heat-lovers, a few tablespoons of chopped jalapeños or a few dashes of hot sauce.

If This Apron Could Talk: The color of this dip will deepen with heating. When first blended, it is quite light without much color, but with heating, more yellow-orange color develops.

Ingredients 411: Extra-virgin olive oil can have a slightly strong flavor for this dip. If you do use it, try just ½ tablespoon of olive with ½ tablespoon of a neutral-flavored oil, or omit altogether. That way, the mild cheese flavor is not overwhelmed.

KD Dip

MAKES ABOUT 2 CUPS

wheat gluten soy **FREE**

Were you one of those kids that put a good ol' squeeze of ketchup on Kraft Dinner? If so, you'll lap up this kid-inspired sauce. Originally, I had made this sauce as a basic cheesy sauce made with only tahini (rather than nuts) so that it could be used in school lunches. One lunchtime, our daughters said, "Mom, this would be good with ketchup in it." Now, my kids can add ketchup to just about anything. But, this time I thought they might be on to something. I added a few squeezes of ketchup—and they were right!

⅔ cup nutritional yeast
2 to 3 tablespoons tahini
½ tablespoon apple cider vinegar (see note)
½ tablespoon freshly squeezed lemon juice (see note)
1 cup + 1 to 2 tablespoons plain unsweetened nondairy milk (almond or soy preferred; see "Plant-Powered Pantry," page xxxiii)
½ teaspoon (scant) sea salt
½ tablespoon arrowroot powder
⅛ teaspoon turmeric (for color)
4 to 5 tablespoons natural ketchup (see note; check ingredients to ensure wheat and gluten free)
1 tablespoon olive oil (optional)

Using a standing blender or an immersion blender and deep cup or jar, puree all the ingredients until very smooth (starting with 1 cup of the milk). Transfer the mixture to a small saucepan and heat over low to medium-low heat for 5 to 8 minutes, until the mixture, stirring frequently, starts to slowly bubble and thicken. Add additional ketchup as desired, to taste (see note). Avoid thickening the sauce over high heat or increasing the heat too fast, as this mixture can scorch quickly. Once sauce has thickened, use as a dip with vegetables, whole-grain pita, or other breads, or (thinned as desired with the remaining 1 to 2 tablespoons of milk) as a sauce for pasta, grains, potatoes, and so forth.

Adult-Minded: Replace a couple of tablespoons of ketchup with salsa, and also add hot sauce or other add-ins (e.g., chopped onions or chopped tomatoes) to taste. You can also try blending a clove of garlic into the sauce.

If This Apron Could Talk: This makes a sizeable batch; you can freeze half for later use, as it thaws and reheats well. Once refrigerated, it also works well as a condiment for school sandwiches.

Ingredients 411:
- If you only have lemon juice on hand (or only apple cider vinegar), feel free to use either in full (1 tablespoon).
- Start with ½ teaspoon of salt. Depending on the brand of ketchup, you may want to add a few pinches afterward. Same goes for the vinegar or lemon juice; you can always add an extra teaspoon or so for a tangier flavor to balance the flavor of the ketchup.
- Start off with about 4 tablespoons of ketchup, and then add more to taste. I like this sauce with 4 to 4½ tablespoons of ketchup, whereas our daughters, of course, like 5 tablespoons (and would take more if they had their way)!

Artichoke and White Bean Dip

MAKES ABOUT 2½ CUPS

wheat gluten soy **FREE**

Artichoke dip is always one of those more-ish kinds of dips, and I've made several recipes over the years. This one borrows creaminess from white beans, and a cheesy flavor from nutritional yeast. It is absolutely delicious, especially gently warmed and slathered on pita or other breads.

2 cups artichoke hearts (I use frozen, blanched in boiling water for 8 to 10 minutes, then drained; see note)

1 (14-ounce) can white beans (navy or cannellini), drained and rinsed (about 1¾ cups)

⅓ cup nutritional yeast

1½ tablespoons freshly squeezed lemon juice

½ tablespoon red wine vinegar

1 small to medium clove garlic (or larger if you love garlic)

2 to 3 tablespoons extra-virgin olive oil

2 tablespoons chopped fresh flat-leaf parsley

½ teaspoon minced fresh rosemary (try not to omit; it adds a lovely subtle flavor)

¾ teaspoon sea salt
Freshly ground black pepper

Combine all the ingredients in a food processor (starting with 2 tablespoons of the olive oil) and process until smooth. Taste, and add additional olive oil for a richer flavor, if you like. Serve immediately, or transfer to an ovenproof dish and heat until just warm and a little golden on top!

Ingredients 411: Frozen artichokes have a much better flavor than canned, so opt for frozen if possible. Don't use the artichokes that are jarred and marinated in oil or a vinegar brine—their flavor is too strong, even if rinsed.

Serving Suggestions: Try using this dip as a layer in lasagne, or to stuff pasta shells.

Grilled Onion Hummus with Hemp Seeds

MAKES 2¼ TO 2½ CUPS

wheat gluten soy FREE

Hemp seeds add a nutritional boost to this hummus, though the real attraction is the caramelized sweet flavor imparted from the grilled onions.

1	medium-size to large onion, sliced thickly (see note)
1 to 2	teaspoons olive oil, to coat onion slices
	A few pinches of sea salt
2	cups cooked chickpeas, drained and rinsed if using canned
½	cup raw or preroasted hemp seeds
4 to 4½	tablespoons freshly squeezed lemon juice
1	medium clove garlic
2	tablespoons extra-virgin olive oil
2 to 3	tablespoons fresh flat-leaf parsley (optional)
½	teaspoon sea salt
	Freshly ground black pepper
1 to 3	tablespoons water (use less/more to thin as desired)

Preheat your barbecue grill to medium-high heat.

Lightly coat the sliced onion with olive oil, and sprinkle with salt. Once the grill is ready, place the onions on the grill and cook (with cover down) for 7 to 10 minutes, then check and flip to cook on the other side for another 4 to 7 minutes (see note). Cook until softened and starting to caramelize, then remove from the grill (see note).

Meanwhile, in a food processor, combine the chickpeas, hemp seeds, 4 tablespoons of the lemon juice, garlic, olive oil, parsley, sea salt, pepper, and 1 tablespoon of the water. Puree until smooth, scraping down the sides of the bowl as needed.

Once the onions are grilled, add to the mixture (reserving a couple of rings for presentation, if desired) and puree. Add extra water to thin to your desired consistency, and the remaining ½ tablespoon of lemon juice, if desired, to taste.

If This Apron Could Talk: If you don't have a barbecue grill (or, if it's the middle of winter and you don't want to grill outdoors!), you can instead sauté and caramelize the onions on your stovetop. Simply add the onions (sliced more thinly to sauté than were you grilling them) to a sauté pan over medium-high heat with a tablespoon or so of oil and a couple of pinches of salt and pepper. Toss to coat the onions in the oil, and cook, stirring frequently, until the onions are softened and golden. This should take 12 to 15 minutes (or longer for fully caramelized onions).

Ingredients 411: Keep the onion slices thick if you are going to grill them. They will be easier to flip and less likely to fall through the grates of the grill. Also, try not to flip them too often, just once or twice, until nicely softened and with good grill marks. After cooking, you should have ¾ to 1 cup of grilled onion rings. I find it easiest to use both tongs and a spatula to turn the onions. If you like, reserve a couple of rings to top the hummus, for a pretty presentation.

Kid-Friendly: My kids aren't fond of onions. Even though the onions are pureed into this dip, your little ones might also pick up on their flavor. You can opt to use half the amount, or omit them altogether, and in place, add some nutritional yeast. Kids usually love the addition of nooch to hummus and other dips, so try adding ¼ to ½ cup to make this a cheesy hemp hummus!

White Bean Pesto Spread

MAKES 5 TO 6 SERVINGS OR MORE,
AS AN APPETIZER WITH CROSTINI,
BREADS, AND/OR CRUDITÉS

wheat
gluten **FREE**
soy

Take the appeal of vibrant summer pesto and churn into a spread that you can enjoy year-round. The toasted nuttiness of the pine nuts with the aromatic basil gives this spread a sophisticated flavor, yet it is incredibly fast and easy to make.

2 cups cannellini beans (white kidney beans), drained and rinsed if using canned

2½ tablespoons freshly squeezed lemon juice

1 medium to large clove garlic

2 to 3 tablespoons extra-virgin olive oil

½ teaspoon sea salt
Freshly ground black pepper

⅔ cup (packed) fresh basil

⅓ cup pine nuts, lightly toasted, then cooled

1 to 3 tablespoons water (use less or more to thin as desired)

In a food processor, combine the beans, lemon juice, garlic, 2 tablespoons of the olive oil, salt, pepper, basil, and about half of the pine nuts. Puree until smooth, scraping down the sides of the bowl several times and adding a little water at first, then more, if desired, to thin it. Add additional olive oil for a richer taste, if desired. Once smooth, add the remaining pine nuts and process lightly to break up the nuts but not fully incorporate them. To serve, this spread is best at room temperature to highlight its flavors. Try spreading on crostini (see note), then serving with a drizzle of olive oil and a sprinkling of coarse sea salt.

If This Apron Could Talk: Crostini is the Italian word for "little toasts." Simply thinly slice a whole-grain baguette (or you can use other whole-grain artisan bread), then lightly toast or grill. Once lightly golden and crispy, crostini are often served drizzled with olive oil and seasonings, or topped with spreads, garnishes, or relishes.

Creamy Grilled Eggplant Dip

MAKES ABOUT 1½ CUPS

wheat
gluten **FREE**
soy

This recipe has my kids *loving* eggplant. This is a variation on baba ghanouj, which is a little creamier and a little smokier than many versions of this popular Lebanese dish. Grilling the eggplant on the barbecue grill makes a big difference in the taste of the eggplant (though you can use your oven if needed; see note), and the addition of the cashews adds a sweetness that is a welcome change to traditional tahini. The smoked paprika just tops everything off making this dip a true family favorite.

---

1 medium-size eggplant (about 1 pound)

1 to 2 teaspoons olive oil, to brush on eggplant
Sea salt

⅓ cup soaked and drained raw cashews (about ⅓ cup unsoaked; see "Plant-Powered Pantry," page xxxiv)

2½ tablespoons extra-virgin olive oil

1 tablespoon red wine vinegar (see note)

2 to 3 tablespoons water (as desired, to thin; see note for oven roasting)

1½ teaspoons freshly squeezed lemon juice

1 small to medium clove garlic

1 to 2 teaspoons fresh thyme (optional, but lovely)

¼ teaspoon (rounded) sea salt (about ¼ + ⅛ teaspoon)

¼ teaspoon (generous) smoked paprika
Freshly ground black pepper

Preheat your barbecue grill to medium-high heat.

Halve the eggplant lengthwise. Score the flesh in two directions to make crisscross grids. Rub or brush the flesh with the teaspoon of olive oil, and sprinkle with sea salt.

Place flesh side down on the grill and cook for 6 to 8 minutes, turn skin side down and cook for 6 to 8 minutes, then turn flesh side down again and cook for another 8 to 10 minutes, or longer, until the eggplant is lightly charred on the outside and the inside flesh has become mostly translucent and very soft. (If needed, turn again and cook for another few minutes.)

Remove from the grill and let cool to the touch. Once cool, scoop out all of the eggplant flesh. Puree with all the ingredients until very smooth and creamy (I use a Blendtec blender for a very creamy consistency). Serve as is, or heat in a 400°F oven for 10 to 15 minutes.

If This Apron Could Talk: If you don't have a barbecue grill, prepare the eggplant by peeling, then cutting into cubes 1 to 1½ inches across. Toss with the 2 teaspoons of oil and a couple of pinches of sea salt. Place on a baking sheet lined with parchment, and bake in a preheated oven at 450°F for 25 to 35 minutes, until tender and golden in spots. If you choose this method, you will need extra water to puree this dip—somewhere between ¼ and ½ cup of water. Add water as needed to blend the dip until smooth, but keeping a thick consistency (don't water down; add a tablespoon at a time as needed).

Ingredients 411: If your eggplant isn't a full 1-pounder, go lighter on the vinegar. Start with ½ tablespoon, then taste and add more, if you like. The vinegar can be overpowering if there isn't enough eggplant flesh.

4 Vegan Soup for the Soul

For me, soup makes a hearty meal. As you'll soon see, most of my soups are chock full of satisfying, nutritious ingredients, such as lentils, beans, sweet potatoes, greens, and of course a variety of good ol' veg. You'll find plenty of nourishment at the bottom of each of these bowls, and some of the best flavors as well.

For earthy flavors, and really hearty bowls try Beans 'n' Greens Soup, Tomato Lentil Soup with Cumin and Fresh Dill, and French Lentil Soup with Smoked Paprika. When something more sophisticated calls, turn to Anise and Coriander–Infused Orange Lentil Soup or Pureed Apple, Celeriac, and Sweet Potato Soup. Both of these sound and taste elegant—and are perfect for a soup starter—but still do not involve elaborate preparation. For exotic-flavored and spicy soups and stews, put Caribbean Fusion Stew, Mexican Bean Soup, Moroccan Bean Stew with Sweet Potatoes, Peanut Thai Vegetable Stew, or White Chili with Roasted Poblano Peppers on your menu. Of course, my kids throw a huge vote in for Kids' Cheesy Chickpea and White Bean Soup, but trust me, it's not just for young palates. There's even more in store; I just want to give you a few teasers to get you pulling out that soup pot. And don't forget to try some of the substitutions and also serving suggestions with the soups—some accompaniments really elevate the flavors to round out a spectacular meal.

These soups will nourish your body *and* your soul . . . better than any chicken soup *ever* could.

Beans 'n' Greens Soup

SERVES 5 TO 8

wheat gluten **FREE**

Forget chicken noodle soup! This is the kind of soup that will keep you glowing inside and out, with nutrient-rich kale and plenty o' beans. Yep, this is proper good comforting soup that laughs in the face of all those "healing chicken soup" theories!

1	tablespoon olive oil or splash of water
1½	cups diced onion
2½ to 3	cups red or Yukon Gold potatoes, cut into chunks 1½ to 2 inches thick
½	cup diced celery
1	cup diced carrot or seeded and diced red pepper (add pepper later; see note)
4 to 5	medium to large cloves garlic, minced
1½	teaspoons dried rosemary
1	teaspoon dried thyme
1	teaspoon dried marjoram or oregano
1½	teaspoons dry mustard
¼	teaspoon freshly grated nutmeg (see note)
1	teaspoon sea salt
	Freshly ground black pepper
1	cup brown (green) lentils, rinsed (see note)
2	cups vegan vegetable stock (see "Plant-Powered Pantry," page xlii)
5	cups water
1	tablespoon red miso
1½	tablespoons blackstrap molasses
2	bay leaves
1	(14-ounce) can cannellini beans (white kidney beans) or other white beans, drained and rinsed
6 to 7	cups (loosely packed) roughly chopped or torn fresh kale leaves (1 smallish bunch of kale)
	Extra-virgin olive oil, for finishing (optional)

In a large pot over medium heat, combine the oil or water, onion, potatoes, celery, carrot (if using), garlic, dried herbs and spices, salt, and pepper. Stir well, cover, and cook for 6 to 8 minutes, stirring occasionally.

Add the lentils, stir, cover, and cook for another few minutes, then stir in the vegetable stock, water, miso, molasses, and bay leaves. Increase the heat to bring to a boil, then lower the heat to medium-low, cover, and cook for 30 to 40 minutes, until the lentils are very soft and fully cooked. (If using the chopped red pepper, add after first 25 to 30 minutes of cooking the lentils; see note).

Turn off the heat, add the cannellini beans (see note) and kale, stir, cover, and let the kale wilt in the soup for about 5 minutes.

Remove the bay leaves before serving. Add additional salt and pepper to taste, if desired, and a drizzle of olive oil.

Ingredients 411:
- Nutmeg seems an unexpected addition to this soup, I know. But it works nicely with bitter greens, giving a subtle, sweet spicy flavor to the soup that is pleasant. Give it a try!
- You can use carrot or red pepper, or a combination of both. I prefer to add the red pepper later in the cooking process, just to preserve some freshness.
- Adding the cannellini beans later in the cooking helps preserve the white color of the beans. You can certainly add them earlier, with the lentils, if you want, but they will absorb the broth and turn a brownish color. Just for visual appeal, I prefer to add them later.
- You can use curly kale or dinosaur kale; keep it in fairly large pieces, as they will wilt significantly.

Savvy Subs and Adds: Mung beans would make a good replacement for the green lentils, if you have those handy.

You can substitute other greens in place of the kale, such as collard greens, Swiss chard, or spinach. If using Swiss chard or spinach, you won't need to cook them; just stir for a minute and serve.

Mexican Bean Soup

MAKES 4 TO 6 SERVINGS

wheat
gluten FREE
soy

This soup has bold, vibrant flavors without being heavy, as a chili can be. Be sure to pair with Chipotle Avocado Cream. And avoid substituting cumin powder for cumin seeds—the whole seeds really add a distinctive flavor element.

½ to 1 tablespoon neutral-flavored oil or splash of water (see "Plant-Powered Pantry," page xxxii)
1½ cups finely chopped red onion
6 to 7 medium to large cloves garlic, minced
¾ teaspoon sea salt
Freshly ground black pepper
1¼ teaspoons cumin seeds
2½ teaspoons dried oregano
½ teaspoon ground cinnamon
1 to 2 tablespoons chopped jalapeño (adjust to taste; see note)
2½ to 3 cups water
1 (28-ounce) can diced tomatoes
1 (14-oz) can black beans, drained and rinsed
1 (14-oz) can pinto or kidney beans, or another can of black beans, drained and rinsed
1 cup frozen corn kernels
1 vegan vegetable-flavored bouillon cube (I use Harvest Sun brand)
1 teaspoon agave nectar or other natural sweetener
1½ tablespoons freshly squeezed lime juice
Chopped fresh cilantro, for serving
Lime wedges, for serving
Chipotle Avocado Cream, for serving (page 58)

In a large pot over medium heat, combine the oil or water, onion, garlic, salt, pepper, cumin seed, dried oregano, cinnamon, and jalapeño (if using). Cover and cook for 6 to 8 minutes, stirring occasionally; lower the heat if the onion is sticking.

Starting with 2½ cups of the water, add the remaining ingredients, except the lime juice, cilantro, lime wedges, and Chipotle Avocado Cream. Stir, increase the heat to high, and bring to a boil. Lower the heat to medium-low, cover, and simmer for 10 to 15 minutes.

Stir in the lime juice and add the remaining water to thin, if desired. Serve in individual portions with cilantro and lime wedges and a dollop of Chipotle Avocado Cream.

Kid-Friendly: If making this soup for a family with young children, you may want to omit the jalapeño so the soup does not have spicy heat. It will still be flavorful, just not spicy hot for the little ones. Also, if you don't have a fresh jalapeño on hand, feel free to add a few pinches of crushed red chili flakes or a few dashes of hot sauce, to taste.

Moroccan Bean Stew with Sweet Potatoes

SERVES 5 TO 6 OR MORE

wheat gluten soy **FREE**

There's something about the warmth and complexity of the spices and seasonings in Moroccan cuisine that inspires me to create new dishes using them. This stew offers a heaping serving of black beans, chickpeas, and lentils, along with sweet potatoes that simmer in a fragrant, intoxicating broth infused with cinnamon, cumin, coriander, ginger, fennel, and garlic. Individual servings can be finished with slices of roasted dried figs—elegant and delicious.

1½ tablespoons olive oil or splash of water
1 teaspoon cumin seeds
¾ teaspoon ground cumin
1½ teaspoons ground cinnamon
1 teaspoon ground coriander
½ teaspoon turmeric
½ teaspoon fennel seeds
1 teaspoon dried basil
¾ teaspoon sea salt
   A few pinches of cayenne pepper (optional; can be omitted for kiddos)
   Freshly ground black pepper
1½ cups diced onion
3 to 4 medium to large cloves garlic, minced or grated
3 to 3½ cups peeled and cubed yellow- or orange-fleshed sweet potato
1 (14-ounce) can black beans, drained and rinsed
1 (14-ounce) can chickpeas, drained and rinsed
1 cup dried red lentils, rinsed
3 cups vegan vegetable stock (see "Plant-Powered Pantry," page xlii)
3½ cups water
1½ tablespoons grated fresh ginger

FIG TOPPING:
½ to ¾ cup sliced dried figs, such as Black Mission (7 to 10 figs)
½ to 1 teaspoon olive oil
   Pinch of sea salt

In a large pot over medium heat, combine the oil or water with the spices, salt, and peppers. Cook for a couple of minutes, then add the onion, garlic, and sweet potato. Stir, cover, and cook for 7 to 8 minutes, stirring occasionally, until the onion starts to soften.

Add all the remaining ingredients except the ginger and figs, and increase the heat to high to bring to a boil. Then lower the heat to medium-low, cover, and cook for 20 to 25 minutes, until the lentils are fully dissolved and the potatoes are cooked through.

Meanwhile, prepare the fig topping: Preheat the oven (or a toaster oven) to 425°F and line a small baking sheet with parchment paper. You can slice figs as you like, keeping mostly whole, or sliced, or julienned. The smaller the slice/cut, the less roasting time needed. Spread the figs on the pan and toss with the olive oil and salt. Bake for 12 to 15 minutes, tossing once or twice during the baking process. Remove from the oven and let cool slightly. The figs will get chewier and crispier as they cool.

Add the ginger to the soup and stir.

Serve in individual portions with a sprinkling of roasted sliced figs.

Make It More-ish! Just before serving, try adding 2 to 3 cups of baby spinach or chopped chard. Stir and cook until just wilted, just a minute or two.

Tomato Lentil Soup with Cumin and Fresh Dill

SERVES 6 OR MORE

wheat gluten soy **FREE**

This soup may surprise you. Looking at it, you wouldn't think it is as delicious as it is! The flavors are not aggressive, but meld in such a way that keeps you coming back for just one more ladleful.

1	tablespoon olive oil or splash of water
1½	cups chopped onion
¾	cup chopped celery
½	cup chopped carrot
4	large cloves garlic
2½	cups white potato, peeled and chopped, or 1½ cups cooked brown rice (add rice later; see note)
1 to 1½	cups cauliflower, chopped
½	teaspoon cumin seeds
1	teaspoon ground cumin
1	teaspoon dill seeds
1	teaspoon dry mustard
1	teaspoon sea salt
	Freshly ground black pepper
2	cups red lentils, rinsed
2	cups vegan vegetable stock (see "Plant-Powered Pantry," page xlii)
3½ to 4	cups water (more if using cooked rice; see note)
1	bay leaf (optional)
1	(28-ounce) can crushed or diced tomatoes
2 to 3	tablespoons finely chopped fresh dill

Heat the oil or water in a large pot over medium or medium-high heat. Add the onion, celery, carrot, garlic, potato (if using), cauliflower, cumin seeds, ground cumin, dill seeds, dry mustard, salt, and pepper. Stir, cover, and cook for 8 to 9 minutes, stirring occasionally.

Add the lentils, stock, 3½ cups of the water, and the bay leaf. Bring the mixture to a boil, then lower the heat to medium-low, cover, and simmer for 25 to 30 minutes, until the lentils have cooked through and are softened. Then, add the tomatoes (and brown rice, if using instead of potato), and turn off the heat.

Remove the bay leaf, and using an immersion blender, puree the soup until completely smooth. Turn on the heat again to medium-high, and cook the soup for another 5 or more minutes to heat through (you can return the bay leaf to the soup or not).

Once reheated, stir in the fresh dill, remove the bay leaf, and serve, sprinkling with extra fresh dill, if desired.

Savvy Subs and Adds: If you have leftover cooked brown rice, it substitutes well for the white potato. Simply omit the potato, and add the cooked rice later in the cooking process, along with the canned tomatoes.

Serving Suggestions: Try with a large Classic Caesar Salad, topped with Brazil Nut Parmezan.

Peanut Thai Vegetable Stew

SERVES 4 TO 5

This beautifully flavored stew is brimming with vegetables and tofu in a creamy peanut-coconut sauce that is not too rich or heavy. Sure to become a favorite!

wheat gluten FREE

½ tablespoon organic extra-virgin coconut oil or neutral-flavored oil or splash of water

2 cups diced onion

5 medium to large cloves garlic, minced

2 to 2½ cups peeled and cubed yellow- or orange-fleshed sweet potato

½ teaspoon sea salt

1 teaspoon whole coriander seeds

¼ to ½ teaspoon crushed red pepper flakes (or more if you like the heat!)

1 stalk fresh lemongrass

1½ to 2 cups zucchini that has been halved or quartered lengthwise and sliced about ¼ inch thick

1 cup seeded and chopped red, orange, or yellow bell pepper

2 cups vegan vegetable stock (see "Plant-Powered Pantry," page xlvi)

¾ to 1 cup water

1 (14-ounce) can "lite" coconut milk

½ cup + 1 to 2 tablespoons natural peanut butter, or almond or cashew butter

1 tablespoon tamari

1½ tablespoons grated fresh ginger

½ to 1 (12-ounce) package firm or extra-firm tofu, cut into ¾-inch cubes (see note)

6 to 8 cups (loosely packed) baby spinach or roughly chopped Swiss chard

2½ to 3 tablespoons freshly squeezed lime juice
Fresh cilantro, for serving (optional)
A few lime wedges, for serving

In a soup pot over medium heat, combine the oil or water, onion, garlic, sweet potato, salt, coriander seeds, and red pepper flakes. Cover and cook for 5 to 7 minutes.

Meanwhile, prepare the lemongrass. Cut off the lower yellow bulbous portion (about halfway up), and discard the outer tough leaves, along with the upper portion of stalk. Using your chef's knife, cut a few shallow slits in the stalk and then use pressure on your knife to open and bruise the stalk, to help release its flavors (do not chop the stalk; keep in one piece).

Add the lemongrass, zucchini, bell pepper, stock, water, coconut milk, ½ cup of the peanut butter, tamari, and ginger to the pot. Stir and increase the heat to bring the mixture to a boil. Once it reaches a boil, lower heat to low or medium-low, cover, and simmer for 10 minutes.

Add the tofu (see note) and stir gently. Simmer, covered, for another 3 to 5 minutes, or longer until the sweet potato has completely softened and can be easily squished. Add the fresh spinach and 2½ tablespoons of the lime juice (add more if desired) and stir. If you'd like a fuller peanut flavor, add the remaining 1 to 2 tablespoons of peanut butter or more, if desired. Remove the piece of lemongrass before serving.

Serve immediately (so the spinach stays a vibrant green) garnished with fresh cilantro, if desired, and with lime wedges to squeeze over individual portions.

If This Apron Could Talk: Do not add the spinach until just ready to serve. If making this soup ahead of time, omit the spinach and then reheat the soup, adding the spinach at the last minute, then serve!

Ingredients 411: You can choose to use either the full package of tofu, or a lesser amount, per your preference. If you'd like a very substantial stew, use the full package (or most of it). If you'd like a lighter stew with fewer pieces of tofu, use roughly half of the package, and refrigerate or freeze the remaining tofu.

Savvy Subs and Adds: If you don't care for tofu, add a 14-ounce can of black beans (drain and rinse before adding) for extra heartiness.

Kids' Cheesy Chickpea and White Bean Soup

SERVES 4 TO 5

This soup isn't just for kids; it has plenty of good flavor to be enjoyed equally by adults. But with its smooth texture and cheesy flavor, your kiddos should surely love it, and ask for seconds or thirds!

wheat gluten soy **FREE**

1 tablespoon olive oil or splash of water

1¼ cups diced onion

½ cup (rounded) diced celery

½ cup diced carrot (optional, but adds a tinge of light orange color to the soup)

4 medium to large cloves garlic, minced

⅛ teaspoon sea salt

1 teaspoon dried basil

½ teaspoon dried rosemary

1 (14-ounce) can chickpeas, drained and rinsed

1 (14-ounce) can cannellini beans (white kidney beans), drained and rinsed

2 cups vegan vegetable stock (see "Plant-Powered Pantry," page xlii)

1 bay leaf

½ cup plain unsweetened non-dairy milk (almond or soy preferred; see "Plant-Powered Pantry," page xxxiii) or water

½ cup + 2 tablespoons nutritional yeast

1 tablespoon freshly squeezed lemon juice

In a large pot over medium heat, heat the oil or water. Add the onion, celery, carrot (if using), garlic, salt, basil, and rosemary. Stir, cover, and cook for 6 to 8 minutes, stirring occasionally.

Add the beans, vegetable stock, and bay leaf. Increase the heat to bring to a boil, then lower the heat to medium-low, cover, and cook for about 15 minutes.

Turn off the heat, remove the bay leaf, and add the milk, ½ cup of the nutritional yeast, and the lemon juice. Using an immersion blender, puree the soup until smooth (see note), then gently reheat on low heat, just to warm everything through again.

Add the remaining 2 tablespoons of nutritional yeast, if desired, for more cheesy flavor, and additional salt to taste.

Adult Minded: My kiddos like this soup fairly well pureed, but you can go with a more rustic puree if you like, blending in spots and keeping the soup a little more textured.

Ingredients 411: Feel free to add another ¼ to ½ cup of water to thin the soup more, if desired. Also, consider adding ½ cup of whole beans to the soup after pureeing (either reserve ½ cup, or add an additional ½ cup).

Make It More-ish! Top with a dusting of Cheesy Sprinkle or Brazil Nut Parmezan.

Anise and Coriander–Infused Orange Lentil Soup

SERVES 4 AS A MAIN DISH, MORE AS A STARTER

wheat gluten soy **FREE**

Coriander is a spice I love and have used many times in whole form in recipes. But, as with many whole spices, my kids will inevitably locate them on their spoon or fork, and try to then pick out each seed. With *every* bite. So I decided to infuse the flavor of coriander, along with star anise, in a tea ball in this soup. The soup has the lingering essence of these enchanting spices, and the tea ball can be left in or removed earlier in the cooking, depending on how much flavor you'd like to impart.

½ tablespoon olive oil or splash of water
1 cup diced white or sweet onion
½ cup diced celery
½ cup diced carrot
¾ teaspoon sea salt
   Freshly ground black pepper
1 teaspoon whole coriander seeds, placed in a tea ball
3 whole star anise, place with coriander in a tea ball
2 cups red lentils, rinsed
2 cups vegan vegetable stock (see "Plant-Powered Pantry," page xlii)
3 cups water
1 cup freshly squeezed or good-quality orange juice
1 bay leaf
1 to 1½ teaspoons orange zest
1½ tablespoons grated fresh ginger

In a large pot over medium heat, combine the oil or water, onion, celery, carrot, salt, and pepper. Stir, cover, and cook for 7 to 8 minutes, stirring occasionally, until the onion starts to soften.

Meanwhile, place the coriander seeds and star anise in a tea ball (or another gadget that will allow you to infuse the spices into the soup and then easily remove). Add the tea ball, lentils, stock, water, orange juice and bay leaf to the pot. Increase the heat to bring to a boil, then lower the heat to medium-low, cover, and cook for 20 to 25 minutes (see note), until the lentils are fully softened and dissolved.

Add the orange zest and ginger, stir, and cook for another few minutes. Remove the bay leaf. Season with additional salt and pepper to taste, if desired, and then serve.

If This Apron Could Talk: I infuse the soup for the full cooking time, but if you aren't sure about how much of this flavor you'd like in the soup, you can remove the tea ball after the first 10 minutes or so, and then taste after it is fully cooked and seasoned. Then you can always return the tea ball to the soup and cook a little longer if you want more of the infusion.

Serving Suggestions: Serve with a crusty whole-grain bread and Cashew Chive Spread, or baked white or sweet potatoes with Raw Aioli.

French Lentil Soup with Smoked Paprika

SERVES 4 TO 5

wheat
gluten **FREE**
soy

French lentils, sometimes called Le Puy lentils, hold their shape nicely, a little more than brown (green) lentils do. They are lovely in this soup, which has deep, smoky, and earthy flavors yet is very quick to prepare and cook.

1	tablespoon olive oil or splash of water
1½	cups diced onion
1	cup carrot that has been cut in disks
4 to 5	medium to large cloves garlic, minced
1½	teaspoons dried thyme
1¼ to 1½	teaspoons smoked paprika
1	teaspoon Dijon mustard
¾	teaspoon sea salt
	Freshly ground black pepper
2	cups French lentils, rinsed (see note)
2	cups vegan vegetable stock (see "Plant-Powered Pantry," page xlii)
5	cups water
¼	cup tomato paste
1	bay leaf
1½	tablespoons freshly squeezed lemon juice (optional, but nice)
2	tablespoons chopped chives, for garnish (optional)

In a large pot over medium heat, combine the oil or water, onion, carrot, garlic, thyme, paprika, mustard, salt, and pepper. Stir, cover, and cook for 6 to 8 minutes, stirring occasionally, until the onion starts to soften.

Add the lentils, stir, then add the vegetable stock, water, tomato paste, and bay leaf. Increase the heat to bring to a boil, then lower the heat to medium-low, cover, and cook for 30 to 35 minutes, or longer if needed, until the lentils are fully cooked through.

Remove the bay leaf. Add the lemon juice, if using, stir, and serve, sprinkling with chopped chives, if desired.

Kid-Friendly: Your little ones might like the smoky flavor, but if you aren't sure, ease off on the smoked paprika, starting with just ¾ to 1 teaspoon. You can also add precooked pasta shapes to this soup, for packing in lunches.

Savvy Subs and Adds: If you can't find French lentils, brown (green) lentils substitute nicely.

Serving Suggestions: Serve with crostini or baguette slices with Truffled Cashew Cheese, or a dollop of Spinach Herb Pistachio Pesto.

Pureed Apple, Celeriac, and Sweet Potato Soup

SERVES 4 AS A MAIN DISH,
MORE AS A STARTER

wheat
gluten FREE
soy

This is a delightful autumn soup, perfect to serve as a starter for a dinner party, but fares equally well as a main course, served with rustic bread and a dip (such as Truffled Cashew Cheese) plus a salad. The yellow-fleshed sweet potatoes lend a sweet creaminess to the soup, and the celeriac, also known as celery root, gives a mellow celery flavor with smoother texture and lighter color. The fresh thyme adds a herbaceous earthiness to round out the flavors, so try to include it if possible!

1 to 1 ½ tablespoons olive oil or splash of water

2 cups sliced leek (bottom white portion only, washed well to remove grit) (see note)

4 cups trimmed and chopped celery root (about 1½ pounds before trimming)

2 to 2½ cups peeled and chopped yellow-fleshed sweet potato

2 cups peeled and chopped apple

¼ teaspoon (rounded) sea salt (about ¼ + ⅛ teaspoon)

2 cups vegan vegetable stock (see "Plant-Powered Pantry," page xlii)

2 cups water

1 to 2 bay leaves (use 2 if small)

½ to 1 teaspoon chopped fresh thyme

¼ teaspoon freshly grated nutmeg

½ teaspoon ground cinnamon

1 tablespoon freshly squeezed lemon juice

In a soup pot over medium heat, combine the olive oil or water, leeks, celery root, sweet potato, apple, and salt. Cook for 9 to 10 minutes, covered.

Add the stock, water, bay leaves, thyme, nutmeg, and cinnamon and bring to a boil. Lower the heat and simmer for 10 to 15 minutes, until the vegetables are tender.

Remove the bay leaves, and using an immersion blender, puree the soup until smooth. If desired, add extra water to thin. Stir in the lemon juice, seasoning with salt to taste, if desired, and serve.

Ingredients 411: To clean the leeks, I slice them lengthwise, then submerge them in a sinkful of water. I then use my fingers to work through the layers and remove any grit.

Savvy Subs and Adds: If you want to substitute onion for the leeks, use a white onion, and use less, 1¼ to 1½ cups.

Caribbean Fusion Stew

SERVES 4 TO 6

wheat gluten soy **FREE**

This stew releases an intoxicating aroma while cooking. It is a very satisfying combination of beans and starchy plantains simmered in a spiced coconut broth. It has an exotic edge, yet is not at all difficult to prepare!

½ tablespoon organic extra-virgin coconut oil or splash of water

1½ cups diced onion

1 to 1½ cups seeded and chopped red bell pepper

2 cups barely ripe plantain that has been peeled and cut into small chunks (see note)

1½ teaspoons sea salt
Freshly ground black pepper

1½ teaspoons ground coriander

¾ teaspoon ground cumin

½ teaspoon ground turmeric

½ teaspoon ground allspice

⅛ teaspoon ground cloves

⅛ to ¼ teaspoon freshly grated nutmeg

¼ teaspoon crushed chili flakes (can adjust less/more to taste, I like the balance of heat at ¼ teaspoon, but you might want it spicier, and you can adjust this later, if you like)

¾ cup red lentils, rinsed

2½ cups cooked black beans or small red beans (about 1½ [14-ounce] cans, drained and rinsed)

2 tablespoons grated fresh ginger

1 (14-ounce) can "lite" coconut milk

3 cups water

1 to 2 bay leaves (1 large or 2 small)

2 cups sliced zucchini (see note)

1 cup broccoli or cauliflower florets

3½ to 4 tablespoons freshly squeezed lime juice

1½ teaspoons fresh thyme, or ½ teaspoon dried, added earlier with other spices
Lemon or lime wedges, for serving
Chopped fresh cilantro, for garnish (optional)

In a large pot over medium or medium-high heat, combine the oil or water, onion, bell pepper, plantains, salt, pepper, and ground spices. Stir, cover, and cook for 8 to 9 minutes, stirring occasionally.

Add the lentils, black beans, ginger, coconut milk, water, bay leaves, and dried thyme (if not using fresh thyme). Bring the mixture to a boil, then lower heat to medium-low, cover, and simmer for 15 to 20 minutes (at the 12-to 14-minute mark, add the zucchini and/or broccoli), until the lentils have cooked through and are softened.

Turn off the heat, add the lime juice and the fresh thyme (if using), and stir. Let sit for a few minutes for the thyme to release its flavor. Remove the bay leaves. Serve with additional lime or lemon wedges, and sprinkled with fresh cilantro if desired.

If This Apron Could Talk: When plantains are less ripe (i.e., more greenish), they are less sweet, and more like a waxy potato crossed with a yellow sweet potato. They can be a bit tricky to get into, though, as you might suspect you can peel them like a banana. No, you will need to cut off those peels. Trim the ends and then use your hands to pry back the peels, or your knife to loosen them. Once you have the plantain flesh, I find it easiest to cut in half lengthwise and then again to get quarters, and then it chop into chunks for this stew.

Slice the zucchini in half lengthwise and then cut into half-moons about ¼-inch thick if the zukes are large, or simply slice into ¼-inch rounds if small.

I prefer to add the zucchini and broccoli a little further along in the cooking process, to retain some of their vibrant color. If added too early, these veggies turn mushy and a gray-green color, but if added in the last 7 to 8 minutes of cooking, they stay beautifully vibrant. If you are making this stew ahead of time, simply reserve these veggies and reheat the stew before serving. While reheating, add the broccoli and zucchini, and heat through until they are tender.

Savvy Subs and Adds: If you can't find plantains, substitute waxy potatoes (Yukon Gold or red), or a combination of white potatoes and yellow-fleshed sweet potatoes (not orange-fleshed sweet potatoes).

Substitute more broccoli for some of the zucchini if you wish.

Serving Suggestions: This is delicious served with brown basmati rice. Rather than placing the cooked rice in the bottom of a soup bowl and then ladling the soup over the top, I like to use a spoon to pack the rice into one-half of the bowl, along the bottom and up the side. Then I fill the other half of the bowl with the stew.

White Chili with Roasted Poblano Peppers

SERVES 4 TO 6

(optionally) wheat
(optionally) gluten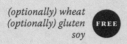
soy

Bulgur and beans give chewy, substantial texture to this tomato-less chili, and roasted poblano peppers elevate the flavors with a mildly spicy smokiness. For a wheat-free version, you can substitute steel-cut oats (or gluten-free steel-cut oats) for the bulgur.

1 tablespoon olive oil or splash of water

1½ to 1¾ cups diced white onion

¾ cup diced celery

4 to 5 large cloves garlic, minced or pressed

1 cup roasted, peeled, and chopped poblano peppers (about 1 large pepper) (see note)

A few pinches of crushed red chili flakes or minced hot peppers (see note)

2½ teaspoons dried oregano, or 2 teaspoons dried + 1½ teaspoons fresh (added later; see directions)

1 teaspoon ground cumin

¾ teaspoon cumin seeds

½ teaspoon ground allspice

¾ to 1 teaspoon sea salt

Freshly ground black pepper

2 cups vegan vegetable stock (see "Plant-Powered Pantry," page xlii)

3½ to 4 cups water

2 (14-ounce) cans cannellini beans (white kidney beans), drained and rinsed

1 (14-ounce) can kidney beans, drained and rinsed, or another can of cannellini beans (see note)

¾ cup dried bulgur (or steel-cut oats for a wheat-free option; ensure they are GF-certified oats for a gluten-free option)

½ cup raw cashews

1 teaspoon Dijon mustard

½ cup fresh or frozen corn kernels (optional)

4 to 6 tablespoons freshly squeezed lime juice

1½ teaspoons finely chopped fresh oregano (optional; see note)

¼ to ½ cup chopped fresh cilantro or flat-leaf parsley, for serving (optional, but adds great color)

Lime wedges, for serving

In a soup pot over medium heat, combine the oil or water, onion, celery, garlic, peppers, dried herbs and spices, ¾ teaspoon of the salt, and the pepper. Cover and cook for 8 to 10 minutes, stirring occasionally, until the onion has softened (lower the heat, if needed, to avoid burning the garlic).

Add the vegetable stock, 2 cups of the water (reserving 1½ cups for blending), and all but 1 cup of the cannellini beans (reserving the rest for the puree), kidney beans (if using), and bulgur. Cover, increase the heat to high, and bring to a boil. Then lower the heat to medium-low and simmer for 20 to 25 minutes, until the bulgur is tender.

Meanwhile, in a blender, combine the 1 cup of reserved cannellini beans (only use white beans for the puree, not the kidney beans) with 1½ cups of the water and the cashews and mustard. Blend until very smooth and uniform.

When the soup is cooked, add the blended mixture and stir. Also add the corn kernels (if using), 4 tablespoons of the lime juice (adjust to taste), and fresh oregano (if using), and let the mixture heat through for a few minutes (enough to heat the corn). For a thinner consistency, add the remaining ½ cup of water. Add the additional lime juice and the extra ¼ teaspoon of salt, if desired.

Serve as individual portions with the cilantro sprinkled on top, and the lime wedges.

Adult-Minded: To bring up the spicy heat, add red chili flakes to taste, or you can add a fresh chopped hot pepper, such as a serrano or jalapeño.

If This Apron Could Talk: Roast the poblano peppers either in your oven or over a gas range. For the oven, leave whole or remove the core and seeds, and slice into a few thick strips, then rub the pepper with a smidgen of oil. Place on a baking sheet lined with parchment. Set the oven to BROIL or GRILL, and place the pan under the broiler (under one of the higher rack settings). Roast for 10 to 15 minutes (turning once or twice while they roast, if using whole), until charred. Remove from the oven and let cool in a bowl covered with plastic wrap. For the gas range, set the flame to high. Place a whole pepper directly on the grate, and use tongs to turn it frequently, charring all sides and edges (this can be a little tedious, but does give a good flavor). Once charred, place in a bowl covered with plastic wrap. Remove the skins with your hands or a towel, by simply rubbing the pepper. Also, if you are able to roast two peppers, reserve the second, then chop the flesh into small chunks to garnish the soup—an attractive finishing touch!

Ingredients 411: Poblano peppers are just mildly spicy, and really add more flavor than heat to this chili.

Savvy Subs and Adds: If you cannot find poblano peppers, substitute green bell peppers, and be sure to roast them as well. Also, be sure to add a little extra flavor and heat with some jalapeños or chili flakes, and maybe a tiny hit of chipotle hot sauce.

Adding just a little pop of color with the kidney beans is very visually appealing. However, if you really want to keep most of the elements in your chili "white," feel free to use another can of cannellini beans.

The fresh oregano isn't crucial, but tastes vibrant and echoes the dried herb in the stew. If using, opt for 2 teaspoons of dried oregano early in the cooking. If you don't use it, use 2½ teaspoons of dried oregano instead.

Pureed Squash, Sweet Potato, and Celeriac Soup

SERVES 5 TO 6 OR MORE

wheat
gluten **FREE**
soy

Squash, sweet potatoes, and celeriac are first roasted whole to concentrate their natural sweetness. Then they are combined with mild curry and other seasonings and pureed until smooth. A delicately seasoned, creamy winter soup that will please a crowd.

2½ to 3	pounds deep orange winter squash (e.g., kabocha, butternut, red kuri; see note)
2 to 2½	pounds yellow- or orange-fleshed sweet potatoes (see note)
1	pound celeriac, or more sweet potatoes or squash (see note)
½	tablespoon coconut or olive oil or splash of water
1½	cups chopped onion
1	cup peeled and chopped apple
3 to 4	large cloves garlic, minced
1	tablespoon curry powder
1	teaspoon ground coriander
½	teaspoon sea salt
	Freshly ground black pepper
1 to 1½	tablespoons grated fresh ginger
3	cups vegan vegetable stock (see "Plant-Powered Pantry," page xlii)
½ to 1	cup water (to thin as desired)
1	bay leaf (optional)
1	(14-ounce) can regular or "lite" coconut milk
1	tablespoon freshly squeezed lemon juice

Preheat the oven to 450°F. Line a baking sheet with parchment paper.

Place the whole squash, sweet potatoes, and celeriac on the prepared pan. Bake for 55 to 75 minutes, or until tender when pierced with a skewer or sharp knife. (The baking time will vary, depending on the size of the vegetables. Smaller sweet potatoes and squash will be tender earlier, whereas larger ones and also the celeriac will take longer time to soften. Remove those that are tender earlier while the others continue to cook.) Once tender, let cool enough to handle.

While the vegetables are cooking and cooling, prepare other ingredients. In a large soup pot, heat the oil or water over medium heat. Add the onion, apple, garlic, curry powder, ground coriander, salt, and pepper. Cover and cook for 7 to 9 minutes, stirring occasionally, until the onion has softened.

Once the roasted vegetables are cool enough to handle, slice the squash and discard the seeds. Scoop the flesh away from the peel and add to your soup pot. Peel the sweet potatoes and trim the celeriac and add these vegetables to the soup pot (if the celeriac remains a touch firm, cut it into smaller chunks so it can more easily soften while the soup simmers).

Add 1 tablespoon of the fresh ginger, the stock, ½ cup of the water, and the bay leaf (if using) to the pot, and bring the mixture to a boil. Lower the heat and simmer, covered, for about 10 minutes, or until all the vegetables are quite tender.

Remove the bay leaf and add the coconut milk and lemon juice. Using an immersion blender, puree the soup until smooth. Taste, and add the remaining fresh ginger if you'd like, and remaining ½ cup of water to thin the soup if desired. Serve.

If This Apron Could Talk: You might find it helpful to roast the vegetables earlier in the day, so they can cool easily and in time to prepare the soup later in the day.

Ingredients 411: You can change the proportions of squash, sweet potatoes, and celeriac as you wish. Simply keep a total weight of 6 to 6½ pounds, which will give you roughly 10 to 11 cups of roasted vegetable flesh (after removing the skins and seeds). Note that some squash (e.g., butternut) will have more flesh and fewer seeds than other squash (e.g., red kuri) that will have a larger seed cavity and less flesh, so measuring out the cups of roasted flesh is helpful to determine how much you are actually using.

Serving Suggestion: Serve with over a wild and brown rice blend, and with Kale-slaw (or other green salad) with Curried Almond Dressing.

5 Side Stars

Some of these sides, my family could eat as a meal. I step in and make sure to add some greens and beans to their plates, but if they had their way, our eldest daughter would eat the Almond Roasted Cauliflower and Roasted O&V Potatoes for dinner (which I'd be okay with, maybe tossing just a few beans her way). Our middle girl would eat the White Bean Mashed Potatoes (pretty okay with this, too, and I don't even need to throw some beans her way, so I'll send some greens, kidding myself because I know they'll come back to me at the end of the meal). Our youngest might eat any of these side dishes as a meal. Or she might be in her mood of throwing it all at me. See, don't complain if your kids only want to eat the side dish. They could be throwing it at you instead.

Dinner games aside, make no mistake: These side dishes are for adults, too. For robust, starchy sides, try White Bean Mashed Potatoes, Roasted O&V Potatoes, and Smashing Sweet Spuds. Creamy Polenta is also a great comfort-food side, but is also very light and somewhat more elegant. Bring some lightly cooked vegetables to the table with Simplicity Asparagus, Oven-Sweetened Beets with Sage, and Gingered Broccolini. Little and big kids alike will also love Almond Roasted Cauliflower, and you might find yourself doubling the batch! There's even more in store—including my ongoing efforts to make fennel as well loved as green beans (ready to try either part of the Duo of Roasted Fennel recipe?) . . . so let your side stars shine!

Almond Roasted Cauliflower

**SERVES 2 TO 3 . . .
OR MAYBE JUST 1!**

*wheat
gluten
soy* **FREE**

Roasting cauliflower is not a new idea, but the addition of almond meal and nutritional yeast makes this side dish something special. Easy . . . and addictive (even if you aren't a huge cauliflower fan)!

4 to 4½ cups bite-size cauliflower florets (about 1 medium-size cauliflower)
1 to 1½ tablespoons olive oil
⅛ teaspoon (rounded) sea salt
Freshly ground black pepper (optional, if making for kids)
2 tablespoons almond meal
1 tablespoon nutritional yeast

Preheat the oven to 425°F. Line a rimmed baking sheet or 8 by 12-inch baking pan with parchment paper.

Toss the cauliflower with the olive oil and sea salt (and pepper, if using). Transfer to the prepared pan. Bake for 20 minutes, tossing once or twice. At the 20-minute mark, check the doneness and color of the cauliflower. If it has started to soften, turning a golden color, add the almond meal and nutritional yeast and toss again. If, at 20 minutes, it isn't at this stage, let it bake for another 10 minutes and then add the almond meal and nutritional yeast.

Bake for another 10 to 15 minutes or more, tossing again once, until the cauliflower is golden brown and fully softened.

Remove from the oven and season with additional salt and pepper, if desired. Serve warm!

Lemon Dijon Green Beans

MAKES 4 SERVINGS
AS A SIDE DISH

wheat
gluten FREE
soy

These beans are cooked until tender and then tossed in a tangy, piquant vinaigrette. If you don't like the taste of fresh tarragon, feel free to substitute flat-leaf parsley, dill, or another fresh herb of choice.

½ pound green beans, yellow wax beans, or dragon tongue beans, ends trimmed (see note)
1 tablespoon freshly squeezed lemon juice
½ tablespoon Dijon mustard
¼ teaspoon sea salt
  Freshly ground black pepper
1 teaspoon pure maple syrup or agave nectar
1 small clove garlic, grated (use kitchen grater)
1½ to 2 tablespoons olive oil
1 teaspoon chopped fresh tarragon, or 1 tablespoon fresh flat-leaf parsley or dill

Place the beans in a pot of boiling, salted water. Cook for 5 to 7 minutes (depending on the thickness of the beans), until just nicely tender to the bite.

Remove from the heat and immediately rinse the beans with very cold water until they have completely cooled. Drain well and set aside.

In a bowl, whisk together the lemon juice, mustard, salt, pepper, agave, and garlic. Continue to whisk and slowly drizzle in olive oil to emulsify. Finally, stir in the tarragon. To serve, toss the beans (pat dry first, if needed) with the vinaigrette.

Ingredients 411: Dragon tongue beans are not always available in grocery stores, but may be found in specialty whole foods stores or at farmers' markets. They are flatter in shape, and have a light yellow base with purplish streaks. They are so fun and colorful, and taste delicious—though most of the purple coloring fades with cooking.

Simplicity Asparagus

SERVES 2 TO 4

wheat gluten soy **FREE**

My sister Dyn'se used to love asparagus sandwiches while growing up. I never understood how she liked asparagus—until I tried it fresh some years later. Asparagus is a vegetable that I like to cook only briefly, rather than add to a longer-cooking casserole or stew. I just think its flavor is best when briefly cooked. A quick roast on an outdoor grill brings fantastic flavor to asparagus, but when it's too chilly outside, turn to this easy recipe.

½ pound asparagus
1 to 1½ teaspoons olive oil
A few pinches of sea salt (less than ⅛ teaspoon)
Freshly ground black pepper (optional)
½ to 1 teaspoon freshly squeezed lemon juice

Set the oven or toaster oven to GRILL or BROIL, and line a small baking sheet with parchment paper.

First trim the thicker, woody ends off the asparagus. You can use a knife for this, or hold the end of each spear in your hands and bend until it snaps at the naturally tender-woody place. If you like, you can also cut the asparagus into bite-size pieces, or leave whole.

Place the asparagus on the prepared pan. Sprinkle with the olive oil, and toss with your fingers to coat the spears. Sprinkle on the salt (and pepper, if using).

Place in the oven and broil for 4 to 6 minutes, tossing once or twice, until the color turns a bright, vibrant green and the asparagus is more tender. Don't overcook. The asparagus will continue to cook some after it is removed from the oven. It will be tender but still have some snap and bite.

Sprinkle on the lemon juice, and serve! That's it!

Serving Suggestions: This side will complement many dishes, including Creamy Barley Risotto with Thyme and Star Anise; "Fit-tuccine Alfredo" with Chanterelle Bread Crumb Topping; Potato, Shallot, and Pepper Frittata; and more. Also try chopping the asparagus, still warm, and adding to a salad.

Oven-Sweetened Beets with Sage

SERVES 4

wheat gluten soy FREE

When beets roast, their sugars intensify and they become much sweeter. Add a touch of balsamic vinegar and just a drop of pure maple syrup, and their natural sweetness is kicked up just a notch. Fresh sage or rosemary contributes a woodsy flavor and aroma, just enough to balance the sweetness.

1½ pounds beets, peeled and cut into 1½-inch cubes (4 to 4½ cups when cut)

1½ tablespoons olive oil

1 tablespoon balsamic vinegar

½ teaspoon pure maple syrup

1 tablespoon finely chopped fresh sage, or ½ tablespoon finely chopped fresh rosemary

¼ teaspoon (rounded) sea salt
Freshly ground black pepper (optional)

3 tablespoons chopped raw or lightly salted pistachios (see note)

Preheat the oven to 400°F.

In a large baking dish, combine all the ingredients, except the pistachios, tossing well.

Bake uncovered for 50 to 60 minutes or more, until the beets are fork tender (be sure to toss the beets a couple of times during the baking process).

Serve sprinkled with extra salt and pepper to taste, and with chopped pistachios.

If This Apron Could Talk: Leftovers can be stored in the fridge and gently reheated; great for salads (see serving suggestions).

Ingredients 411: Although the pistachios aren't essential to this dish, they really add great texture and a beautiful contrasting color.

Serving Suggestions: Pair with Yellow Sweet Potato Chickpea Pie with Basil or pasta with gluten-free White Sauce. Also try this warm on top of a spinach or other green salad; the heat will gently wilt some of the greens, and the sweetness of the beets and sauce will balance out the bitterer greens.

Duo of Roasted Fennel

SERVES 3 TO 4

wheat
gluten **FREE**
soy

I am a little fond of fennel. I think it's one of those very underused and unloved vegetables, but it is actually one of the most delicious—especially when roasted or sautéed or otherwise coaxed to caramelize, which draws out its natural sweetness while also mellowing its anise flavor. Here are two ways to roast fennel for an easy yet impressive side dish. Give them a try—give fennel some love!

ROASTED FENNEL WITH ORANGE AND THYME:

2 small to medium-size fennel bulbs (or 1½ large), stalks and fronds trimmed (reserve fronds), cut in half, and core trimmed out and discarded (about 1 pound *after* trimming)

1½ to 2 tablespoons olive oil

2 tablespoons freshly squeezed orange juice

½ teaspoon orange zest

2 teaspoons chopped fresh thyme, or ½ teaspoon (scant) dried (fresh thyme is preferable here)

¼ teaspoon (scant) sea salt
Freshly ground black pepper

1 to 2 tablespoons lightly toasted pine nuts or chopped almonds, for serving (optional)

Preheat the oven to 400°F.

Slice the fennel lengthwise into ½- to 1-inch-thick wedges or strips.

In a shallow baking dish or pie plate, toss the fennel with the olive oil, orange juice, zest, thyme, salt, and a pinch of pepper. Bake for 40 to 50 minutes, or until golden in areas and softened.

In the meantime, take some of the fronds and chop them roughly, to yield about 2 teaspoons.

Remove the fennel from the oven, sprinkle with nuts (if using) and the chopped fronds, and serve, seasoning to taste with more salt and/or pepper, if desired.

ROASTED FENNEL WITH
BALSAMIC VINEGAR:

- 2 small to medium-size fennel bulbs (or 1½ large), stalks and fronds trimmed (reserve fronds), cut in half, and core trimmed out and discarded (about 1 pound *after* trimming)
- 1½ to 2 tablespoons olive oil
- 1½ teaspoons balsamic vinegar
- ¼ teaspoon (scant) sea salt
  Freshly ground black pepper
- 1 to 2 tablespoons lightly toasted walnuts, for serving (optional)

Preheat the oven to 400°F.

Slice the fennel lengthwise into ½- to 1-inch-thick wedges or strips.

In a shallow baking dish or pie plate, toss the fennel with the olive oil, balsamic vinegar, salt, and a pinch of pepper. Bake for 40 to 50 minutes, or until golden in areas and softened.

In the meantime, take some of the fronds and chop them roughly, to yield about 2 teaspoons.

Remove the fennel from the oven, sprinkle with nuts (if using) and the chopped fronds, and serve, seasoning to taste with more salt and/or pepper, if desired.

If This Apron Could Talk: Fennel is also delicious sliced very, very thinly, tossed with nothing more than a smidgen of oil, salt, and pepper, and baked at about 425°F on a sheet lined with parchment, until golden and roasty-toasty (35 to 45 minutes). Makes a great topping for salads, soups, and other dishes. The fennel will really lessen in volume when roasted this thin, but becomes so caramelized and delicious that it is irresistible!

Ingredients 411: Fennel gets crispier with longer roasting, and caramelizes even more. If you bake closer to the 50-minute mark, the fennel will become more golden and deliciously caramelized! The longer you roast, the more golden and reduced the fennel becomes. It will also become slightly chewy with longer roasting.

Serving Suggestions: Pair either version with Lemon-Infused Mediterranean Lentils, or Yellow Sweet Potato Chickpea Pie with Basil. For a beautiful autumnal salad, try the warm fennel (including the pine nut, almond, or walnut topping) tossed in a baby spinach salad along with cranberries, and maybe some finely sliced apple (tossed in lemon juice to preserve its color).

Gingered Broccolini

SERVES 2 TO 3

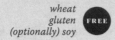

wheat
gluten
(optionally) soy
FREE

Although steaming is often the cooking direction for broccolini (and broccoli), I prefer to steam it via a light sauté, adding some ginger and seasonings that create flavor-encapsulated rather than water-logged florets. This is a simple, quick side dish, and broccoli florets can of course be substituted.

1 bunch broccolini (6 to 8 ounces)
1 tablespoon olive oil
⅛ teaspoon sea salt
Freshly ground black pepper
1½ to 2 teaspoons grated fresh ginger
½ teaspoon tamari (omit for soy-free option)
½ teaspoon toasted sesame oil (or more olive oil)
½ teaspoon pure maple syrup or agave nectar (optional)

Clean and trim the broccolini (see note), and cut lengthwise into smaller sections.

Place the olive oil, salt, and pepper to taste in a sauté pan (ideally, one with a lid) over medium-low heat. Add the broccolini, toss with the oil, and cover the pan. You will need to have a good seal to keep in the steam, so use the pan's lid, or a heatproof plate that will fit.

Cook over medium-low heat for 5 to 8 minutes, tossing once midway through the time, until the broccolini has turned bright green (turn down the heat if the broccolini is scorching, and add a few drops of water if it's getting dry). Check for tenderness. If the broccolini is still a bit firm, continue to steam for another few minutes, until still bright green but tender.

Toss with the ginger, tamari, sesame oil, and maple syrup, and serve.

Ingredients 411: You may want to peel the tougher outer layer on the stalks of the broccolini. It will make them more tender and easier to chew.

Serving Suggestions: Try with Thai Almond Chickpea Curry, with brown rice and Wonder Bean Puree, or all on its own with quinoa drizzled with Peanut Tahini Sauce.

Sunshine Fries with Rosemary and Coarse Sea Salt

SERVES 4 TO 6

wheat gluten soy FREE

Many of us have tried sweet potato fries, but these are usually made with orange-fleshed sweet potatoes. Try another variety of sweet potatoes—the yellow-fleshed kind—for home fries. They have a delightful sweet flavor that you expect, but hold up a little firmer than the orange variety. Of course, you could also combine both varieties in this recipe, for a very colorful side dish! (p.s. Tanya, you'll love these!)

4 to 4½ pounds yellow-fleshed sweet potatoes
2 to 2½ tablespoons extra-virgin olive oil
2 teaspoons finely chopped fresh rosemary
½ teaspoon (scant) coarse sea salt (see note)

Preheat the oven to 400°F and line a baking sheet or two with parchment paper.

First wash and peel the sweet potatoes. Then cut the whole potatoes into wedges, starting by cutting in half lengthwise, then working wedges out of the halves, 1 to 1½ inches at the thick edge (see note).

Toss the wedges in the olive oil and fresh rosemary, and place on the prepared pan(s). Sprinkle with the coarse salt (see note). Bake for 50 to 65 minutes, flipping the fries and rotating the pan(s) a couple of times during the baking process, until the sweet potatoes have softened and are also caramelized (delicious!) in spots.

Taste and season with extra salt, if needed. Serve!

If This Apron Could Talk: If the potatoes are taking longer to cook than you'd like and dinner is nearing, bump the temperature up to 425°F. Just let the fries bake at 400°F for the first 20 minutes or so, then go ahead and increase the heat.

This makes a large batch. If you want to make enough to serve just two, it is easy enough to cut all the measurements in half. You may also find the potatoes cook a little faster with less on a large pan.

Ingredients 411: Depending on the girth of the sweet potatoes you have, you might get three or four wedges out of each half, but if the potatoes are on the small side, you might get just four wedges out of the whole potato.

Coarse sea salt is wonderful because you notice the taste and texture of the salt just a little more than you do regular sea salt. It is tricky to measure, so you can eyeball it if you want, or grind it and properly measure it out. I like to use a scant ½ teaspoon, to underseason the fries, and then add a fresh grind of coarse sea salt just before serving.

Roasted O&V Potatoes

SERVES 4 TO 5

 wheat gluten soy FREE

I had been making these potatoes for my family and never thought much about detailing them in recipe form. But after making them for a potluck once, and having guests ask how to make them, I thought, "Okay, time to put pen to paper." These are very easy to prepare and please adults and kids alike.

3 pounds nugget, red, or Yukon Gold potatoes (see note)

2½ tablespoons extra-virgin olive oil

2 to 2½ teaspoons balsamic vinegar

¼ teaspoon sea salt or coarsely ground sea salt (see note)

¼ teaspoon minced fresh rosemary, or 2 to 3 tablespoons chopped fresh basil, dill, or flat-leaf parsley (optional)

Preheat the oven to 400°F.

Pierce the potatoes with a skewer or knife, and place directly on the oven rack (or on a baking sheet, if you prefer). Bake for 40 to 60 minutes, depending on size, until tender when pierced with a knife or skewer and skins are becoming blistered.

Remove from the oven and transfer to a large bowl. Let cool for 5 to 10 minutes, then add the olive oil, vinegar, salt, and herbs (if using). Toss to coat.

If you have used larger potatoes, cut through them roughly, slicing into halves or quarters (carefully, they will be very hot inside)—just enough to allow some of the seasonings to cover some surface area of the flesh of the potatoes. If using nugget potatoes, leave some whole and just lightly score the rest (don't need to fully cut through).

This is a rustic dish; just toss and see how well the taters are coated, and season to taste as needed with extra salt (using coarsely ground salt is especially tasty; see note).

Ingredients 411: It is easiest to measure fine sea salt for this recipe. But when I prepare these at home, I prefer to use a coarse grind of sea salt and approximate the measure, adjusting to taste. Coarse salt with tender potatoes is just a beautiful thing, so give it a try if you have a salt grinder.

Serving Suggestions: These make a happy addition to just about any veggie burger or loaf recipe (see Chapter 7). Also try with BBQ Sunflower Tofu or Jerk Chickpeas.

White Bean Mashed Potatoes

SERVES 4 TO 6

wheat gluten soy **FREE**

This recipe wasn't designed for ingenuity but nutrition. I mean, who doesn't love creamy mashed potatoes? But why not bump up the nutritional profile of your whipped spuds by adding protein from white beans and vitamin-rich butternut squash? The beans are pureed before mixing, so no one will know they are in there, and the butternut squash adds a beautiful golden color. Of course, you can have the satisfaction of knowing how much more nutritious each mouthful is!

1½ pounds Yukon or red potatoes, peeled and cut into large chunks

½ to ¾ pound peeled butternut squash, cut into cubes the same size as the potatoes chunks (or use only potatoes, 2 to 2¼ pounds total)

1 (14-ounce) can cannellini beans (white kidney beans), drained and rinsed

½ cup plain unsweetened nondairy milk (almond or soy preferred; see "Plant-Powered Pantry," page xxxiii)

1⅛ to 1¼ teaspoons sea salt

3½ to 4½ tablespoons extra-virgin olive oil

¼ teaspoon freshly grated nutmeg

1 teaspoon finely chopped freshly rosemary (optional; see note)

Freshly ground black pepper (optional)

Place the potatoes and butternut squash (if using) in a large pot and cover with cold water. Heat over high heat and bring to a boil, then lower the heat to medium-low and simmer for 15 to 18 minutes, or longer, until tender throughout when pierced with a skewer (try to avoid overcooking because the potatoes will become watery; also, the squash may cook faster than the potatoes).

While the potatoes are cooking, using an immersion or standing blender), combine the white beans with the milk and puree until very smooth, then set aside.

Drain the potatoes and squash in a colander. Using a potato ricer, press the potatoes and squash back in your cooking pot.

Combine with the white bean mixture, as well as 1⅛ teaspoons of the salt, 3½ tablespoons of the olive oil, the nutmeg, and the rosemary or other fresh herbs (if using), and mix well until smooth. Add additional olive oil, and salt and/or pepper to taste.

Serve immediately, or transfer to an ovenproof dish to keep warm in the oven until serving.

Kid-Friendly: I love the addition of butternut squash to this dish. It adds a lovely color, a slight nutty squash flavor, and of course, extra nutrition. If, however, you think your crew will be picky about the color, feel free to substitute more potatoes.

Make It More-ish! I often serve these potatoes with Rosemary Gravy. Because this gravy is already infused with rosemary, I omit the rosemary from these potatoes. But if serving without the gravy, the addition of fragrant rosemary is quite lovely. Other options to mix into the potatoes include chopped chives or green onions, grated or roasted garlic, or some nutritional yeast.

Serving Suggestion: This is an ideal side dish for any holiday menu, including as a side for Festive Chickpea Tart. Also try it with Braised Tempeh in a Lemon, Thyme, and Caper Sauce, or Tofu Baked in an Olive, Grape, and Herbed Marinade.

Smashing Sweet Spuds

SERVES 4 TO 6

wheat
gluten **FREE**
soy

Cooking confession: I really dislike making mashed potatoes. There. Said it. Much to my family's dismay, as they all love a good side of mashed potatoes. But between peeling the potatoes, boiling and draining them, putting them through a ricer, and dealing with all the mess through those steps . . . not fun! One night, I baked up some sweet potatoes alongside some Yukon Golds, smashed them all up with some seasonings, and the crew lapped them up. Score! Not only more nutritious using some sweet potatoes, these smashed spuds are much, much easier.

1¾ to 2 pounds red or Yukon Gold potatoes
1½ pounds yellow- or orange-fleshed sweet potatoes
1 to 2 tablespoons extra-virgin olive oil
½ teaspoon (rounded) sea salt
Freshly ground black pepper (optional)
Fresh herbs (optional, for garnishing or to work into potatoes; see note)

Preheat the oven to 400°F.

Pierce the red or Yukon Gold potatoes with a skewer or knife, and place directly on an oven rack (or on a baking sheet, if you prefer). You don't need to pierce the sweet potatoes; in fact they will ooze and drip if you do—just place those on the oven rack or pan. Bake for 50 to 65 minutes (or longer, depending on size), until tender when pierced with a knife or skewer.

Remove from the oven and let cool enough to handle. Carefully remove the skins from the sweet potatoes and place in a large bowl with the red or Yukon Gold potatoes (leaving the skins of these on). With a potato masher, or even a wooden or other large spoon, mash/smash the potatoes, adding the oil, salt, and pepper (if using), and incorporating the white potatoes with the sweets, until well smooshed together! This is very casual, so work with it as you prefer . . . leave more chunky, or mash smoother. Work in fresh herbs, if desired, and season to taste with additional salt or oil, as you wish.

Adult-Minded: The addition of fresh herbs is delish. Try chopped fresh thyme, dill, basil, parsley, or chives (or the leafy green portion of green onions).

If This Apron Could Talk: If you are short on time, bump up the oven temp to 425° or 450°F for part of the baking time, to speed things up.

This makes a decent batch of spuds. Be sure to have friends to share (or be prepared to eat leftovers, which work well in wraps, BTW)!

Savvy Subs and Adds: I love the clean, simple flavor of olive oil in this dish, but if you're partial to Earth Balance margarine, you can substitute it for the oil. Just be sure to omit the salt (as there is usually enough seasoning in the Earth Balance).

Serving Suggestions: Bring a new twist to mashed potatoes for your next holiday dinner with this dish. Also try it with "No-fu Love Loaf," topped with Rosemary Gravy.

Indian-Inspired Rice

SERVES 4 TO 6

wheat gluten soy **FREE**

This rice has a light, fragrant spice that does not dominate; rather, it elevates this side dish. While this contains some traditional spices used in Indian cuisine, it has enough of a balanced flavor to pair with a wide array of dishes.

2 tablespoons organic extra-virgin coconut oil

1 tablespoon brown mustard seeds

½ teaspoon cumin seeds (optional)

1 cup diced onion

¼ teaspoon sea salt

½ teaspoon ground cardamom

2 teaspoons ground coriander
A few pinches of ground cinnamon

1¼ cups brown basmati rice

3 cups water

1½ to 2 tablespoons freshly squeezed lime or lemon juice (I prefer lime)

Pour the oil into a medium-size pot. Turn the heat to high, add the mustard seeds and cumin seeds (if using). Cook for a couple of minutes, until you hear the mustard seeds popping. Then lower the heat to medium, add the onion, and cook for 7 to 8 minutes, until turning golden. Add other spices, and stir.

Rinse the rice, then add it to the pot, stirring to coat with the spices and oil, and cooking for another minute. Add the water and increase the heat to high, to bring to a boil. Once at a boil, lower the heat to low and cover the pot. Keep covered and cook for 35 minutes.

Remove the lid to check the rice. If water is still visible, return the lid to the pot and cook for another 5 minutes or more. If the rice has absorbed the water, turn off the heat and remove the pot from the stove.

Stir in the lime or lemon juice, and serve.

Serving Suggestions: Try serving with Fragrant Kidney Bean Lentil Dal, Pumpkin Chickpea Cauliflower Curry, or Pureed Squash, Sweet Potato, and Celeriac Soup.

Creamy Polenta

SERVES 3 TO 4

wheat
gluten **FREE**
soy

I like freshly made polenta kept fairly simple, with just a few seasonings. This version is creamy with some help from nondairy milk and olive oil, and just a touch of lemon zest helps lift the flavors (really try to include it)! Feel free to add some fresh rosemary or thyme, for a fresh herbaceous touch.

1½ cups water (or 2 cups of water and only 1 cup of milk)
1½ cups plain unsweetened nondairy milk (almond or soy preferred; see "Plant-Powered Pantry," page xxxiii)
½ teaspoon sea salt
1 cup dried polenta (corn grits; I use Bob's Red Mill brand)
2 to 2½ tablespoons extra-virgin olive oil
2 tablespoons nutritional yeast (optional, but give it a try!)
½ to 1 teaspoon lemon zest
Freshly ground black pepper (optional)

Bring the water, milk, and salt to a boil in a medium-size pot over high heat, then lower the heat to low and begin to whisk in the polenta. Add it somewhat slowly, whisking as you go. Cook, stirring, for about 5 minutes, until thickened. Add the oil, nutritional yeast, lemon zest, and pepper, if desired, and stir. Taste, and add additional salt, if desired.

Serve immediately. To thin, add a little extra water or milk (see note).

Adult-Minded: I love the mellow, soft flavors and pillowy texture of this polenta just as is. But if you're one to bump up the seasonings and textures, there are plenty of things you can try. If you have fresh rosemary or thyme on hand, a small amount would be a nice touch. Try ½ to 1 teaspoon of minced rosemary or 1½ teaspoons of chopped thyme, added just at the last minute or two of cooking. Other add-ins you might consider are: chopped roasted red peppers, chopped sun-dried tomatoes, very slightly cooked and chopped asparagus (it will cook more in the polenta), roasted garlic, chopped green onions, sliced olives, a few tablespoons of pesto (e.g., Brazil Nut Pesto or Spinach Herb Pistachio Pesto), or sautéed or roasted mushrooms. All of these can be stirred in during the last minute or two of cooking.

If This Apron Could Talk: After adding the full 3 cups of liquid (1½ cups milk and 1½ cups water), the polenta will be thick and creamy. As it continues to set, however, you may want to thin it more to your desired consistency. If so, keep the heat at low and stir in another 2 to 4 tablespoons of water or milk, or more, as needed. After the polenta has sat (after serving), you can also loosen it again by gently reheating and whisking in a touch more water.

Serving Suggestions: Two of my favorite dishes to serve over this polenta are Lemon-Infused Mediterranean Lentils and Tofu Baked in an Olive, Grape, and Herbed Marinade.

6 Your Main Squeeze: Casseroles, One-Pot Wonders, and Tarts

A few go-to casserole recipes seem to be essential in a vegan's cooking repertoire. I used to think this need for casseroles centered around potlucks. But I think folks talk about potlucks more than they actually go to them! No, I think our quest for good casseroles goes back to the comfort food of our childhood. I grew up eating my mom's macaroni and cheese, cod au gratin, lasagne, and other very hearty, comforting meals. Yes, those casseroles we remember as kids were entirely comforting. But think back . . . they were rarely very healthy. Usually they included ground beef or other meat, as well as cheese and/or dairy-based sauces. How many do you remember that contained a can or two of cream of mushroom soup?

Vegan casseroles can still be comforting, they can still be delicious, but with a big

difference from those you remember—they can be wholesome and nourishing, too! You can get plenty of flavor from such ingredients as herbs, spices, vegetables, or legumes, no cholesterol, and far less fat and salt than in Mom's old standbys!

In this section you'll find savory, creamy crowd-pleasing dishes such as Winter Veg Chickpea Potpie, Boulangerie Potatoes with Sautéed Fennel and White Beans, and No-fu Love Loaf (a lentil-based dinner loaf). Please note that there are more casseroles in Chapter 8. I kept those with their pasta peers, but you must try Mac-oh Geez! or Baked Macaroni with Broccolini in a Creamy Walnut Gravy—and then tote them along to those ever-popular (but elusive) potlucks!

You'll also find "One-Pot Wonders" here. These are sort of like stews, sometimes with bold, spicy, and exotic flavors (try Thai Chickpea Almond Curry, Pumpkin Chickpea Cauliflower Curry with Fresh Cream Sauce, or Jerk Chickpeas); but other times, with more of a simplified yet flavorful lentil or bean preparation (e.g., Lemon-Infused Mediterranean Lentils or Wonder Bean Puree). Or they might be a tofu or tempeh entrée (e.g., Tempeh Tickle or BBQ Sunflower Tofu) that comes together lickety-split by combining everything in one baking pan. These kinds of dishes make eating deliciously a little easier.

Want something a bit more sophisticated? Well, tarts (no, not that kind) to the rescue! Okay, it's been pointed out more than once that I like using the word *tart*. It's the "Corrie" coming out in me. (For those of you out of the loop, that's the British soap opera *Coronation Street*—and my guilty pleasure.) Festive Chickpea Tart is the perfect holiday centerpiece, and Yellow Sweet Potato Chickpea Pie with Basil is the perfect way to sneak chickpeas and sweet potatoes into a pie shell—it's a tasty balance of sweet and savory!

Before you go on, don't forget that your "main squeeze" might just be a soup or stew—or a pasta or burger. So be sure to check out those chapters, too, for some good dinner lovin'!

Thai Chickpea Almond Curry

SERVES 4 TO 5, DEPENDING
ON ACCOMPANIMENTS

*wheat
gluten* **FREE**

While this bakes, you will be enchanted with the aromatic mingling of nutty coconut sauce infused with lime, ginger, and curry. It is a deeply flavorful dish that is also almost effortless in preparation. Everything comes together lickety-split and you have an exotic bean entrée to serve over rice.

SAUCE:

- 1 medium to large clove garlic, minced
- ½ teaspoon sea salt (plus another few pinches, if desired)
- 2½ to 3 tablespoons freshly squeezed lime juice
- 1 (14-ounce) can "lite" coconut milk
- ¼ cup almond butter
- ½ tablespoon tamari
- 1½ tablespoons peeled and roughly chopped fresh ginger
- 1½ to 2 teaspoons red curry paste (I use Thai Kitchen brand)
- ⅛ to ¼ teaspoon crushed red pepper flakes (optional; or use more if you like the heat!)

CHICKPEA MIXTURE:

- 2 (14-ounce) cans chickpeas, drained and rinsed (3¾ to 4 cups)
- 2 cups zucchini that has been halved or quartered lengthwise (depending on thickness) and sliced about ¼ inch thick (see note)
- ¾ cup green onion (mostly white bottom portion, but some green as well)
- 2 dried or fresh kaffir lime leaves (optional)
- 2 to 3 tablespoons chopped fresh Thai basil, basil, or cilantro, for garnish (optional)
  A few lime wedges, for serving

Preheat the oven to 400°F.

First prepare the sauce: In a blender, or using a deep large cup and an immersion blender, combine the garlic, ½ teaspoon of the salt, lime juice, coconut milk, almond butter, tamari, ginger, and curry paste. Puree well. Pour the sauce into a baking dish (8 by 12-inch, or similar size) and stir in the red pepper flakes. Add the chickpeas, zucchini, green onions, and lime leaves (if using), and stir well.

Cover the dish with foil and bake for 35 minutes. Then remove the foil, stir, and bake for another 5 to 10 minutes uncovered. (Note that the sauce should thicken but can become too thick, so keep an eye on it, and remove once it begins to thicken, so it is does not become pasty.)

Add a few pinches of salt to taste, if desired. Serve, topping the portions with fresh herbs, if desired, and with a lime wedge on the side.

Savvy Subs and Adds: Almond butter is my first choice in this recipe, but consider switching it up occasionally with natural peanut or cashew butter in place of the almond.

Feel free to substitute other veggies in part or in whole for the zucchini. I love zucchini, so it is a natural choice for me. Other veggies to consider are sliced red peppers (and these add a lovely color), chopped cauliflower, steamed potatoes, or snow peas.

Winter Veg Chickpea Potpie

SERVES 4 TO 6, DEPENDING ON ACCOMPANIMENTS

(optionally) wheat
(optionally) gluten **FREE**
soy

This is a homey dish, with plenty of winter vegetables mingling in a light cream sauce with chickpeas, herbs, and seasonings, capped with a pastry topping. The potpie is much easier to prepare if using a premade whole-grain pastry shell (see below), but you can also use my spelt and oat Gluten-Free Piecrust (page 242).

2 tablespoons olive oil

1 cup finely chopped onion, or 1½ cups sliced leek (white portion only, rinsed well)

1 cup sliced celery (cut about ¼ inch thick)

¾ cup sliced carrot (cut into rounds about ¼ inch thick)

3½ to 4 cups cubed combination of yellow-fleshed sweet potato, Yukon Gold or red potato, and/or parsnip (see note)

1 to 1½ chopped cups fennel (stalks and core removed)

1 to 2 medium to large clove garlic, minced

½ teaspoon dried thyme

¼ teaspoon dried rosemary

½ teaspoon poultry seasoning (or increase the thyme to ¾ teaspoon and add ¼ teaspoon sage)

½ teaspoon dry mustard

1 teaspoon sea salt

¼ teaspoon freshly grated nutmeg

⅛ to ¼ teaspoon freshly ground black pepper

⅓ cup millet flour (for gluten-free), spelt flour, or whole wheat pastry flour (I prefer millet)

2¾ cups plain unsweetened nondairy milk (almond or soy preferred; see "Plant-Powered Pantry," page xxxiii)

½ to ¾ cup trimmed and sliced green beans (cut into bite-size pieces) or frozen peas

2 cups cooked chickpeas, or 1 (14-ounce) can, drained and rinsed

1 to 2 frozen whole wheat (or wheat- or gluten-free) pastry shells, thawed, or other vegan pie pastry (I use Wholly Wholesome brand; see directions)

Preheat the oven to 375°F. Lightly oil a baking dish (I use an 8-inch square glass dish; you can use another, similar size).

Place the olive oil, onion, celery, carrot, potato mixture, fennel, garlic, thyme, rosemary, poultry seasoning, dry mustard, salt, nutmeg, and pepper in a large pot over medium to medium-low heat. Cover and let cook for 12 to 15 minutes, stirring occasionally, until the vegetables are somewhat tender when pierced.

Sprinkle the flour into the pot, and immediately stir in. Cook for a couple of minutes, stirring, and then drizzle in the milk, still stirring. Scrape the bottom of the pot while stirring, to bring up all the caramelized flavors. Increase the heat to bring to a boil, let bubble for a minute or two to thicken, then remove the mixture from the heat. Add green beans and chickpeas and stir well.

Transfer the mixture to the prepared baking dish and let cool.

Cut the pastry shells in to strips or blocks to place on top of the mixture (a cookie cutter can be used to cut out attractive shapes). You can layer the pastry thinly, using just one pie shell, or layer more thickly, using up to two shells. Arrange the dough over the cooled mixture.

Bake for 30 to 35 minutes, or until the crust is golden brown and the sauce is bubbling around the edges. Remove from the oven and let cool for 5 to 10 minutes before serving.

Ingredients 411: Use no more than 1 cup of parsnips for the combination, as they have a very pronounced flavor. About 2½ cups of yellow-fleshed sweet potatoes is tasty.

Savvy Subs and Adds: Chopped cauliflower would work well here; add in place of some of the fennel or sweet potatoes. You can also add broccoli, but because it discolors with cooking, stir it into the mixture after cooking on the stovetop, just before transferring to the baking pan.

Serving Suggestion: A dollop of cranberry sauce works with this potpie; it adds a sweet-and-sour contrast and bright bite.

"No-fu Love Loaf"

SERVES 5 TO 6

(optionally) wheat
(optionally) gluten 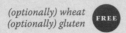 **FREE**

Many vegan versions of meat loaf are made with tofu, veggie ground round, TVP, or even seitan. Those tofu-averse will be happy to know no tofu or veggie meat analogues are in this loaf. This savory version uses only lentils, cracked wheat, quick oats, and white chia seed, along with a mix of seasonings to make it all magically come together!

½ cup brown (green) lentils, rinsed

1 cup vegan vegetable stock (see "Plant-Powered Pantry," page xlii)

⅓ cup water

1 bay leaf

¾ cup bulgur (use GF-certified steel-cut oats for gluten-free version)

1 cup water, boiled

¼ cup natural ketchup

1 cup rolled or quick oats (ensure GF-certified for gluten-free version)

3 tablespoons tamari (use wheat-free for wheat- or gluten-free version)

2 tablespoons nutritional yeast

2 tablespoons ground white chia or flax meal

2 tablespoons vegan Worcestershire sauce (see note for gluten-free version)

2 tablespoons tahini or sunflower seed butter

2 teaspoons blackstrap molasses

¼ teaspoon dried thyme

¼ to ½ teaspoon dried oregano

1 teaspoon dried basil

⅛ teaspoon ground fennel (optional)

Freshly ground black pepper

TOPPING:

3 to 4 tablespoons ketchup

1 teaspoon vegan Worcestershire sauce (optional), or 2 teaspoons vegan barbecue sauce (optional)

Combine the lentils, vegetable stock, ⅓ cup of water, and bay leaf in a saucepan. Bring to a boil, then lower heat to medium-low, cover, and cook for 25 to 30 minutes, until just about tender. Once done, add the bulgur and boiling water, cover, and cook on medium-low heat for another 8 to 9 minutes.

Meanwhile, preheat the oven to 375°F. Lightly oil an oven-proof glass loaf pan and line the bottom of the pan with a strip of parchment paper to cover (place it in to protrude along the short ends of the pan; this helps for easier removal of the veggie loaf from the pan). Combine the topping ingredients in a small bowl.

Once the bulgur is cooked, remove the bay leaf and add all the remaining ingredients (except topping). Stir very well. Transfer the mixture to prepared pan and pack it in. Spread the topping mixture over the top.

Cover the dish with aluminum foil and bake for 25 to 28 minutes. Remove the foil and bake for another 7 to 8 minutes. Remove from the oven and let stand for 10 to 15 minutes or so, before cutting to slice and serve.

Allergy-Free or Bust! Despite its not having any tofu, tempeh, or TVP, I cannot technically categorize this recipe as "soy free" because of the inclusion of tamari and vegan Worcestershire sauce. These are important seasonings in the loaf.

That said, to replace the Worcestershire for a gluten-free version, use instead an extra ½ tablespoon of wheat-free tamari, along with an extra ½ teaspoon of molasses, and 2 teaspoons of apple cider vinegar.

Savvy Subs and Adds: If you'd like to add some veggies to the loaf, try adding ½ cup of seeded and finely chopped green pepper, or ¼ cup of finely chopped celery (stir into the mixture with the seasonings).

Serving Suggestions: Rosemary Gravy is excellent with this loaf, but this dish is equally delicious served with condiments as a burger of sorts: Pop slices of the loaf into pita or a folded tortilla, along with ketchup and vegan mayonnaise (or "Almonnaise").

Jerk Chickpeas

SERVES 4, WITH RICE AND/OR
OTHER ACCOMPANIMENTS

wheat
gluten **FREE**

Why not combine the exciting flavors of a jerk marinade with healthy chickpeas? This dish is a snap to bring together, and bakes in about a half hour, so you can have it topped over rice and on the dinner table with little fuss.

3 to 4	tablespoons freshly squeezed lime juice (see directions)
2	tablespoons tamari
1	tablespoon extra-virgin olive oil
1	tablespoon tomato paste
1½	tablespoons pure maple syrup
1¼ to 1½	teaspoons dried thyme
1	teaspoon ground allspice
1	teaspoon ground cinnamon
¼	teaspoon ground cloves
¼	teaspoon ground black pepper
1	tablespoon grated fresh ginger
2	large garlic cloves, grated
	A few pinches of red chili flakes (⅛ to ¼ teaspoon; I find ⅛ teaspoon is just right, but up the spice ante if you want!)
2½	cups cooked chickpeas
¾ to 1	cup seeded, chopped or sliced red bell pepper (see note)
¾	cup sliced green onion (white and green portions; see note)
2	tablespoons finely chopped fresh cilantro or flat-leaf parsley, for garnish (optional; see note)

Preheat the oven to 375°F.

In a baking dish (I use an 8 by 12-inch), combine all the ingredients (starting with 3 tablespoons of the lime juice) except the chickpeas, red bell peppers (see note), green onions, and cilantro. Stir until well mixed. Then add the chickpeas, red peppers, and green onions and stir again.

Cover the dish with foil and bake for 25 minutes. Remove the foil, stir, and bake uncovered for another 5 to 8 minutes, stirring again about halfway through, until the marinade has partially absorbed into the chickpeas.

Taste; if you'd like more tang, add another ½ to 1 tablespoon of lime juice, and stir well, along with any reserved green onions and fresh cilantro. Serve over rice, or in pita breads or tortillas with sliced avocados and with extra squeezes of lime juice, if desired.

If This Apron Could Talk: If you'd like to keep the texture and color of the red pepper a little firmer and vibrant, add after about the first 10 to 15 minutes of baking, and stir in. Ditto for the green onions.

Ingredients 411: If you reserve 1 to 2 tablespoons of the greenish portion of the green onions, chop them finely and use to sprinkle over the finished dish. Or you can use 2 tablespoons of fresh cilantro or parsley to add a perk of color and freshness.

Chickpea and Artichoke "Bliss in a Dish"

SERVES 4 TO 6

wheat gluten soy **FREE**

I love artichokes and I love chickpeas. I also really love Mediterranean seasonings and briny olives with a touch of sweetness thrown in. So, when I make this dish, it's like a little bit of bliss in a dish!

2	tablespoons + 1 teaspoon olive oil
2½ to 3	cups cubed red or Yukon gold potatoes (¾ to 1 pound; see note)
3 to 3½	cups cooked chickpeas, or 2 (14-ounce) cans, drained and rinsed
3	cups frozen artichokes (thawing optional)
4	medium to large cloves garlic, minced or grated
3	tablespoons water
½	cup seeded and chopped red bell pepper
⅓ to ½	cup pitted kalamata olives, sliced in half
1	cup chopped tomatoes
3 to 4	tablespoons sultana or other raisins
1	teaspoon dried oregano
1	teaspoon dried basil
½	teaspoon dried rosemary
½	teaspoon sea salt
	Freshly ground black pepper
1½	tablespoons balsamic vinegar
⅓ to ½	cup julienned fresh basil (optional), or ¼ cup chopped fresh flat-leaf parsley

Preheat the oven to 400°F. Use 1 teaspoon of the olive oil to oil a large casserole dish (about 8 by 12 inches).

Place the potatoes in a saucepan, cover with water, and bring to a boil. Lower the heat to medium-low and boil for 15 to 20 minutes, or until fork tender (see note).

When potatoes are ready, drain well and add to the prepared dish along with the other ingredients, except the vinegar and the fresh basil.

Toss the mixture well, cover the dish with foil, and bake for 40 minutes (stirring about halfway through the baking process), until the potatoes are fully tender and the other vegetables have heated through and somewhat softened. Add the vinegar, toss again, and bake for another 10 to 15 minutes uncovered.

Remove from the oven, sprinkle with the fresh basil, and season to taste with salt and pepper as desired. Serve on its own, with bread for dipping in olive oil and balsamic vinegar, or over quinoa, brown rice, or pasta, topped with Basil Lemon Pistou.

If This Apron Could Talk: If you already have the ingredients prepped and are waiting on the potatoes, go ahead and starting baking the casserole. You can add the potatoes to it once they're ready.

This makes a fairly large casserole, enough for a meal one night for 3 to 4 people, and leftovers for another night (it's also good for a potluck)!

Savvy Subs and Adds: Another delicious variation on this dish is to omit the potatoes and use 1 to 2 fennel bulbs instead. No parboiling step involved; simply toss the fennel with all the other ingredients as directed and bake for the same amount of time.

Boulangerie Potatoes with Sautéed Fennel and White Beans

SERVES 4 TO 5, OR MORE
AS A SIDE DISH

wheat
gluten **FREE**
soy

I've adapted this recipe from a version of Boulangerie Beans and Potatoes from Mark Bittman's *How to Cook Everything Vegetarian*. Bittman's recipe was an adaptation of a classic French dish, Boulangerie Potatoes, in which thinly sliced potatoes are layered and baked in a broth. My version combines sautéed fennel, which adds a sweet and mellow flavor . . . as well as a few other customizations.

4   cups cooked navy or cannellini beans (or measure from 3 [14-ounce] cans, drained and rinsed)

2½ to 3 teaspoons minced fresh thyme

¼ + ⅛ teaspoon sea salt

2½ to 3½ tablespoons olive oil

3½ to 4 cups thinly sliced fennel, core and stalks removed, (about 2 medium-size bulbs)

A few pinches of freshly ground black pepper

4½ to 5 cups very thinly sliced potato (peeling optional; see note)

1   cup vegan vegetable stock (see "Plant-Powered Pantry," page xlii)

½   cup white wine or good-quality apple juice (I use So Nice organic juice)

A few of pinches of freshly grated nutmeg (optional)

A few tablespoons chopped chives, for garnish (optional)

Preheat the oven to 400°F. Lightly oil a large, shallow casserole dish (e.g., 8 by 12-inch).

Place the beans in the pan. Sprinkle the thyme and ⅛ teaspoon of the salt over the beans.

In a skillet over medium heat, combine 1½ tablespoons of the olive oil, the fennel, the remaining ¼ teaspoon of salt, and the pepper. Cook for 11 to 14 minutes, tossing occasionally, until the fennel is caramelized and softened. Layer the fennel over the white beans, and then layer the thinly sliced potatoes over the top.

In a cup or small bowl, stir together the vegetable stock and wine or juice. Pour the mixture slowly over the casserole, trying to cover most of the surface area while pouring. Brush or drizzle 1 tablespoon of the olive oil over the potatoes, and sprinkle the mixture with the nutmeg (if using).

Cover the dish with aluminum foil and bake for 40 minutes. Remove the foil and bake for another 20 to 35 minutes (this may vary, depending on the type of dish you are using), until the potatoes are tender when pierced with a sharp knife.

Set oven to BROIL, and then broil the casserole for 2 to 3 minutes, to give the potato topping an extra bit of color.

Remove from the oven, drizzle with the remaining 1 tablespoon of olive oil (this is optional; you can omit), let cool for 5 to 10 minutes, then cut and serve, sprinkling with chopped chives, if using.

Ingredients 411: Red, Yukon Gold or even russet potatoes can be used. With russets, I recommend peeling; whereas with red or Yukon Gold, the peels can be left intact. Prepare the spuds last so that they do not discolor before baking. If prepping potatoes in advance, place in a bowl of cold water after slicing. Drain the water and pat the potatoes dry before layering.

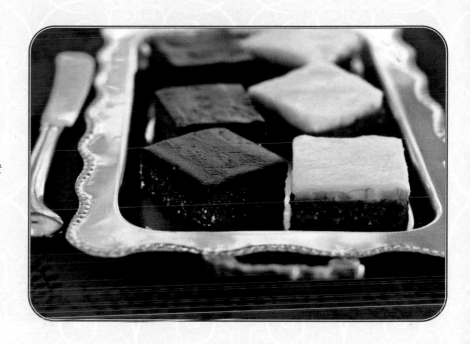

Frosted "B-raw-nies" (page 204); Raw Banana Nut Squares with Coconut Cream Cheese Frosting (page 202)

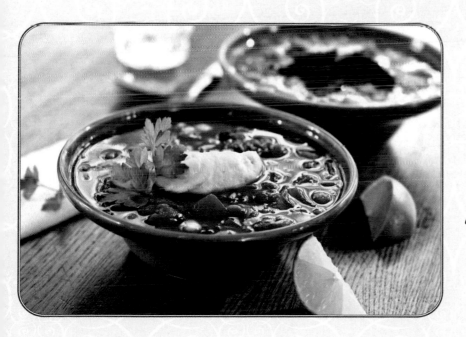

Mexican Bean Soup (page 77) topped with Chipotle Avocado Cream (page 58); Moroccan Bean Stew with Sweet Potatoes and Roasted Figs (page 78)

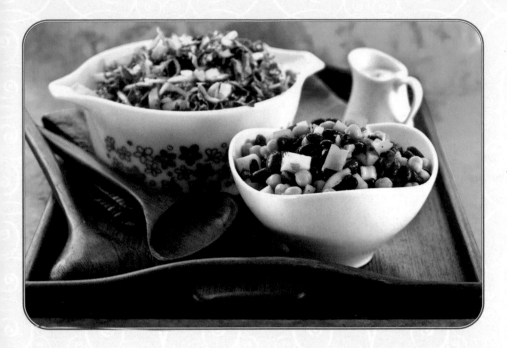

Kale-slaw with Curried Almond Dressing (page 37); Three-Bean Salad (page 36)

Black Bean, Quinoa, and Sweet Potato Spicy Croquettes (page 146) topped with Pumpkin Seed Chipotle Cream (page 59)

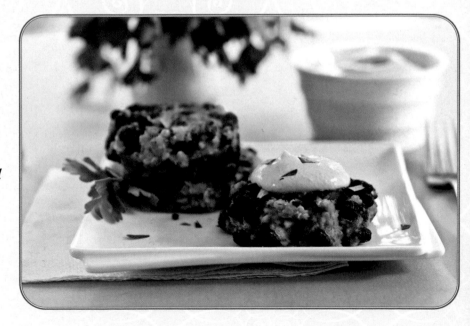

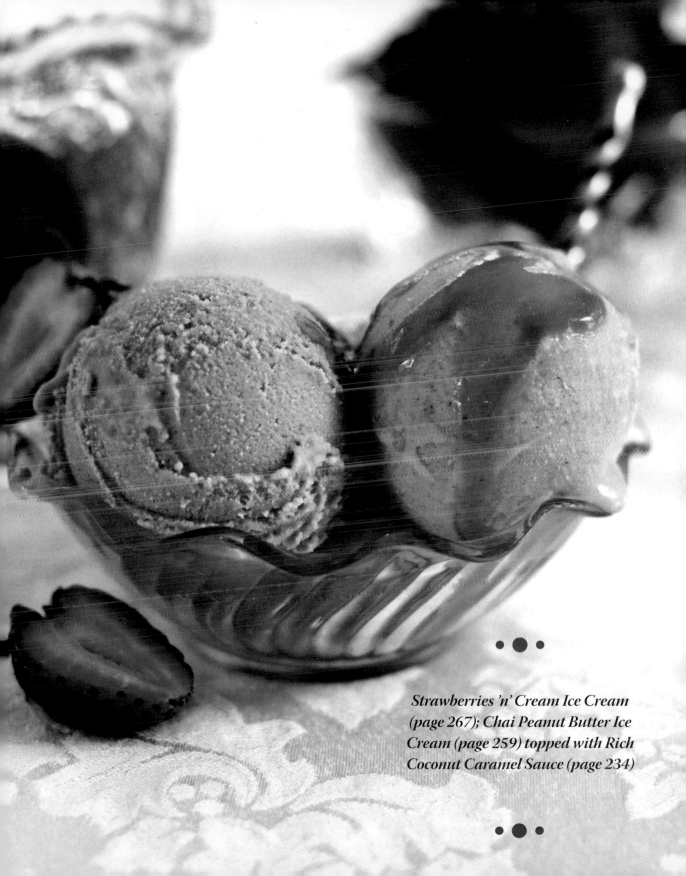

Strawberries 'n' Cream Ice Cream (page 267); Chai Peanut Butter Ice Cream (page 259) topped with Rich Coconut Caramel Sauce (page 234)

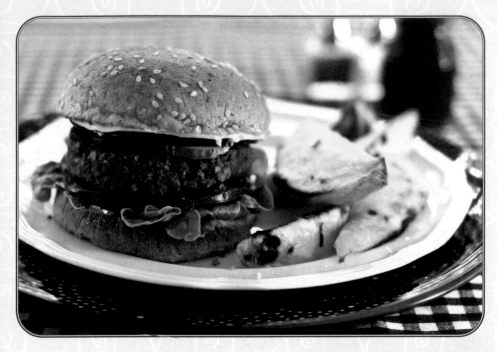

Nutty Veggie Burgers (page 135); Sunshine Fries with Rosemary and Coarse Sea Salt (page 101)

Pumpkin Cake (page 211) with Cooked Vanilla Frosting (page 226)

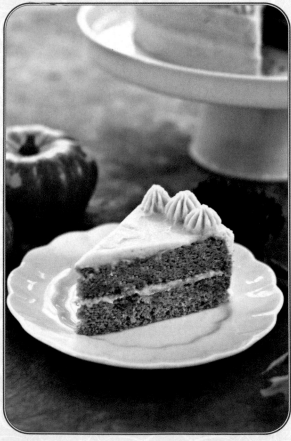

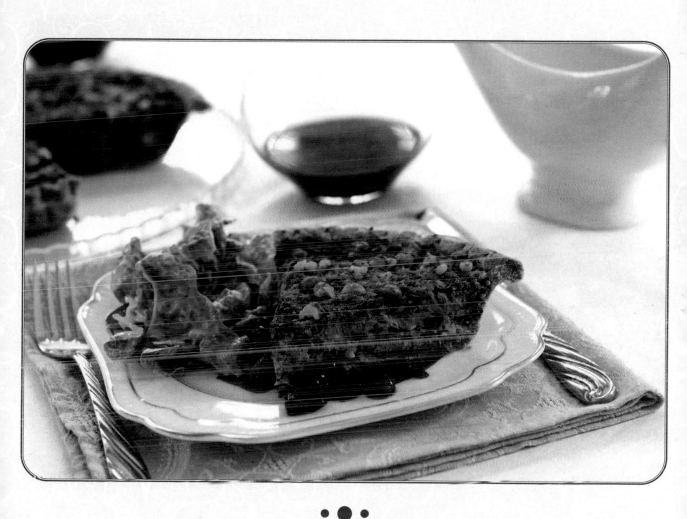

Festive Chickpea Tart (page 128)

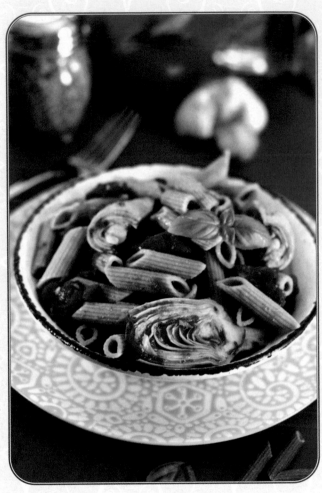

Apple-A-Day Green Smoothie (page 31); Citrus-Scented Almond Muffins (page 6)

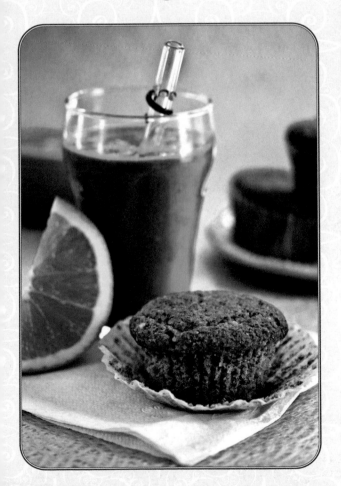

Tomato Artichoke Pasta (page 158); Brazil Nut Parmezan (page 62)

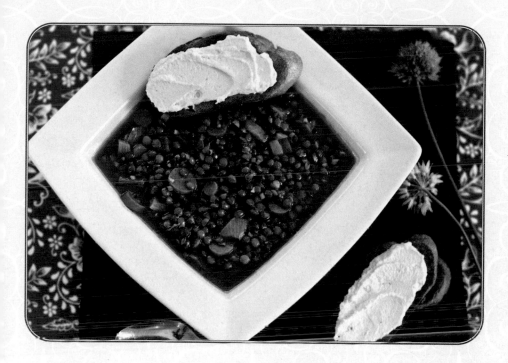

French Lentil Soup with Smoked Paprika (page 84); Truffled Cashew Cheese (page 64)

Jerk Chickpeas (page 114)

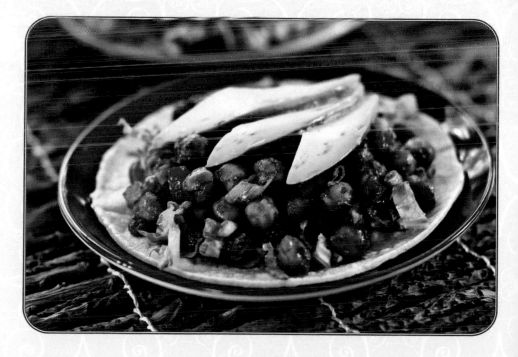

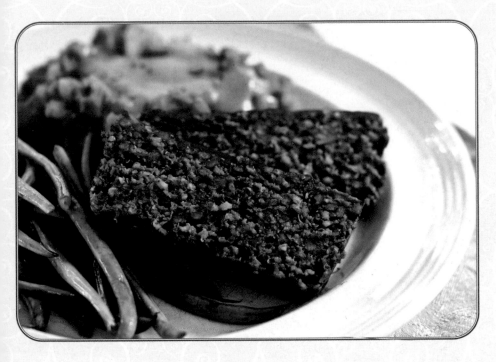

*"No-Fu Love Loaf"
(page 112); Smashing
Sweet Spuds
(page 104); Rosemary
Gravy (page 61)*

*White Bean Pesto
Spread (page 72);
Romesc-oat Sauce
(page 157)*

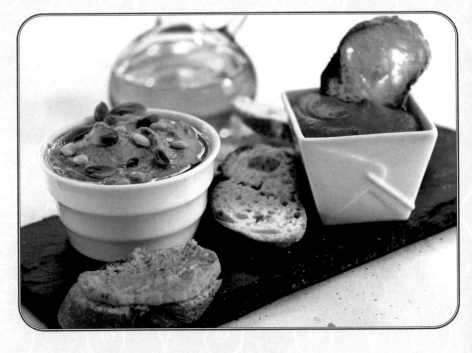

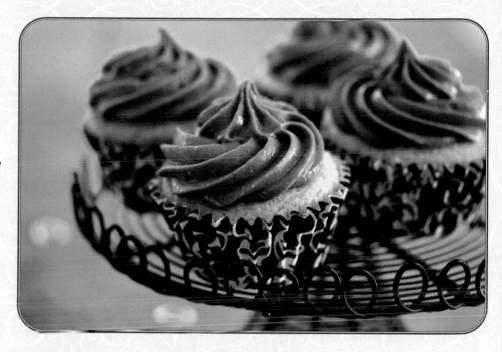

Banana-Scented Vanilla Cupcakes (page 215) with Cooked Chocolate Frosting (page 228)

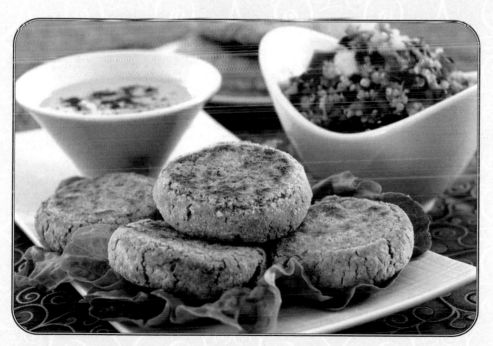

Pan-fried Falafel Patties (page 145); Smoky Spiked Tahini Sauce (page 54); Quinoa Taboulleh with Olives (page 40)

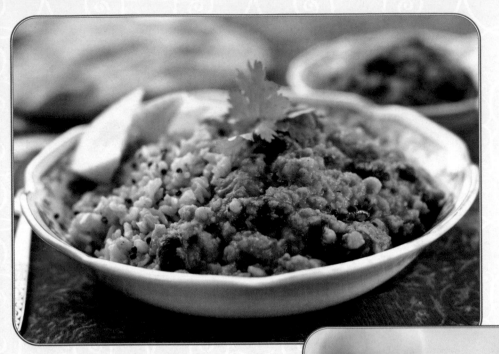

*Fragrant Kidney
Bean Lentil Dahl
(page 119);
Indian Inspired Rice
(page 105)*

*Raw Lemon-Lime
Cheesecake with
Coconut Nut Crust
and Fresh Mango Sauce
(page 246) topped with
Lemon-Scented Whipped
Cream (page 231)*

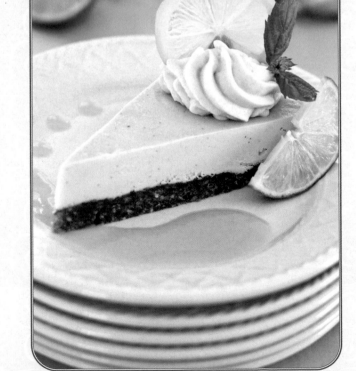

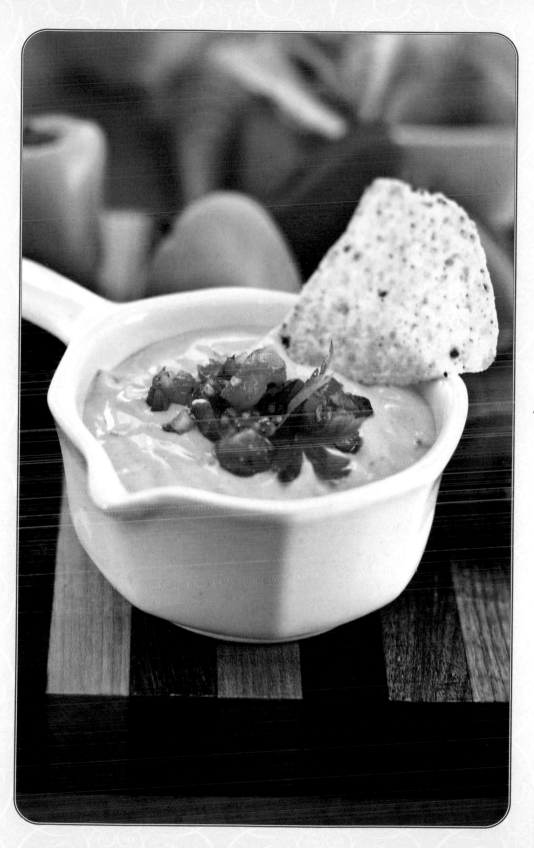

"Vegveeta" Dip
(page 67)

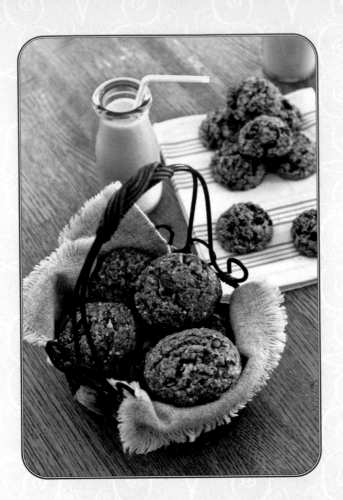

Monsta! Cookies
(page 22);
Wholesome Oat
Snackles! (page 17)

Thai Chickpea
Almond Curry
(page 109)

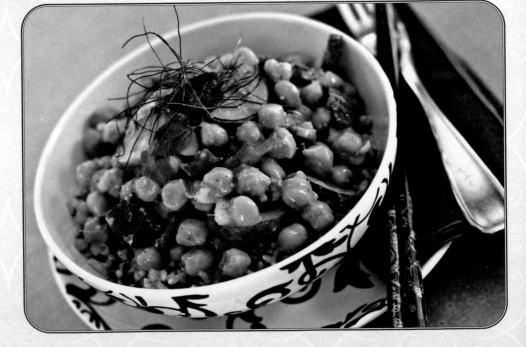

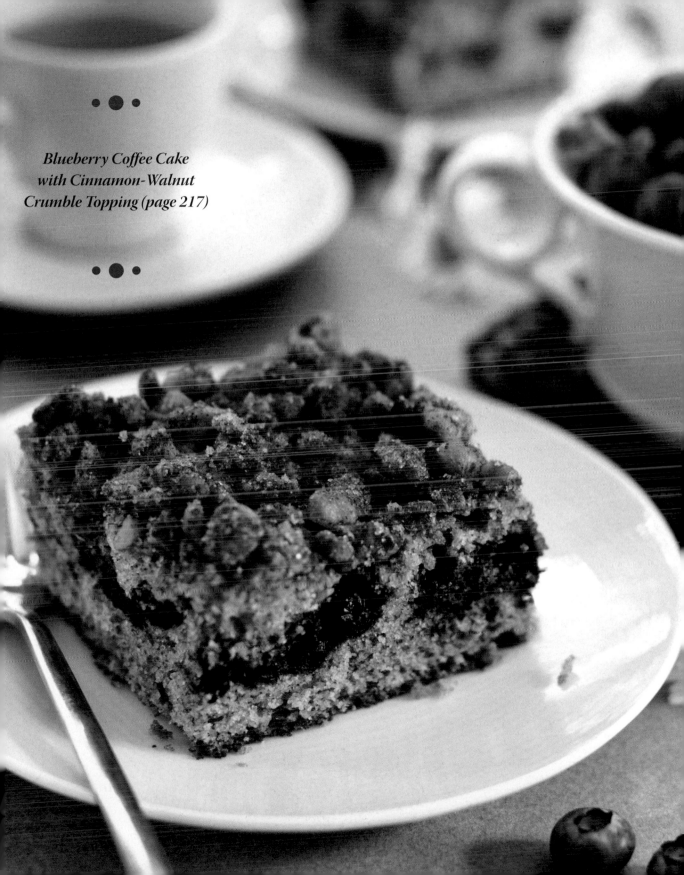

*Blueberry Coffee Cake
with Cinnamon-Walnut
Crumble Topping (page 217)*

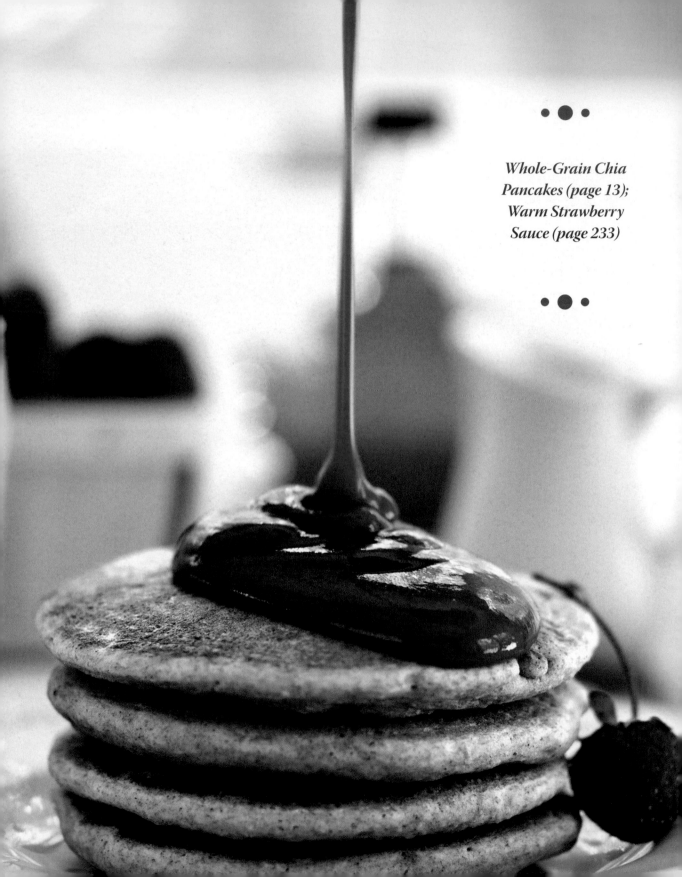

Whole-Grain Chia Pancakes (page 13);
Warm Strawberry Sauce (page 233)

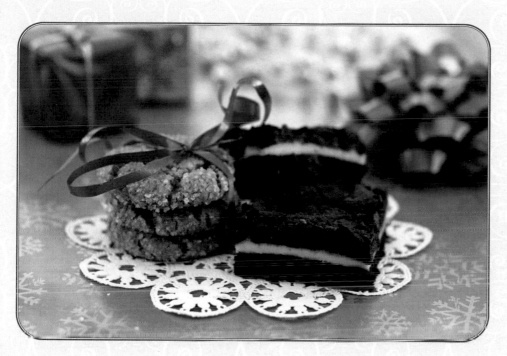

Gingery Cookies (page 191); Creamed Cheese Brownies with Salted Dark Chocolate Topping (page 200)

Creamy Barley Risotto with Thyme and Star Anise (page 127); Simplicity Asparagus (page 96)

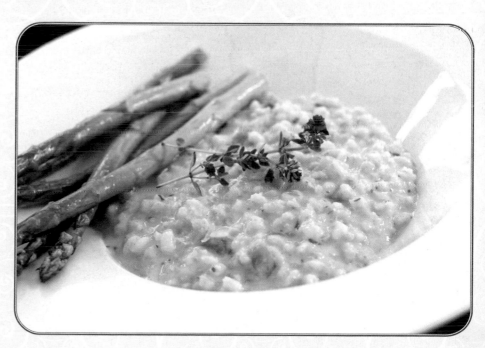

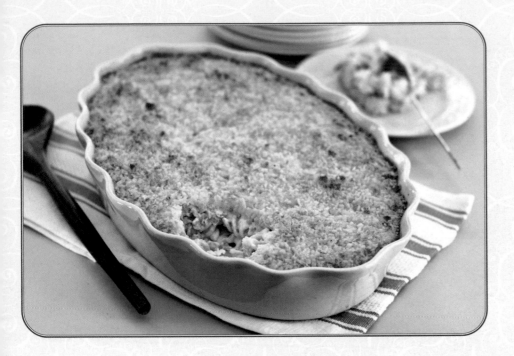

Mac-oh-geez!
(page 164)

Tempeh Tickle
(page 122); Spinach-
Herb Pistachio
Pesto (page 154);
Almond Roasted
Cauliflower (page 94)

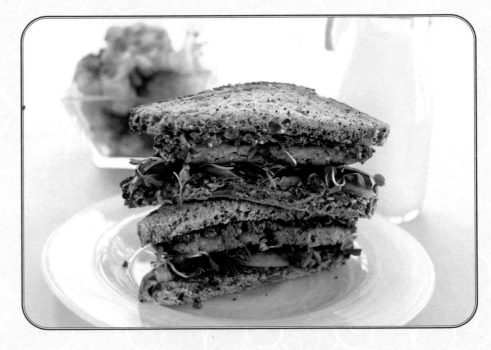

Corn Chowder Quinoa Casserole

SERVES 4 TO 5

wheat
gluten **FREE**
soy

Here corn chowder meets beans and quinoa in a casserole! This is a comforting homey kind of dish, and if you like some heat in your corn chowder, go ahead and add the optional hot sauce.

2 cups plain unsweetened nondairy milk (almond or soy preferred; see "Plant-Powered Pantry," page xxxiii)

1½ cups frozen or fresh corn kernels

1 cup uncooked, rinsed quinoa or millet (see note for millet)

1 cup vegan vegetable stock (see "Plant-Powered Pantry," page xlii)

½ cup finely chopped onion

¾ cup seeded and diced red bell pepper

2 tablespoons extra-virgin olive oil

1 teaspoon dried basil

½ teaspoon Dijon mustard

1 large bay leaf

1 (14-ounce) can cannellini beans (white kidney beans) or navy beans, drained and rinsed

½ teaspoon (rounded) sea salt
Freshly ground black pepper
A few pinches of cayenne, or a few dashes of hot sauce (optional; don't use for a kid-friendly version)

1 to 2 tablespoons freshly squeezed lime juice (optional)

3 to 4 tablespoons finely chopped fresh flat-leaf parsley (optional)

1 to 3 tablespoons extra nondairy milk (if needed)

Preheat the oven to 400°F.

Combine 1 cup of the milk with ¾ cup of the corn kernels in a large, deep cup (reserving other ¾ cup of corn to add later). Puree with an immersion blender or in a blender.

In a large casserole dish (about 8 by 12 inches), combine this mixture with the reserved corn plus all the other ingredients, except the lime juice, parsley, and extra milk, and stir well.

Cover with foil and bake for 30 minutes. After this time, remove from the oven to stir again. Put the foil back on and return to the oven to bake for another 20 to 25 minutes, until the quinoa is cooked through.

Remove from the oven and remove the bay leaf. Add the lime juice and parsley (if using), stir well, add the milk if you would like the mixture to be a little thinner, and serve.

If This Apron Could Talk: Whether using the quinoa or millet (but especially with the millet), as this casserole sits, the moisture will continue to be absorbed. It is helpful to add another tablespoon or two of milk while the casserole sits, and to keep the dish covered with foil after removing from the oven so moisture stays in the casserole.

Ingredients 411: Be sure to rinse the quinoa before cooking, to remove its bitter saponins.

Make It More-ish! If you'd like to add some textural crunch to garnish this casserole, try some toasted nuts, such as almonds or walnuts, crushed or chopped.

Savvy Subs and Adds: If using millet, add another ⅓ cup of nondairy milk and another ½ cup of water to the casserole before cooking, and cook for an additional 10 to 15 minutes.

Lemon-Infused Mediterranean Lentils

SERVES 4 TO 5

wheat gluten soy **FREE**

Lentils are a favorite of mine; they cook quickly, taste fresh and clean, and are easy to digest. What makes these lentils even better is infusing them with fresh lemon and herbs during cooking, and finishing off the dish with tomatoes, pine nuts, and dry olives. The sour lemon juice works nicely against the richness of the pine nuts and olives, for a satisfying flavor finish.

2 tablespoons extra-virgin olive oil

1 cup brown (green) lentils, rinsed

3 to 4 tablespoons freshly squeezed lemon juice (see directions)

1 large clove garlic, grated or minced (optional)

1 teaspoon dried basil

1 cup vegan vegetable stock (see "Plant-Powered Pantry," page xlii)

1 cup water

1½ teaspoons fresh thyme

¾ to 1 cup cherry or grape tomatoes, left whole if small, or cut in half if larger (see note)

1 tablespoon capers, rinsed

3 tablespoons sliced or chopped Moroccan dried olives, or kalamata or green olives

1 teaspoon lemon zest

1 teaspoon pure maple syrup or agave nectar

¼ cup pine nuts (preferably toasted), for garnish
Freshly ground black pepper (optional)

In a medium-size or large saucepan over medium-high heat, combine the olive oil and lentils. Stirring, sauté for a couple of minutes. Add 3 tablespoons of the lemon juice, and the garlic, basil, vegetable stock, and water. Bring to a boil, then lower the heat to medium-low, cover the pot and cook for 35 to 45 minutes, until tender.

Turn off the heat and stir in the thyme, tomatoes, capers, olives, lemon zest, and maple syrup. Cover and let sit for 4 to 5 minutes, then stir again and taste, adding an additional ½ to 1 tablespoon of lemon juice (or more), if desired, for extra tang! Serve, sprinkling portions with pine nuts and with freshly ground black pepper, if desired.

Ingredients 411: I add the tomatoes quite late in the cooking process, to preserve more of their freshness—basically just warming them through rather than cooking them. If you aren't fond of uncooked tomatoes, feel free to add them earlier, about 20 minutes into the lentil cooking time.

Serving Suggestions: Serve over quinoa, brown rice, or with pasta. Also works well as a filling for wraps, or as a pizza topping (under sliced fresh tomatoes and a sprinkling of vegan cheese). Alternatively, chill and toss with a whole grain, plus a little extra olive oil, lemon, salt, and pepper, for a chilled lentil salad.

Fragrant Kidney Bean Lentil Dal

SERVES 4 OR MORE

wheat
gluten **FREE**
soy

This dish is a dal of sorts, and is especially fragrant and flavorful, rich with spices, and yet not spicy in a hot sense. I enjoy how this dish is not hot-spicy, however, you can always add a few splashes of hot sauce if you like.

2 to 2½ tablespoons organic extra-virgin coconut oil or neutral-flavored oil (see "Plant-Powered Pantry," page xxxii)
1 cup onion, diced
1¼ teaspoons sea salt
Freshly ground black pepper
2 teaspoons cumin seeds
2 teaspoons mustard seeds
½ teaspoon fennel seeds (see note)
1 teaspoon coriander powder
1 teaspoon turmeric
½ teaspoon ground allspice
Pinch or two of crushed red pepper flakes (more/less to taste; see note)
1 cinnamon stick, or ½ teaspoon ground cinnamon
2½ to 3 cups water (see note)
½ cup freshly squeezed or good-quality orange juice (see note)
2 large cloves garlic, minced
1½ tablespoons grated fresh ginger
1 cup red lentils, rinsed
1 (14-ounce) can red kidney beans or black beans, drained and rinsed
2 bay leaves
Hot sauce (optional; see note)
Chopped fresh cilantro, for garnish (optional)

Heat the oil in a large pot over high or medium-high heat. Add the onion, salt, pepper, spices, and cinnamon stick. Stir, cover, and cook for 4 to 5 minutes, stirring occasionally. Add 2½ cups of the water, and the orange juice, garlic, ginger, lentils, kidney beans, and bay leaves. Stir, bring the mixture to a boil, then lower the heat to medium or medium-low, cover, and cook for 10 to 12 minutes.

Remove the cinnamon stick (leaving the stick in will impart a stronger cinnamon flavor, but this can be overpowering), and cook for another 10 to 15 minutes, until the lentils are fully dissolved and the mixture has thickened. For a thinner consistency, add the extra water, anywhere from ¼ to ½ cup, or more, if desired.

Remove the bay leaves before serving. Season with additional salt, if desired. Add hot sauce to taste and sprinkle with fresh cilantro (if using).

If This Apron Could Talk: The consistency of this dish can be kept thicker, for scooping with roti bread or even whole-grain tortillas, or made thinner to serve over rice, or to eat more like a stew. Start with the 2½ cups of water and then thin out later to your desired consistency.

Ingredients 411: I am a fennel lover. The flavor of fennel, anise, licorice—all resonate very favorably for me. If you also love fennel, go ahead and use a full 1 teaspoon (I usually do). But if you are a little more tentative about the fennel flavor, use just ½ teaspoon. Just don't leave it out altogether; it really combines beautifully with the spice profile in the dish.

Kid-Friendly: If serving this to children, you might want to omit the crushed red pepper flakes and reserve the hot sauce for the adult individual portions. If you like things spicy, feel free to add hot sauce to the dal to taste, or add more crushed red pepper flakes earlier in the cooking process with the other spices.

Savvy Subs and Adds: The orange juice brings a lovely flavor to this dish, but if you don't have any oranges or juice on hand, feel free to replace with water.

Serving Suggestions: Serve with Indian-Inspired Rice, roti bread, and chutney (if you like).

Pumpkin Chickpea Cauliflower Curry with Fresh Cream Sauce

SERVES 4 TO 6

wheat gluten soy FREE

Pumpkin is so often used in desserts yet sometimes overlooked for savory recipes. This stew highlights pumpkin, along with vegetables and beans, in a curry that is flavorful without being too hot-spicy. Topped with the Fresh Cream Sauce, this is one of my favorite autumnal dishes.

1 tablespoon organic extra-virgin coconut oil or neutral-flavored oil or splash of water (see "Plant-Powered Pantry," page xxxii)

1½ to 2 cups chopped onion

1 tablespoon curry powder

1¼ teaspoons sea salt

1 teaspoon brown or yellow mustard seeds

1 teaspoon garam masala

2 teaspoons ground coriander

½ teaspoon cumin seeds

½ teaspoon turmeric
A pinch or two of crushed red pepper flakes (or more to desired heat)

2 to 3 cloves garlic, grated or minced

2 cups cauliflower that has been cut in florets (see note on timing)

2 cups chopped zucchini (see note on timing)

3½ to 4 cups cooked chickpeas, or a combination of chickpeas and kidney beans (2 [14-ounce] cans total, drained and rinsed)

1 (15-ounce) can pumpkin puree (not pumpkin pie filling; see note)

1 cup water

1½ to 2 tablespoons grated fresh ginger

1½ to 2 tablespoons freshly squeezed lemon juice
Fresh Cream Sauce (page 57), for serving (see note)
Lemon wedges, for serving

In a large pot over medium-high heat, combine the oil or water, onion, curry powder, salt, mustard seeds, garam masala, coriander, cumin seeds, turmeric, and crushed red pepper. Cook for 5 to 7 minutes, covered, and then lower the heat to medium and add the garlic. Stir, and cook for another 2 to 3 minutes, adding a splash of water if needed to prevent the garlic from sticking or burning.

Add the cauliflower and zucchini, and toss, followed by the beans, pumpkin, and water. Bring the heat up to a boil, then lower the heat to medium-low and simmer for 15 to 20 minutes, until the cauliflower and zucchini have become tender (if you want more texture in the veggies, hold off adding them until the last 10 minutes or so of simmering). Add the ginger, lemon juice, and stir.

Add additional salt and pepper to taste, if desired. Serve drizzled with Fresh Cream Sauce, with lemon wedges on the side for extra squeezing!

Ingredients 411: Canned pumpkin varies in moisture and consistency. I use just 1 cup of water in this curry, using the Farmer's Market brand of organic canned pumpkin. It makes for a fairly thick curry, with the veggies also releasing some moisture during simmering. You may want to add more water, depending on whether you substitute other vegetables, and also depending on the consistency of the canned pumpkin.

Savvy Subs and Adds: Other veggies you can use in place of the zukes and cauliflower include chopped red pepper and green beans cut into bite-size pieces.

The cream sauce really is superb drizzled over this curry. It adds a color contrast, and a creamy texture against a spicy dish. If you don't make the sauce, consider adding about ½ cup of raw cashews to the curry when adding the zucchini and cauliflower. They will soften with cooking and bring more interest to every bite.

Wonder Bean Puree

**SERVES 4 TO 5
WITH ACCOMPANIMENTS**

*(optionally) wheat
(optionally) gluten* **FREE**

You might call yourself Wonder Woman (or Wonder Man!) after preparing this easy dish. It came together one night when I wanted beans on the menu—and fast. I got to work and served up a warm seasoned kidney bean puree on top of brown rice that my family loved. It was surprising that something relatively simple in preparation could impress my lot as it did! So, when you are multitasking and feel somewhat like a superhero managing everything, reinforce your well-earned status with this recipe!

1	tablespoon olive oil or splash of water
1 to 1¼	cups chopped onion (see note)
¾	teaspoon sea salt
1¼	teaspoons dried oregano
	Freshly ground black pepper
2	(14-ounce) cans kidney beans, drained and rinsed
½	cup water
2	teaspoons vegan Worcestershire sauce (for wheat- or gluten-free options, see note)
2½ to 3	teaspoons balsamic vinegar
1	tablespoon blackstrap molasses
2 to 3	tablespoons finely chopped fresh flat-leaf parsley
	Lime wedges, for serving

In a saucepan over medium heat, combine the oil or water, onion, salt, oregano, and pepper to taste. Cover and cook for about 10 minutes, until the onion is softened.

Turn off the heat and add the beans, water, Worcestershire sauce, vinegar, and molasses. Then, using an immersion blender, blend the mixture until it is fairly well pureed (does not have to be completely smooth). Turn heat back on to medium, return the cover to the pot, and heat through for about 10 minutes.

Stir in parsley, and season to taste with additional salt and pepper, if desired. Serve over brown rice, or layer in whole-grain tortillas. Serve with lime wedges, to squeeze over the top.

Adult-Minded: For a little more sophisticated flavor, add ¼ cup red wine after sautéing the onions and before adding the beans and other ingredients. After adding the wine, turn the heat up to high to let the alcohol burn off, cooking for a couple of minutes, and then turn off the heat and follow the directions to add the beans, water, and so on. Also, add a splash of hot sauce, if that's your thing!

Allergy-Free or Bust! For a wheat-free option, omit the Worcestershire sauce and add 1 teaspoon tamari and increase the balsamic vinegar to 3 to 3½ teaspoons, or opt for a gluten-free Worcestershire.

If This Apron Could Talk: Although the final color of this dish isn't the most appetizing, it truly tastes great. Adding the chopped fresh parsley helps to brighten and liven up the color of the dish, as well as to provide extra flavor. Fresh cilantro can be used in place of the parsley, if you wish.

Tempeh Tickle

SERVES 2 TO 3

wheat gluten **FREE**

Tempeh is not always approachable for folks. It looks strange, sounds strange, and can even taste strange. But when prepared with a little TLC (and yet still simply), it can taste phenomenal! This recipe will tickle your taste buds, and get you past the tempeh fear factor—fast!

1 (8-ounce) package tempeh
2 tablespoons white or red wine
1 tablespoon tamari
1½ tablespoons extra-virgin olive oil
½ tablespoons balsamic vinegar
1 teaspoon Dijon mustard
1 teaspoon dried oregano
1½ teaspoons pure maple syrup
½ teaspoon garlic powder

First prepare the tempeh, by simmering in 2 to 3 cups of water for about 20 minutes. Drain the tempeh in a colander and leave it in the colander to cool slightly while preparing the marinade (see note).

In a baking dish, combine remaining the ingredients, stirring or whisking to blend fully.

When the tempeh has cooled enough to handle, remove from the colander and gently pat or press with towels to remove any excess moisture. Slice the tempeh, first cutting the block into quarters, and then slice each quarter in half lengthwise (to make thinner) to make eight slices. Place the slices in the marinade. Cover the dish, and if marinating for more than ½ hour, be sure to refrigerate after this time.

I like to barbecue the tempeh, grilling it over medium-high heat on the first side for 4 to 5 minutes, and then the second side for 2 to 3 minutes, until grill marks appear and it is heated and firmed slightly, but not drying out. But you can also bake or panfry the tempeh.

To bake, preheat the oven to 400°F, cover the dish with foil, and bake for 12 to 15 minutes. Remove the foil, flip the slices, then cook for another 6 to 8 minutes, until the marinade is absorbed and the tempeh is lightly browned.

To panfry, place on a nonstick skillet over medium-high heat. Let the tempeh cook without flipping for 5 to 6 minutes. Then check the underside and if golden brown, flip to the other side (if not, cook on the first side for another couple of minutes to gain color). Cook on the other side for another 4 to 5 minutes, or longer if necessary, until golden brown.

If This Apron Could Talk: The trick with this marinade is to get the slices of tempeh soaking while still warm. After boiling it, let it drain in a colander until just warm (don't rinse!), then pat dry and get it into the marinade while warm so it can soak up the flavors.

Serving Suggestions: In addition to serving hot as an entrée, this is delicious in sandwiches, still warm or cooled, with a thick spread such as Spinach-Herb Pistachio Pesto, Raw Aioli, or "Almonnaise."

Braised Tempeh in a Lemon, Thyme, and Caper Sauce

SERVES 3 TO 4

wheat gluten **FREE**

. . . and if you don't like capers, you can omit them altogether, the tempeh and sauce will still be tremendously delicious. This cooking technique helps seal the flavorful juices in the tempeh—lemony, savory, scrumptious!

3 tablespoons extra-virgin olive oil

¼ teaspoon (rounded) sea salt

⅛ teaspoon (roughly) freshly ground black pepper

¾ to 1 cup thinly sliced red onion or shallot

1 (8-ounce) package tempeh, cut in 8 or more pieces (see note)

¾ cup white wine

1½ tablespoons freshly squeezed lemon juice

2 tablespoons capers, drained

1½ tablespoons tamari

1½ tablespoons pure maple syrup or agave nectar (see note)

1½ tablespoons roughly chopped fresh thyme

1 small lemon, seeds squeezed out, sliced into rounds or half-moons (about ¼ cup)

Preheat the oven to 425°F.

Heat 2 tablespoons of the olive oil, and the salt, pepper, and onion in an ovenproof skillet or Dutch oven over medium-high heat on the stovetop. When the oil mixture is hot, add the tempeh and cook on one side for 4 to 5 minutes, to brown lightly. Carefully turn the pieces of tempeh and cook for a few minutes on the other side. Add the wine, turn the heat to high, and let boil for a couple of minutes. Turn off the heat, and add the remaining ingredients, including the remaining tablespoon of olive oil.

Place in the oven and bake, partially covered, for 20 to 25 minutes.

Remove from the oven and serve, spooning some of the sauce, capers, and lemon over each portion (the lemon slices are mostly to season the dish while cooking, and for an attractive appearance; however, you may not want to eat them, as they are bitter).

If This Apron Could Talk: When I first created this recipe, I liked using larger pieces of tempeh that were easy to work with and get browned, and then also to serve two or more with brown rice or other accompaniments. But, I soon realized when my husband wasn't devouring the "cutlets" as I was, that he—like many others—prefers tofu and tempeh cut into thinner slices to absorb more of the flavor and also just not be as "meaty." So, if you are one of these people (or your loved one is!), then feel free to cut the tempeh in smaller cubes, or even slice it thinly.

Ingredients 411: I use a white wine that isn't very dry, so if you are using a very dry white wine, add another 1 to 2 teaspoons of maple syrup or agave nectar to the marinade.

BBQ Sunflower Tofu

SERVES 4

wheat
gluten **FREE**

This mix of seasonings and spices gives tofu a thick, flavorful coating that has a barbecue-like flavor, but with the ease of using your oven and a baking dish. Simply stir everything in your dish, add your tofu, and get baking!

½ tablespoon sunflower seed butter, or tahini or pumpkin seed butter

2 tablespoons ketchup

1 tablespoon tamari

2 tablespoons balsamic vinegar

1 tablespoon extra-virgin olive oil

2 medium cloves garlic, grated or very finely minced

½ teaspoon pure maple syrup (optional)

⅛ teaspoon poultry seasoning (optional)

½ teaspoon dried oregano

¼ teaspoon smoked paprika

1 (12-ounce) package extra-firm organic tofu (see note)

Preheat the oven to 375°F.

While it heats, get your sauce together, and do so straight in your baking dish (I use an 8 by 12-inch). Use a spoon or small whisk to work the sunflower seed butter, ketchup, tamari, and balsamic together, until well combined. Then, incorporate the olive oil, garlic, maple syrup, and spices.

Pat the tofu with towels to remove the excess moisture, cut in half lengthwise, then slice into ¼- to ½-inch-thick squares. Pat again to remove excess moisture. Place the tofu slices in the marinade, and turn them over to get both sides coated. Bake for 20 minutes covered (flipping halfway through the baking process), then for another 8 to 10 minutes uncovered.

Ingredients 411: If you use the tofu straight from the package, the consistency will be firm, but still soft after baking. For a firmer consistency, you can first freeze and thaw the tofu, or press it. Both methods will extract excess water to make the tofu firmer and "meatier," though they do require some advance planning. For more details, see notes, page xli.

Serving Suggestions: Serve with a whole grain, or with baked potatoes or sweet potatoes, or use in a burger bun or in sandwiches.

Tofu Baked in an Olive, Grape, and Herbed Marinade

SERVES 4

wheat gluten **FREE**

This could be the most scrumptious way to eat tofu! The marinade is divine, combining salty, pungent flavors with a sweet and tangy balance. You'll want to make this again . . . and when served over Creamy Polenta . . . yet again!

¼ cup white wine
1 tablespoon pure maple syrup or agave nectar
2 teaspoons dried oregano
1½ teaspoons dried basil
2½ tablespoons balsamic vinegar
⅓ cup pitted and roughly chopped kalamata or Moroccan dried olives (see note)
¼ to ⅓ cup chopped sun-dried tomatoes
⅓ cup quartered seedless red or purple grapes, or ¼ cup raisins
¼ teaspoon (rounded) sea salt
⅛ teaspoon ground allspice
Freshly ground black pepper
2 to 2½ tablespoons extra-virgin olive oil
1 (12-ounce) package firm or extra-firm tofu
1 tablespoon minced flat-leaf parsley, for garnish (optional)
1 to 2 tablespoons pine nuts (preferably toasted), for garnish (optional)

Preheat the oven to 400°F.

In an 8 by 12-inch baking dish, combine the wine, maple syrup, oregano, basil, vinegar, olives, sun-dried tomatoes, grapes, salt, allspice, pepper to taste, and olive oil, and stir well.

Cut the tofu into half lengthwise and then into squares ¼ to ½ inch thick (24 to 28 slices). Pat gently with towels to remove excess moisture (no need to freeze and thaw). Add the tofu to the baking dish and turn to coat each side.

Bake covered for 15 minutes. Turn the tofu over, and continue to bake uncovered for another 12 to 15 minutes, until the tofu has soaked up most of the marinade.

Remove from the oven and let cool a little before serving; pour any remaining oil, spices, and seasonings over the tofu. Serve with a light sprinkle of fresh parsley and pine nuts, if desired.

Ingredients 411: Moroccan dried olives are special in this dish. You can purchase them in the deli section of your supermarket. Be sure to use them (or kalamata olives) in the dish, rather than opting for regular canned black olives, which do not have the same complexity of flavor.

Warmly Spiced Quinoa Chickpea Stew with Figs

SERVES 4 TO 5 OR MORE,
DEPENDING ON ACCOMPANIMENTS

*wheat
gluten* **FREE**
soy

This dish is a cross between a casserole and a stew. It is cooked on the stovetop, much like a stew, but is much more like a casserole in consistency. The quinoa and chickpeas are simmered with warm, earthy spices, and balanced with the sweetness of dried figs and sautéed fennel.

1	tablespoon olive oil or splash of water
1	cup chopped onion
¾ to 1	cup seeded and chopped red bell pepper (see note)
1 to 1½	cups chopped fennel, core and stalks removed (see note)
3	large cloves garlic, minced or grated
1	teaspoon sea salt
	Freshly ground black pepper
1½	teaspoons curry powder
1	teaspoon fennel seeds
1½	teaspoons paprika
1½	teaspoons dried basil
¾	teaspoon ground cinnamon
¼	teaspoon freshly grated nutmeg
⅛	teaspoon ground allspice
½	cup white wine
¾	cup quinoa, rinsed (see note)
2	cups cooked chickpeas, or 1 (14-ounce) can, drained and rinsed
2 to 2¼	cups water (+ another 2 to 4 tablespoons if needed; see directions)
	1 bay leaf
⅓	cup chopped dried Black Mission figs or dried apricots, or whole raisins
1½ to 2	tablespoons extra-virgin olive oil, for finishing (optional)
½	cup pine nuts (preferably toasted) or pistachios (optional)

In a large pot over medium heat, combine the oil or water, onion, red pepper, fennel, garlic, salt, black pepper to taste, curry powder, fennel seeds, paprika, basil, cinnamon, nutmeg, and allspice. Stir, cover, and cook for 6 to 8 minutes, stirring occasionally.

Add the wine, bring to a boil, and let boil for a couple of minutes. Then add the quinoa, chickpeas, 2 cups of the water, and the bay leaf and stir. Bring back to a boil, then lower the heat to medium or medium-low, cover, and cook for 18 to 22 minutes.

Once the quinoa is cooked and most of the liquid is absorbed (see note), stir in the figs, remove from the heat, and let sit for 3 to 4 minutes.

Remove the bay leaf. Season to taste with additional salt and pepper, if desired. Serve, drizzling individual portions with extra-virgin olive oil and a sprinkling of nuts, if desired.

If This Apron Could Talk: If the liquid is absorbed but quinoa isn't tender, add the extra ¼ cup of water and cook another few minutes.

After this dish is cooked, keep it covered before and after serving portions. It will get a little dry if left uncovered. Also, as it stands, the heat from the pot will continue to cook the quinoa and so it will absorb more water and get drier. If needed, have on hand some water boiled in your kettle, so you can stir a couple of tablespoons before getting a second helping!

Savvy Subs and Adds: If you don't have red pepper, you can substitute chopped carrot or winter squash (e.g., butternut), though the red pepper adds a nice color contrast with the other ingredients.

Creamy Barley Risotto with Thyme and Star Anise

SERVES 4

wheat soy **FREE**

This risotto is lightly fragranced with star anise and cardamom, which get cozy with the Fresh Cream Sauce. Much like how a cream or fat such as whipping cream or butter is folded into traditional risotto just before serving, the Fresh Cream Sauce adds a lot of body and flavor to this whole-grain risotto. This version of risotto is much heartier and chewier than traditional ones using arborio rice, and is also more nutritious.

2 tablespoons olive oil
1½ cups diced onion
½ cup diced carrot
½ teaspoon (scant) sea salt
1⅓ cups pearl or pot barley (see note)
2 to 3 cloves garlic, minced or grated
¼ teaspoon (rounded) ground cardamom
1 whole star anise (see note)
Freshly ground black pepper
⅓ cup white wine
2 cups vegan vegetable stock (see "Plant-Powered Pantry," page xlii)
4 cups water (helps to boil in advance so it's good and hot)
2½ to 3 teaspoons minced fresh thyme
1½ teaspoons lemon zest
½ to ⅔ cup Fresh Cream Sauce (page 57; see note)
Lemon wedges, for serving
Fresh thyme, minced, for serving

In a heavy skillet, heat the oil over medium-heat. Add the onion, carrot, and salt, and let cook for a minute or two, then add the barley, garlic, cardamom, star anise, and pepper and cook another 2 to 3 minutes, stirring frequently. Add the wine, turn up the heat to high, and stir while letting the alcohol in the wine burn off, for a minute or so. Lower the heat to medium or medium-low, and add the vegetable stock, stirring, until most of the liquid is absorbed, 10 to 15 minutes.

Add 2 cups of the hot water, and cook, stirring occasionally, for 25 to 30 minutes, until the water has been absorbed and the barley is starting to become tender and the sauce thicker. Add another cup of hot water, and cook until absorbed, 7 to 8 minutes. Then add another ½ to 1 cup of hot water (depending on how tender your barley is, whether you are using pearl vs. pot barley, and whether you want your risotto soupier or a little thicker) and cook for another 6 to 8 minutes, or until absorbed.

Remove the star anise, then add the thyme, lemon zest, and ½ cup of the cream sauce. Taste, and if you'd like more cream, go ahead and add extra, as desired. Serve, garnished with the thyme and with a lemon wedge for squeezing.

If This Apron Could Talk: Risotto is typically served and eaten right after preparing. If, however, you have to put it on hold, you will probably want to add a little extra water, as the risotto will thicken with standing. To thin out again, add ½ to ⅔ cup of hot (boiled) water, and/or another 1 to 2 tablespoons of the cream sauce (as much as needed and to your taste).

Ingredients 411: Pot barley is less processed than pearl barley, with more of the grain and thereby nutrients left intact. If you are used to eating pearl barley, you will notice pot barley is much heartier and chewier. Pearl barley will still be chewy, but a little smoother and softer. It will also cook a little quicker than pot barley, and you may need less water.

If you are unsure how much of the star anise flavor you'd like to infuse in the risotto, you can remove it after 15 to 20 minutes of cooking, so the flavor is less intense.

Festive Chickpea Tart

SERVES 4 TO 5

(optionally) wheat
(optionally) gluten **FREE**

Move over, faux turkeys! This savory tart takes center plate with its combination of chickpeas, crunchy walnuts, spinach, and seasonings nestled together. This dish is elegant enough to serve for holiday gatherings, but also easy enough to make for a family dinner any time of the year.

FILLING:

- 1 tablespoon olive oil
- 1 cup diced onion
- ½ cup diced celery
- 4 to 5 medium to large garlic cloves, minced
- ½ teaspoon sea salt
  A few pinches of freshly ground black pepper
- 2 cups cooked chickpeas (or measure from 2 [14-ounce] cans, drained and rinsed)
- 2 tablespoons freshly squeezed lemon juice
- 2 teaspoons tamari
- ½ teaspoon ground sage
- ¾ cup walnuts, toasted
- ⅓ cup rolled oats (use GF-certified for gluten-free option)
- 1 (10-ounce) package frozen chopped spinach, thawed and squeezed to remove excess water (about 1 cup after squeezing)
- ¼ cup dried cranberries
- ¼ cup chopped fresh flat-leaf parsley
- 1 tablespoon chopped fresh thyme, or 1 teaspoon dried

Preheat the oven to 400°F.

Prepare the filling: Combine the oil, onion, celery, garlic, ¼ teaspoon of the salt, and the pepper in a skillet over medium-high heat. Cook for 9 to 10 minutes, stirring occasionally, until softened and turning golden.

In a food processor, combine 1⅔ cups of the chickpeas (reserve the rest), lemon juice, tamari, sage, the remaining ¼ teaspoon of salt, and the sautéed mixture, and partially puree (not fully like hummus, but leaving some chunkier consistency). Add the toasted walnuts and oats, and pulse briefly to lightly break up the nuts. Transfer to a bowl, and stir in the spinach, cranberries, parsley, thyme, and reserved chickpeas.

TO ASSEMBLE:

1 prepared whole wheat pastry pie crust, thawed (for wheat- or gluten-free options, see note)

½ tablespoon olive oil

1 teaspoon tamari

2 tablespoons chopped walnuts (no need to toast beforehand) Cranberry sauce, an oil and balsamic vinegar slurry, or Rosemary Gravy (page 61), for serving (see note)

Transfer the mixture to the pie shell (or a lightly oiled pie plate; see note), smoothing to evenly distribute. Combine the oil and tamari, and brush over the top. Sprinkle the tart with the walnuts. Bake for 30 to 35 minutes, until the tart is golden on the edges and top.

Let cool for 5 to 10 minutes, then serve with your sauce of choice.

Allergy-Free or Bust! This tart can be made with a wheat- or gluten-free pastry crust, or without any pastry crust, if preferred. Do not overbake without a crust, as the tart can become dry.

Ingredients 411: The rolled oats, while lending some structure to the tart, can easily be omitted.

Serving Suggestions: Serve with Smashing Sweet Spuds. A dollop of cranberry sauce makes a nice condiment to this pie. I use my Traditional Cranberry Sauce from *Eat, Drink, & Be Vegan.* Or, try Rosemary Gravy.

Potato, Shallot, and Pepper Frittata

SERVES 4 TO 6

wheat (optionally) gluten 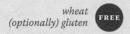 **FREE**

This might better be named "Frit-not-ta," as this quichelike dish contains no eggs, yet has a great texture from the cashews and tofu. The oat bran topping lends a slightly crunchy texture. For gluten-free options, ensure GF-certified oat bran is used.

POTATO MIXTURE:
- 1 tablespoon olive oil
- ¾ cup chopped shallot
- 2 cups cubed red or Yukon Gold potatoes (peeling optional)
- ¼ teaspoon sea salt
  Pinch of freshly ground black pepper
- 1 to 1¼ cups seeded and chopped combination of red, yellow, or orange bell pepper

TOFU MIXTURE:
- ½ cup raw cashews
- ¾ cup + 1 to 2 tablespoons plain unsweetened nondairy milk (almond or soy preferred; see "Plant-Powered Pantry," page xxxiii)
- 1 tablespoon freshly squeezed lemon juice
- 1 large clove garlic
- 2 teaspoons brown rice miso (or other light miso)
- ½ teaspoon dry mustard
- ½ teaspoon (scant) sea salt
  Freshly ground black pepper
- 1 (12-ounce) package extra-firm tofu
- ¼ teaspoon dill seeds
- ½ teaspoon agar powder
- 2 teaspoons chopped fresh thyme or oregano

TOPPING:
- ¼ cup oat bran (for gluten-free option, use GF-certified or substitute gluten-free bread crumbs)
- 1 tablespoon olive oil
- 1 tablespoon nutritional yeast
  A few pinches of sea salt

Preheat the oven to 375°F. Lightly oil an ovenproof glass pie plate or other baking dish.

Prepare the potato mixture: In a skillet over medium heat, combine the olive oil, shallots, potatoes, salt, and pepper. Cook, stirring occasionally, until the potatoes are cooked through and golden, 15 to 20 minutes (add a teaspoon or two of water if the potatoes are sticking, to deglaze the pan). Add the bell pepper and cook for another couple of minutes.

Meanwhile, prepare the tofu mixture: In a blender (see note), combine the cashews, milk, lemon juice, garlic, miso, dry mustard, salt and pepper, tofu, dill seeds, and agar. Blend until smooth and creamy.

Once the potato mixture is cooked, transfer to a bowl and stir in the tofu mixture (scrape out as much of the tofu batter as possible, and use another 1 to 2 tablespoons of milk, if needed, to help loosen the mixture), as well as the fresh thyme. Transfer the mixture to the prepared pan and smooth out. In a small bowl, combine the topping ingredients and sprinkle over the top of the frittata.

Bake for 40 to 45 minutes, then set the oven to BROIL and bake for another couple of minutes, to crisp up the topping slightly.

Remove from the oven and let cool for 10 to 15 minutes, then cut in wedges or scoop portions to serve.

If This Apron Could Talk: I use a Blendtec for the pureeing, and so it easily and quickly smooths out the tofu, along with the cashews and other ingredients. If you don't have a Blendtec, you will need to first blend the cashews with the milk and lemon juice until smooth, using an immersion blender or regular blender. Then add the tofu and remaining ingredients to the blender (or a food processor, if you are having trouble smoothing with the blender) and blend until very smooth.

Yellow Sweet Potato Chickpea Pie with Basil

SERVES 4 TO 6

(optionally) wheat
(optionally) gluten **FREE**
soy

This pie is somewhat like a quiche in appearance, but not so much in taste and texture. The sweet potatoes and chickpeas work as the base for the pie, giving both body and flavor, along with seasonings and herbs, including fresh basil. Use a wheat- or gluten-free pastry crust for those dietary options.

1	tablespoon olive oil
1 to 1¼	cups diced onion
3	large cloves garlic, minced
¾	teaspoon + ½ (scant) teaspoon sea salt
⅛	teaspoon freshly ground black pepper
1	(14-ounce) can chickpeas, drained and rinsed (about 1¾ cup)
1	cup cooked yellow-fleshed sweet potato
¼	cup chickpea flour
2	tablespoons tahini
1	tablespoon freshly squeezed lemon juice
1	teaspoon Dijon mustard
½	teaspoon dried oregano
⅛ to ¼	teaspoon turmeric (optional, for color)
½	cup (packed) fresh basil
2 to 3	tablespoons pine nuts, for sprinkling (optional; slivered almonds are also nice)
1	(9-inch) prepared whole wheat pastry crust, thawed (I used Wholly Wholesome; you can use a wheat- or gluten-free crust, for those options)

Preheat the oven to 425°F. In a skillet over medium heat, combine the oil, onion, garlic, ½ (scant) teaspoon of salt, and pepper. Cook for 9 to 12 minutes, until the onion has softened and is golden in spots (reduce the heat, if needed, to prevent the garlic from burning).

Meanwhile, in a food processor, combine all the remaining ingredients, including the remaining ¾ teaspoon of salt, except the basil and pine nuts (and pie shell!). Puree until very smooth. Once the onion mixture is cooked, add it to the food processor and puree again until smooth. Add the basil and puree fairly well, but leave a little more unprocessed with green flecks. Transfer to the pie shell, scraping out all of mixture.

Bake at 425°F for 15 minutes, then lower the heat to 375°F, sprinkle on the pine nuts, and bake for 20 to 22 minutes.

Remove from the oven and let cool for about 10 minutes before slicing.

If This Apron Could Talk: I cook the sweet potato in advance by baking it whole in the oven. Simply scrub the potato, leaving the peel intact, and place on a baking sheet lined with baking parchment. Bake at in a preheated 400°F oven for about 45 to 60 minutes, until tender throughout (time depends on size of the potato).

The first couple of wedges of pie will be the trickiest to cut and serve; the pie is much easier to slice and remove from the pie plate after it has been allowed to cool for 10 to 15 minutes.

Savvy Subs and Adds: You can use cannellini beans or other white beans in place of the chickpeas. The pie will be a touch looser with white beans, as chickpeas are firmer, but still great!

Serving Suggestions: Serve the pie with a fresh salad, and another vegetable such as Simplicity Asparagus or steamed broccoli. A side of long-grain brown rice or roasted potatoes is also good, and the pie can be topped with a sauce or gravy of choice, such as Smoky Spiked Tahini Sauce or Rosemary Gravy.

7 When Burgers Get Better

Whenever I hear someone mockingly reference a tofu or veggie burger on TV or elsewhere, it irks me. I want to pick up my ingredients, processor, and sauté pan, and head straight to whip up a proper, delicious, veggie burger to hush them up! Truth is, though, some veggie burgers *have* given veggie burgers a bad name. Some commercial brands from the past (and present) that folks have tried as a healthy alternative have disappointed. With strange flavors and textures, sometimes trying to mimic meat, these burgers fall flat.

Rather than try to imitate hamburgers, I've always preferred to "distract and replace"! Bring on something completely different, not trying to taste or chew like meat, but that has scrumptious flavors and new textures to waken up those tired taste buds.

Common complaints I've heard about veggie burgers are that they "don't hold together" or are "too spicy for our kids."

There are at least two burger recipes here that fix this glitch! Nutty Veggie Burgers and Chickpea Pumpkin Seed Burgers are both nicely firm and seasoned well enough, but without any overpowering flavors and no noticeable bits of things such as peppers that the little ones try to pick out! The Mushroom Pecan Burgers, Take II, Too-Good-to-Be-Tofu Burgers, and Lentil Walnut Burgers are also great firm patties, though the seasonings are just a touch more pronounced (though certainly not "hot") for little taste buds. But who knows, your kids might just surprise you and love them as much as you do. And when you don't want to prep much at all, nature has given you the ultimate burger— just a little seasoning love and Juicy Grilled Portobellos will become a favorite, as they have for us!

I've also included some more delicate croquettes and patties (try Black Bean,

Quinoa, and Sweet Potato Spicy Croquettes with Pumpkin Seed Chipotle Cream) for special dinners, and Walnut Pecan Balls for serving on pasta (though these are equally delicious formed into patties and served burger style). And for some Middle Eastern infusion, make an entire dinner platter with Panfried Falafel Patties. . . . details follow!

Now you are armed with the goods the next time you hear some ridiculous quip about veggie burgers. How you choose to use that patty in defense is up to you.

Nutty Veggie Burgers

MAKES 5 TO 6 PATTIES

wheat (optionally) gluten 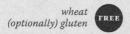 FREE

I came up with these burgers after realizing how fussy children can be with veggie burgers. Many recipes (mine included) are too savory for them, or have onions and other veggies that they feel the need to pick out. Also, sometimes the patties are too delicate for kids eating them on a hamburger bun. I got to work and made this recipe, which is very nutritious and delicious without being too heavy in herbs or spices. Perfect for kids *and* adults, and, yes, you can serve it with confidence on a burger bun!

1½ cups raw almonds
½ cup raw walnuts
½ cup raw pecans (or more walnuts)
1 small clove garlic, cut into quarters
¼ teaspoon sea salt
1 tablespoon ketchup
2 tablespoons nutritional yeast
1 tablespoon tamari
¼ teaspoon poultry seasoning, or ⅛ teaspoon each of dried thyme and dried sage
½ cup (packed) finely grated carrot
½ cup (packed) finely grated zucchini
½ to 1 cup rolled oats (use certified gluten-free oats for that option)
A smidgen of oil, for panfrying

In a food processor, combine the almonds, walnuts, pecans, garlic, and salt. Puree until the nuts are finely ground. Then add the ketchup, nutritional yeast, tamari, poultry seasoning, carrot, and zucchini, and pulse until the mixture becomes dense and is starting to hold together. Pulse in the oats. Remove the blade and shape the mixture into patties.

To cook, lightly oil a nonstick skillet over medium heat. Cook the patties for 5 to 7 minutes on the first side, and then another 3 to 5 minutes on second side until golden brown, working in batches, if necessary.

Serve with lettuce, tomatoes, and fixings of choice (and try "Almonnaise" as an alternative to vegan mayonnaise).

If This Apron Could Talk: If you'd like to make this into a loaf, it works pretty well. Press into a lightly oiled and lined (with a strip of parchment paper, for easy removal) loaf pan. Cover with foil and bake in a preheated 375°F oven for 25 minutes, uncovering for the last 5 to 10 minutes, just to lightly brown the top. Let cool for 5 to 10 minutes in the pan, and then use the parchment to lift the loaf out of the pan to slice.

Ingredients 411: Using ½ cup of oats will firm the patties up nicely enough, and you can use up to 1 full cup of oats for even firmer patties.

Chickpea Pumpkin Seed Burgers

MAKES 5 TO 6 PATTIES

(optionally) wheat
(optionally) gluten 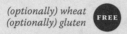 **FREE**

This is another burger recipe that can be made in a jiff, and is firm enough to serve up on a bun. There's no sautéing of onions, garlic, or other seasonings; just a few simple whizzes in the food processor will do the trick! These are also kid-friendly, especially if yours enjoy Goddess Dressing (though substitutions can be made if you don't have this product).

1 (14-ounce) can chickpeas, drained and rinsed
1 medium clove garlic, chopped roughly
½ teaspoon sea salt
 Freshly ground black pepper (optional)
2 tablespoons nutritional yeast
2 tablespoons Annie's Goddess Dressing (see note for wheat- or gluten-free options)
1 tablespoon ground white chia seeds, or 1½ tablespoons flax meal
1 tablespoon red wine vinegar or apple cider vinegar
2 teaspoons Dijon mustard
⅓ to ½ cup sliced green onions (mostly green portion, and less white)
¼ cup fresh basil (see note)
1 cup cooked brown rice, preferably cooled or chilled (see note)
½ cup raw pumpkin seeds (see note)
1 cup rolled or quick oats (use certified gluten-free for that option)
 A smidgen of oil, for panfrying

In a food processor, combine the chickpeas, garlic, salt, nutritional yeast, Goddess Dressing, chia seeds, vinegar, and mustard. Pulse until pureed. Add the green onions and basil, and pulse to break up and incorporate. Then add the rice, pumpkin seeds, and oats and pulse to incorporate and to break up seeds somewhat.

Remove blade and shape the mixture into patties (you can refrigerate the mixture for about 30 minutes before frying, to make it firmer and easier to shape, but it's not essential).

To cook, lightly oil a nonstick skillet over medium or medium-high heat. Cook the patties for 6 to 8 minutes on each side, or until golden brown, working in batches, if necessary.

Adult-Minded: For grown-ups, you can kick up the seasonings with another clove of garlic or even a dash of hot sauce, if you like.

Allergy-Free or Bust! Annie's Goddess Dressing makes a quick fix, but contains wheat. To adapt for a wheat-free or gluten-free version, replace the dressing with 2 teaspoons of tahini, 2 teaspoons of red wine vinegar (in addition to the 1 tablespoon), 1 teaspoon of tamari, and ¼ teaspoon of dried oregano. Voilà—gluten-free!

If This Apron Could Talk: To make these patties quick to prepare, cook the rice a day or so in advance. I typically cook larger batches of rice on any given night, so that leftovers can be refrigerated for another meal, or to use in burgers, burritos, and so on.

If you want to double the burger batch, you can do so. Just be sure to stop the food processor several more times to work the mixture up from the bottom of the processor bowl, as it can get heavier on the bottom and need some coaxing to incorporate the ingredients on the top and sides.

You can make a dinner loaf out of this recipe. Lightly oil a loaf dish (I use an ovenproof glass one), and bake in a preheated 400°F oven for 25 minutes covered, and then for another 5 to 10 uncovered, until lightly browned. Remove from the oven and let sit in pan for 5 to 10 minutes before slicing and serving.

Ingredients 411: If using chickpeas you have cooked yourself from dried, use about 1¾ cups. You may need a tablespoon of water to moisten the mixture, as home-cooked chickpeas are sometimes are drier than canned.

Savvy Subs and Adds: If you don't have fresh basil, you can substitute a small amount of dried basil. About 1 teaspoon works well; add along with chickpeas and condiments.

If you don't have cooked rice handy, you can substitute with another ½ cup of chickpeas (or white beans) and another ½ cup of oats.

No pumpkin seeds? Try sunflower!

Serving Suggestions: Try pairing with Roasted O&V Potatoes, a salad drizzled generously with Citrus Tahini Dressing or as a loaf (see note above) drizzled with Rosemary Gravy.

Mediterranean Bean Burgers

MAKES 6 OR 7 PATTIES

*wheat
(optionally) gluten* **FREE**
soy

Kalamata olives, fresh oregano, and other Mediterranean-inspired seasonings give a perky twist to veggie burgers. These are also way healthy, made with kidney beans, rolled oats, and no added oil.

2 (14-ounce) cans kidney beans, drained and rinsed

1 to 2 medium to large cloves garlic, chopped roughly (use 1 for kid-friendly)

2½ tablespoon tomato paste

1½ tablespoon red wine or balsamic vinegar

1 teaspoon Dijon mustard

¾ cup sliced green onions (using mostly green portion, and less white)

¼ cup roughly chopped fresh parsley

2 to 2½ tablespoons chopped fresh oregano

½ teaspoon (lightly rounded) sea salt

Freshly ground black pepper

1¼ cups rolled oats (use certified gluten-free for that option)

⅓ to ½ cup roughly chopped kalamata olives (see note)

¼ cup seeded and diced red bell pepper (optional; see note)

In a food processor, combine the kidney beans, garlic, tomato paste, vinegar, and mustard. Pulse until pureed. Add the green onions, parsley, oregano, salt, and pepper to taste, and process to break up and blend. Add the oats and pulse to begin to incorporate.

Transfer the mixture to a large bowl (or remove the blade) and stir in the olives and red pepper (if using; see note).

Refrigerate the mixture for 30 to 45 minutes, then shape into patties with your hands (see note). To cook, add a smidgen of oil to a nonstick skillet over medium or medium-high heat. Cook the patties for 6 to 8 minutes per side, or until golden brown.

If This Apron Could Talk: If you have family members that don't care for olives, simply remove a scoop of the mixture before adding the olives and form into a patty or two. And the red peppers add a touch of freshness and texture to the burgers, but can be easily omitted—or, as with the olives, you can make some patties without them before adding the diced peppers.

Refrigerating the mixture is important as it helps the burger mixture firm up. When you first start to pulse in the oats, the mixture will appear somewhat loose. But, the oats absorb moisture as the mixture sits and refrigerates, and once you remove to shape into patties you'll notice the mixture has firmed up some.

Ingredients 411: If you dislike olives and want to omit them altogether, note that you may want to add another few pinches of salt to season the mixture, as the olives contribute a salty bite.

Mushroom Pecan Burgers, Take II

MAKES 5 TO 6 PATTIES

(optionally) wheat
(optionally) gluten FREE

I had a mushroom pecan burger in my first cookbook, *The Everyday Vegan*. My husband always loved these burgers, and I received great feedback on them from other folks. The only thing was that they were a tad delicate. Fine for stuffing in a pita, but to properly put on a burger bun, they could fall apart. I reworked this recipe, changing the cooking technique and also tweaking the seasonings just slightly. Now these burgers truly hold their shape, and are still moist and flavorful—a must-make!

1 tablespoon olive oil
1 pound cremini or white button mushrooms, stems trimmed, chopped
Freshly ground black pepper
1¼ cups diced onion
A few pinches of sea salt
3 to 4 large cloves garlic, grated or minced
1 tablespoon balsamic vinegar
2 to 2½ tablespoons tahini
1 tablespoon light miso (e.g., brown rice miso)
½ teaspoon ground sage
1 teaspoon dried oregano
1½ tablespoons balsamic vinegar
1 tablespoon tamari
1¾ cups quick oats (use GF-certified for gluten-free option)
½ cup fresh flat-leaf parsley
1 teaspoon vegan Worcestershire sauce (optional; omit or use gluten-free vegan Worcestershire for wheat- or gluten-free version)
½ cup pecans, toasted lightly (see note)
A smidgen of oil, for panfrying

In a large skillet (as large as you have) over high heat, combine the oil, mushrooms, and pepper. Cook, stirring occasionally, until the mushrooms have started to brown and shrink down (9 to 10 minutes). Push most of the mushrooms to the outer edges of the skillet (creating a well in the center), turn the heat down to medium or medium-low, and add the onion and salt. Cook for a couple of minutes, then add the garlic (adding the garlic later helps prevent it from burning). Stir the mushrooms into the onion mixture and cook for another 6 to 7 minutes, until the onion is softened and translucent. Add the 1 tablespoon of the balsamic vinegar to the pan, stir, and then remove from the heat.

In a food processor, combine about three-quarters of the mushroom mixture with the tahini, miso, sage, oregano, the remaining 1½ tablespoons of balsamic vinegar, and the tamari, oats, fresh parsley, and Worcestershire sauce (if using). Process until it just comes together. Add the pecans, pulse once or twice (to break up but not fully process), and then add the remaining mushroom mixture, pulsing once or twice just to incorporate.

Remove the blade, and shape mounds of the mixture into patties with your hands (yielding six, or five larger patties). The patties can be refrigerated or cooked immediately. To cook, lightly oil a nonstick skillet over medium or medium-high heat and cook the patties for 6 to 8 minutes, then flip and cook for another 4 to 5 minutes until a golden sear has formed on each side, working in batches, if necessary. Serve up!

Serving Suggestions: Because these burgers take a little more prep than others, pair with the simplest of spuds, such as baked whole sweet or white potatoes. But if you're up to just a little more prep, try Lemon Dijon Green Beans or Sunshine Fries with Rosemary and Coarse Sea Salt. A green salad will round out the meal and add freshness; try one loaded with raw veggies and drizzled with Walnut Mustard Vinaigrette.

Lentil Walnut Burgers

MAKES 9 TO 11 PATTIES

These savory burgers will surprise you with little bites of sweetness, courtesy of fresh apple. Plus, they hold together quite well, without being too starchy or heavy.

(optionally) wheat
(optionally) gluten 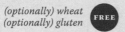 FREE

1 tablespoon olive oil (optional, omit by cooking onions and garlic with lentils, see note)

1½ cups chopped onion

3 medium to large cloves garlic

⅛ + ¼ teaspoon sea salt
Freshly ground black pepper (generous is good)

2 cups cooked green lentils (see note)

½ tablespoon vegan Worcestershire sauce (omit for wheat- or gluten-free version or use a gluten-free vegan Worcestershire for wheat- or gluten-free version)

1½ tablespoons mild miso (I use Genmai brown rice miso)

1¼ teaspoons dried thyme, or 1½ to 2 tablespoons fresh

½ to ¾ teaspoon dried sage

½ teaspoon dried basil

1 cup rolled or quick oats (use GF-certified oats for gluten-free option; see note)

¾ cup raw walnuts (toast to enhance the flavor)

1 cup peeled and diced apple (choose firm, crisp varieties such as Gala, Fuji, or Yellow Delicious), tossed with a squeeze of lemon juice (see note)
Splash of neutral-flavored oil, for frying (see "Plant-Powered Pantry, page xxxii)

Pour the olive oil into a skillet over medium-high heat. Add the onion, garlic, ⅛ teaspoon of the salt, and pepper to taste, and cook for 7 to 8 minutes, until the onion has softened (see note for a shortcut on cooking the onion and garlic with the lentils).

Meanwhile, in a food processor, combine the cooked lentils, Worcestershire sauce, miso, thyme, sage, basil, and ¼ teaspoon of salt and blend. When the onion mixture is ready, add this to the food processor and puree again, scraping down the sides of the bowl as needed. Add the oats and walnuts, and pulse a few times to break up the walnuts (do not fully pulverize; leave in a rough chop). Transfer the mixture to a large bowl. Add the apple and mix well.

At this point, you can refrigerate the mixture until ready to fry (refrigerating for at least 30 minutes will make it firmer and easier to shape). To cook, take scoops of the mixture and form into patties with your hands. In a skillet over medium-high heat, heat the neutral oil. Add the patties, flatten gently on the pan, and fry for 6 to 9 minutes on each side, until golden and a crust has developed; flipping them over only once or twice (the second side will cook quicker than the first), working in batches as needed.

If This Apron Could Talk: Some days you might want to skip the step of sautéing the onion and garlic. If you're having one of those days, simply toss the onion and garlic in with the dried lentils and water (see lentil cooking note below); they will cook while the lentils simmer. You can omit the oil and salt, and simply add a smidgen more salt with the puree (lightly round the ¼ teaspoon salt in the pureed mixture).

If refrigerating for more than 30 minutes, reserve the apples. This mixture can be refrigerated up to a day or two in advance; however, the apples will lose their texture and taste if they sit in the mixture that long. So, if preparing burgers in advance, omit the apples and refrigerate, then stir in the chopped apple while getting ready to panfry the patties.

These burgers form patties that will hold together but are still fairly soft. For firmer burgers, add another ¼ cup or so of oats.

Use leftover patties in sandwiches, much like a pâté, or crumble and add to other fixings in a pita or wrap sandwich.

Ingredients 411: If cooking the lentils yourself, use about ¾ cup of dried lentils to 1¾ to 2 cups of water. Add a bay leaf, bring to a boil, then lower heat to low and simmer covered for about 35 minutes, until the lentils are tender and the water is absorbed. If the lentils are tender but there is extra water, either drain off the water, or remove the cover and simmer until the water has evaporated. Feel free to use canned cooked lentils, in a pinch (drain and rinse first).

You can also grate the apple, if you prefer. Use a large-holed grater, and then toss the grated apple with the lemon juice, per the directions.

Serving Suggestions: Instead of whole wheat burger buns, try serving in pita, or a folded whole-grain tortilla with your favorite fixings! Try a dollop of Raw-nch Dressing, or a large romaine salad tossed with Classic Caesar Dressing.

Too-Good-to-Be-Tofu Burgers

MAKES 6 TO 7 BURGERS

wheat (optionally) gluten 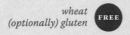 FREE

Enough jokes about tofu burgers already. Yes, there are some bland, uninteresting tofu burgers out there. But don't let them give all tofu burgers a bad rap. These burgers are flavorful with herbs and seasonings, and just all-out yummy.

½ tablespoon olive oil

1½ to 1¾ cups chopped onion,

½ cup chopped celery or seeded red bell pepper

⅛ teaspoon sea salt
Freshly ground black pepper

1 (14-ounce) package extra-firm tofu (squeeze lightly to remove excess water)

2½ to 3 tablespoons brown rice miso (or other light miso)

3 tablespoons tomato paste or natural ketchup (see note)

2 teaspoons red wine vinegar (see note)

1 medium to large clove garlic, cut into quarters

1 to 1½ teaspoons Dijon mustard

2 teaspoons dried basil

1½ teaspoons dried oregano

1 teaspoon dried savory

½ teaspoon dried rosemary

1½ cups rolled or quick oats (use GF-certified for gluten-free option)
A smidgen of oil, for panfrying

In a skillet over medium to medium-high heat, combine the oil, onion, celery, salt and pepper to taste, and cook 9 to 12 minutes, until the onion and celery have softened.

In a food processor, combine the tofu, miso, tomato paste, vinegar, garlic, mustard, and herbs, and process until the tofu becomes crumbly and then starts to smooth somewhat (stop to scrape down the sides of the processor as needed). Try not to overprocess, as tofu becomes sticky. Add the sautéed mixture, and process again, followed by the oats, pulsing to incorporate briefly but not overprocessing.

Remove the blade and shape the mixture into patties (you can refrigerate the mixture for about 30 minutes to make it firmer and easier to shape, but it's not essential). To cook, lightly oil a nonstick skillet over medium or medium-high heat. Cook the patties for 8 to 12 minutes on each side, or until golden brown, working in batches, if necessary.

Savvy Subs and Adds: Sometimes I don't have tomato paste on hand. Ketchup makes a good stand-in, and it will also add a touch of sweetness. If using ketchup, reduce the red wine vinegar to 1 teaspoon.

Serving Suggestions: This are hearty burgers, so you might want to lighten up the sides with a smallish portion of spuds (Roasted O&V Potatoes come to mind) and/or a generous salad tossed in a light vinaigrette, such as Citrus Tahini Dressing.

Walnut Pecan Balls

MAKES 17 TO 20 BALLS

(optionally) wheat
(optionally) gluten **FREE**

These savory balls have a buttery taste from a combination of walnuts, pecans, and sautéed vegetables. They are delicious topped on pasta with a good-quality pasta sauce, but can also be used as finger foods to dip in a warmed marinara sauce, or formed into patties and eaten as veggie burgers.

1 tablespoon olive oil
1 cup chopped onion
½ cup chopped celery
1¼ teaspoons dried oregano
½ teaspoon dried thyme
¼ teaspoon sea salt
Freshly ground black pepper
¾ cup raw pecans
¾ cup raw walnuts
1 cup + 2 tablespoons rolled or quick oats (use GF-certified for gluten-free option)
2 tablespoons vegan Worcestershire sauce (use gluten-free Worcestershire for wheat- or gluten-free option)
1 tablespoon tamari
½ tablespoon balsamic vinegar
1 teaspoon blackstrap molasses
1 to 2 tablespoons olive oil, for frying (optional; you can omit and bake, see note)

In a skillet over medium heat, combine the 1 tablespoon of olive oil, onion, celery, oregano, thyme, salt, and pepper to taste. Cook for 10 to 14 minutes, stirring occasionally, until the onion and celery are nicely softened and golden brown, then transfer them to a food processor with the remaining ingredients, except the olive oil for frying, and process until the mixture becomes crumbly. Stop and scrape down the sides of the bowl. Process again to incorporate any larger pieces, and just as mixture becomes sticky and/or forms a ball, stop the processor.

Refrigerate for at least 30 minutes (refrigerating the mixture will make it firmer and easier to shape). Take small spoonfuls of the mixture, about 1 tablespoon (using a small cookie scoop is helpful, but otherwise use your hands, rinsing hands when needed to keep the mixture from sticking to your palms), and form into balls. If cooking on the stovetop (see note for oven baking), heat the oil in a nonstick skillet over medium-high heat. Add the balls and fry for 5 to 7 minutes (lower the heat if burning), shifting the pan to turn the sides of balls every minute or two, to form a golden crust fairly evenly around the balls. Remove from the heat and serve

If This Apron Could Talk: If you prefer baking these in the oven, place the balls on a baking sheet lined with parchment paper. Bake in a preheated 400°F oven for 12 to 15 minutes, turning once or twice during the baking process, until golden brown. These mixture can also be formed into patties and panfried as a burgers. Or it can be placed in a loaf dish and baked. Don't know what to do with leftovers? Refrigerate them and use another day as a sandwich filling, simply mashing and stirring in vegan mayonnaise, plus chopped veggies, if you like.

Serving Suggestions: Most obviously, serve these warm with tomato sauce and pasta. But also try as an hors d'oeuvre with a warmed sauce (e.g., marinara or other pasta sauce) or Raw Yellow Tomato Sauce or Classic Caesar Dressing for dipping, Or add them to a salad to turn it into a more substantial meal.

Juicy Grilled Portobellos

MAKES 5 TO 7 BURGERS

wheat gluten soy **FREE**

This is one of the simplest veggie burgers you can make, and in my opinion, one of the most delicious! Use fresh, plump portobellos, and you will have delectable, juicy burgers that are satisfying without being heavy.

5 to 7   portobello mushrooms (7 medium-size or 5 to 6 large; 1¼ to 1½ pounds)
2   large cloves garlic
2 to 2½   tablespoons balsamic vinegar
2½ to 3   tablespoons extra-virgin olive oil
A few pinches of sea salt and freshly ground black pepper

First, clean mushrooms, using a damp (not wet) towel or paper towel to wipe the tops. You can also use a spoon to scrape the gills from the underside of the mushrooms (I like to, as they release a lot of black juice after cooking).

Grate the garlic (I use a kitchen grater) in a large, shallow dish. Add the vinegar and oil and stir to incorporate. Add the mushrooms, and gently flip and move around in the marinade to cover most of the surface area of each. Cover the dish and let mushrooms marinate for at least 30 minutes (1 to 2 hours, if you have the time), flipping the mushrooms once during the marinating time.

To cook, preheat a barbecue grill to high or medium-high heat. Once the grill is ready, place the mushrooms on the grill, and then sprinkle with a few pinches of salt and pepper over. Grill for 4 to 7 minutes on each side (the first side usually needing longer than the second), until grill marks have formed and the mushrooms have softened slightly (but not too wilted; they should still be juicy). Remove from the grill and serve.

Kid-Friendly: One of our daughters really loves these burgers. But I go easy on the pepper for her portion. You may also want to have a light hand with the garlic, depending on your children's tastes.

Savvy Subs and Adds: Did you know that cremini mushrooms (also called baby bellas) are essentially "baby" portobellos? Use an equivalent amount of cremini (or even white button mushrooms) in place of portobellos, and serve as a side or hors d'oeuvre.

Serving Suggestions: Try on burger buns with such fixings as vegan mayonnaise (try "Almonnaise"), tomato slices, and grilled onions (especially delicious!) Because these burgers are not as heavy as bean- and grain-based patties, try serving with a heartier side salad, such as Three-Bean Salad or Smoky Sweet Potato and Black Bean Salad. Of course, you can always team up with spuds, such as Roasted O&V Potatoes or Sunshine Fries with Rosemary and Coarse Sea Salt.

Panfried Falafel Patties

MAKES 20 TO 24 FALAFELS

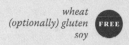

wheat
(optionally) gluten **FREE**
soy

Falafels are scrumptious, flat out. But most are deep-fried. Here, I take falafels in a new, fresher, and lighter direction. The ingredients are all swiftly combined in a food processor and then lightly dusted with flour to panfry in just a wipe of oil. Here, all the flavor comes from the herbs, aromatics, and seasonings—rather than the oil!

2 (14-ounce) cans chickpeas, drained and rinsed

½ cup (packed) fresh flat-leaf parsley leaves (not chopped, just torn from stems)

½ to ¾ cup (packed) fresh cilantro leaves and tender stems

½ cup chopped green onions (mostly white but some green portion)

¼ cup chopped celery

2 tablespoons freshly squeezed lemon juice

½ tablespoon red wine vinegar or apple cider vinegar

2 to 3 medium to large cloves garlic (use 3 large if you love a garlicky kick)

2 teaspoons ground cumin

1 teaspoon turmeric

1½ teaspoons ground coriander

1¼ teaspoons sea salt

¼ teaspoon (rounded) freshly ground black pepper

¼ to ½ teaspoon crushed red pepper flakes (I use ¼ teaspoon; use more if you like things spicy)

¾ cup rolled oats (use GF-certified oats for gluten-free option; see note)

⅓ cup millet flour, or other flour, seasoned with a few pinches of sea salt

Splash of oil for panfrying (use less or more per personal preference)

In a food processor, combine the chickpeas, parsley, cilantro, onion, celery, lemon juice, vinegar, garlic, and spices, and process until the mixture is well incorporated and starting to smooth out, scraping scrape down the sides of the bowl as needed. Then add the oats and pulse a few times to work them in. Refrigerate the mixture for 30 minutes if possible (refrigerating will make it firmer and easier to shape).

Take small scoops of the mixture, 1½ to 2 tablespoons (using a cookie scoop is helpful, but you can use your hands, rinsing when needed to keep the mixture from sticking to your palms) and form into balls. Once finished, place the seasoned millet flour in a bowl. Add the falafel balls to the bowl and lightly toss, then toss a moment in your hand to remove any excess clumping of flour.

Lightly oil a nonstick skillet over medium or medium-high heat. Place the falafel balls in the pan, flattening them slightly with a spatula, and cook for 6 to 9 minutes on each side, until golden brown and crisped on the outside, working in batches, if needed. Serve.

If This Apron Could Talk: You can also bake these falafels. Spray the balls with a spritz of olive oil, if you have a spritzer; otherwise you can leave them as is or very lightly coat with oil with your hands. Bake in a preheated 400°F oven for 20 to 22 minutes, flipping once through the baking process, until a little browned and crispy in spots.

Ingredients 411: I like these falafels soft and tender. Feel free to add another ¼ to ⅓ cup of oats (and another pinch of salt) to make a little firmer.

If you'd like to use more oil for crispier patties, feel free to do so, using 1 to 2 tablespoons, if desired.

Serving Suggestions: Serve in pita with fixings, or on their own drizzled with tahini sauce (try Smoky Spiked Tahini Sauce or Peanut Tahini Sauce). Up the ante by making a falafel platter, including Quinoa Tabbouleh with Olives.

Black Bean, Quinoa, and Sweet Potato Spicy Croquettes

MAKES 8 TO 11 CROQUETTES

wheat gluten soy FREE

These are more delicate than a burger, and meant to be eaten with a fork as a patty or croquette (rather than on a bun). The sweet potatoes balance the smoky and savory elements of cumin, oregano, chile, garlic, and the infusion of lime to heighten all the flavors. Be sure to serve with Pumpkin Seed Chipotle Cream—the combination is dynamite.

1 tablespoon organic extra-virgin coconut oil or olive oil

1¼ teaspoons cumin seeds (not ground cumin)

¾ to 1 cup diced onion

½ tablespoon (roughly) finely chopped serrano chile (about 1 chile), or jalapeño or red chile, or a few pinches of crushed red pepper (optional)

2 medium to large cloves garlic, chopped finely

1 teaspoon dried oregano

⅛ teaspoon ground allspice

¼ (lightly rounded) teaspoon + ½ teaspoon sea salt
Freshly ground black pepper

1 cup (packed) skinned, mashed, cooked orange-fleshed sweet potato (see note)

1 (14-ounce) can black beans, drained, rinsed, and patted dry

1½ cups cooled, cooked quinoa (see note)

1 tablespoon ground white chia seeds (see note)

2 tablespoons freshly squeezed lime juice (first zest the limes; see below)

½ to 1 teaspoon lime zest

¼ cup chopped fresh cilantro

½ to 1 tablespoon organic extra-virgin coconut oil or olive oil, for panfrying)
Pumpkin Seed Chipotle Cream (page 59), for serving

In a skillet over medium-high heat, heat the oil. Add the cumin seeds and cook for a minute or two, stirring. Lower the heat to medium and add the onion, chopped chile, garlic, oregano, allspice, ¼ teaspoon of the salt, and the pepper to taste, and cook for 8 to 10 minutes, until onion is very soft (be sure to lower the heat if the garlic starts to brown, so it doesn't burn and develop a bitter taste). Once the onion is soft, transfer the mixture to a large bowl.

Add the remaining ingredients, except the coconut oil and Pumpkin Seed Chipotle Cream, and mix well. At this point, you can refrigerate the mixture until ready to fry (refrigerating for at least 30 minutes will make it firmer and easier to shape). Take scoops of the mixture and form into small patties with your hands. These are not firm patties; they will be soft and more delicate, so simply shape in relatively neat patties, repeating until you have used all of the mixture. In a nonstick skillet over medium-high heat, heat the ½ to 1 tablespoon of oil. Add the patties, flatten gently on the pan, and fry for 6 to 9 minutes on each side, until golden and a crust has developed, flipping them over only once or twice (the second side will cook quicker than the first), working in batches, if necessary. Serve with a generous drizzle of Pumpkin Seed Chipotle Cream.

If This Apron Could Talk: When cooking grains such as quinoa, it is helpful to cook extra so that you have leftovers refrigerated for another day. One cup of dried quinoa yields roughly 3 cups cooked. Using cooled precooked quinoa also helps with forming the croquettes, as freshly cooked quinoa is moist and can make the patties too wet. So, cook your quinoa in advance, and refrigerate until ready to prep this recipe.

Ingredients 411: Cook the sweet potatoes in advance by baking whole. Simply place one or two sweet potatoes (depending on size) on a baking sheet lined with a little parchment paper (to catch drippings). Bake in a preheated 400°F oven for 40 to 50 minutes, until very soft when pierced with a knife or skewer.

The ground white chia helps the patties hold together. They can be made without the chia, but will be a little fragile and more difficult to flip. If you use the chia, be sure to use ground, not whole, white chia.

Kid-Friendly: For kids, omit the chile in the sauté stage, and then before making the patties, remove a portion for your children. You can add the chile (raw, or cook it) or another spice to the remaining mixture to be served to the adults.

Fab Cakes with Smarter Tartar Sauce

MAKES 11 TO 12 PATTIES

(optionally) wheat
(optionally) gluten 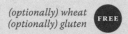 FREE

These patties are a faux crab cake of sorts, but aren't trying to emulate them other than imparting a briny sea flavor and pairing them with a smarter kind of tartar sauce!

SMARTER SAUCE:

½ cup "Almonnaise" (page 55) or vegan mayonnaise of choice (see note)

1½ tablespoons unseasoned rice wine vinegar, red wine vinegar, or apple cider vinegar)

1 tablespoon finely chopped fresh flat-leaf parsley,

¼ cup seeded and minced cucumber

1 tablespoon capers, drained

¾ teaspoon pure maple syrup or agave nectar

⅛ to ¼ teaspoon dry mustard (use full ¼ teaspoon for more "bite")

¼ teaspoon (rounded) onion powder

1 teaspoon lemon zest

⅛ teaspoon sea salt
Freshly ground black pepper

Prepare the sauce: Combine all the ingredients in a small bowl and stir until well mixed. Refrigerate (covered) until serving.

CAKES:

8 ounces tempeh

1 to 1⅛ cups cooked potatoes, chopped roughly (can use leftover boiled or roasted potatoes)

2 tablespoons freshly squeezed lemon juice

1½ tablespoons vegan Worcestershire sauce (use gluten-free Worcestershire for wheat- or gluten-free option)

1 tablespoon Dijon mustard

1 teaspoon kelp granules

½ teaspoon sea salt

¼ teaspoon freshly ground black pepper

½ teaspoon paprika

½ teaspoon dried thyme
Pinch of cayenne pepper

½ cup seeded and diced red bell pepper

⅔ cup peeled and diced apple, tossed with a squeeze of lemon juice to prevent browning

⅓ cup sliced green onions (both greener and whitish portions) or chives
Dash of hot sauce (optional)

⅓ cup (roughly) potato starch, for frying (optional)

1½ to 2 tablespoons olive oil, for frying

Prepare the tempeh: Simmer the tempeh in 2 to 3 cups of water or vegetable broth for about 20 minutes, then let cool. Then squeeze the excess water from the tempeh with your hands (it's okay to squish as the tempeh will be processed next).

In a food processor, first pulse the tempeh with the potatoes, lemon juice, Worcestershire sauce, mustard, kelp granules, salt, pepper, paprika, thyme, and cayenne (pulse until combined and broken up, but not fully pureed—alternatively, you can mash these ingredients by hand). Add the bell pepper, apple, green onions, and hot sauce (if using), and stir.

Take small scoops of the mixture (about ¼ cup) and form into small cakes with your hands. Place the potato flour in a shallow dish. Lightly coat each side of the patties in the potato flour. Repeat until you have used all of the tempeh mixture.

In a nonstick skillet over medium-high heat, heat the oil. Add the patties, flatten gently on the pan, and fry for 7 to 9 minutes on each side, until golden and a crust has developed, flipping them over only once or twice (the second side will cook quicker than the first), working in batches, if necessary. Serve with dollops of Smarter Sauce.

Savvy Subs and Adds: "Almonnaise" is my homemade version of a vegan mayonnaise that is not overly oily, using raw almonds as the base. If you'd like a shortcut, try a vegan mayonnaise. While I generally prefer Vegenaise as a vegan mayonnaise, in this sauce I like to use something like NatureNaise or Nayonnaise as they are creamier and lighter.

8 Good Pasta Belongs on a Plate— Not the Wall!

While pasta might traditionally be a "starter" in Italy, we know that it can make the best main course. This chapter gives you a range of pasta sauces and dishes, from fresh, bright, and light fare such as Raw Yellow Tomato Sauce, and Tomato Artichoke Pasta, to richer, heartier sauces such as "Fit-tuccine Alfredo" and White Bean Sweet Potato Pasta Sauce. There are also casseroles, such as my signature Mac-oh-geez! and nut-based sauces, including two vibrant basil pestos and a Romesc-oat Sauce. I have even included a simple, quick gluten-free White Sauce for those who are aching to have one for their pasta and pasta casseroles. All these sauces and casseroles can be made with a variety of whole-grain pastas (see "Plant-Powered Pantry," page xxxv) for meals that are as nutritious as they are delicious.

And should you be tempted to followed that old tip (as I did as a teenager, throwing random spaghetti noodles at my mother's walls!), here's a better way to check if it's done: Remove a noodle from the cooking water . . . and bite into it. Newfangled science, huh?! Hey, there are enough fingerprints and other goop on my walls that I don't need pasta stains, to boot (and I'm sure my mother didn't, either—sorry, Mom!).

Raw Yellow Tomato Sauce

SERVES 4

wheat gluten soy **FREE**

This sauce is fresh and vibrant, and can be served tossed into your pasta of choice, or topped on a whole grain, or kept virtuous in its raw capacity to accompany raw noodles or toss into a raw salad. Yellow tomatoes are usually less acidic and a little sweeter than red, and as they are such a glorious color, make the ideal ingredient for this sauce. Plus, with the addition of extra garlic and some jalapeño peppers, this sauce quickly transforms into a salsa (see note)!

2½ cups chopped yellow tomatoes (see note)
1 to 2 medium to large cloves garlic, cut in half or into quarters (adjust to taste; see note)
½ cup sliced green onions (green portion mostly)
2 tablespoons extra-virgin olive oil
¾ to 1 teaspoon sea salt (adjust to taste; see note)
Freshly ground black pepper
¼ cup (loosely packed) flat-leaf parsley (optional; you can use less or omit)
⅓ cup (tightly or loosely packed) fresh basil (don't substitute dried)
½ cup seeded and diced red bell pepper
Extra olive oil, for serving (optional, but very good!)

In a bowl, gently squeeze the chopped tomatoes to remove most of their excess juice. It will help keep the sauce from being too thin and runny (remove as much as you can, but no need to fret or excessively squeeze to remove it all; some tomatoes are naturally juicier than others). Then transfer the tomatoes along with the remaining ingredients, starting with ¾ teaspoon of salt, excluding the bell peppers and optional olive oil, to a food processor or blender, and pulse to partially break up the sauce. Add the peppers and pulse again, maintaining chunkier bits of peppers rather than pureeing. Add additional salt and pepper to taste . . . then serve as you wish, in pasta, on rice, drizzled on a wrap sandwich, and so on.

Adult-Minded: To switch this into a salsa, add another clove of garlic (if you like), along with ½ to 1 jalapeño pepper, seeded and diced, and 1 tablespoon of freshly squeezed lime juice. Substitute cilantro for the parsley or basil, and you can add more green onions, if you like. When processing, keep much chunkier than you would for a sauce.

If This Apron Could Talk: I like one average clove of garlic in this sauce. You can add more if you like, but keep in mind that too much garlic can overpower the other subtle flavors unless converting sauce to a salsa.

You may want less or more salt depending on how you use the sauce. If tossing with cooked pasta, you may need extra; however, if drizzling over rice or grains, it will taste stronger and so you may opt for less.

If serving this on cooked pasta, it helps to bring the sauce to room temperature (if previously refrigerated) just so you aren't tossing a very cold sauce into the pasta. Also, you can gently warm it by transferring the sauce to a covered container and letting sit in a few inches of hot water until it is has become warmed through.

Ingredients 411: At our local farmers' market in the summer, there is a stall with beautiful organic bell peppers, eggplant, and a variety of tomatoes. I tried a variety of yellow tomatoes one week, and it became a favorite. The Hugh's Beefsteak variety in particular is amazing in this sauce (and all on its own!), and the Lemon Boy variety is also quite lovely.

Savvy Subs and Adds: If you keep dehydrated (raw) tomatoes on hand, try substituting about ⅓ cup, chopped, for the red bell pepper.

Spinach Herb Pistachio Pesto

MAKES ABOUT 1½ CUPS

wheat
gluten FREE
soy

Normally, for me, pesto is all about the basil. But fresh basil is abundant for only a brief period of the year. Still, it *is* available in modest amounts at grocery stores year-round. Here, I use a smaller amount of basil, along with parsley, to bring life to spinach via pesto. Pistachios offer sweetness to balance the more astringent spinach. While I'm usually loyal to my full-on basil pesto, this recipe competes for my affection!

1	cup raw, unsalted pistachios
2	tablespoons pine nuts (optional, or more pistachios)
1 to 2	medium to large cloves garlic, quartered (see note)
1½ to 2	tablespoons freshly squeezed lemon juice
½	teaspoon sea salt (see note) Freshly ground black pepper
2	tablespoons olive oil
1½ to 3	tablespoons water (see note)
3½	cups (loosely packed) baby spinach leaves
¾ to 1	cup (loosely packed) fresh basil leaves
¼	cup (packed) flat-leaf parsley leaves
¾ to 1	pound dried pasta of choice (see "Plant-Powered Pantry," page xxxv, and note) Extra olive oil, salt, pepper, and lemon wedges, for serving (optional) Crushed pistachios, for garnish

In a food processor, combine the nuts, garlic, 1½ tablespoons of the lemon juice, salt, pepper to taste, olive oil, 1½ tablespoons of the water, and the spinach, basil, and parsley. Puree until fairly smooth, less for a chunkier consistency or longer for a smoother one. Add and blend in additional water if you need to, for the consistency you desire.

At this point, you may refrigerate the pesto in a covered container until ready to use it. If you are serving this immediately with pasta, set the pesto aside and cook the pasta according to the package directions.

Just before draining the pasta, remove and reserve about ½ cup of its cooking water. Drain the pasta (don't rinse it!) and toss with the pesto, using as much or as little pesto as you like. If the pasta is a little dry, add more pesto plus a tablespoon at a time of the reserved cooking water.

Season to taste with additional salt, black pepper, and fresh lemon juice, as desired. Serve garnished with a sprinkle of crushed pistachios.

Adult-Minded: I typically use one clove of garlic, because when the pesto is warmed by the pasta rather than cooked, the garlic maintains a raw taste. Our kids tend to quickly pick up on the zing of raw garlic, so one clove works best. If you like a stronger garlic flavor, by all means, add another clove!

If This Apron Could Talk: If you are serving this pesto with the greater amount of pasta, you may need to add extra cooking water or oil to help spread the pesto through the pasta.

You may want to add more salt to this pesto after tossing with the pasta. The seasoning depends very much on how you use this pesto, and also how much of it you use! For instance, if you like just a light coating of pesto with your pasta, you may find the seasoning a touch bland, and in that case you can add a touch more salt to your pasta, to taste. If you like a thick, generous coating of pesto on those noodles (as I do!), then adding extra salt will be just too much. Also, if you like using pesto as a spread for breads or vegetables, this amount of salt is just right.

Serving Suggestions: This pesto is also great to spread on pizza crusts, slather on crusty breads, dollop on soups, or mix with sandwich fillings!

Brazil Nut Pesto

MAKES ABOUT 1¼ CUPS

wheat gluten soy **FREE**

Brazil nuts take this pesto down a new delicious path! They offer a nutritional dose of selenium and protein. And the raw walnuts offer those important omega-3 fatty acids. But beyond all these healthy benefits, this pesto tastes terrific, and is a complete breeze to make!

½ cup raw Brazil nuts
½ cup raw walnuts
1 medium to large clove garlic, quartered
2½ to 3 tablespoons freshly squeezed lemon juice
¾ teaspoon sea salt
  Freshly ground black pepper
2 tablespoons olive oil
3½ to 5 tablespoons water (see note)
3 cups (lightly packed) fresh basil (tender leaves and stems only)
  A few pinches of freshly grated nutmeg
¾ to 1 pound dried pasta of choice (see "Plant-Powered Pantry," page xxxv, and note)
  Extra olive oil, salt, pepper, and lemon wedges, for serving (optional)

In a food processor, combine the nuts, garlic, lemon juice, salt, pepper to taste, olive oil, 3½ tablespoons of water, basil, and nutmeg. Puree until fairly smooth, less for a chunkier consistency or longer for a smoother one. Add and blend in additional water if you need to, for the consistency you desire.

At this point, you may refrigerate the pesto in a covered container until ready to use it. If you are serving this immediately with pasta, set the pesto aside and cook the pasta according to the package directions.

Just before draining the pasta, remove and reserve about ½ cup of its cooking water. Drain the pasta (don't rinse it!) and toss with the pesto, using as much or as little pesto as you like. If the pasta is a little dry, add more pesto plus a tablespoon at a time of the reserved cooking water or olive oil.

Season to taste with additional sea salt, black pepper, and fresh lemon juice, as desired. In the summer, top this salad with fresh, sliced ripe cherry tomatoes!

If This Apron Could Talk: If you use the greater amount of pasta, you may need to add extra cooking water or oil to help spread the pesto through the pasta.

Ingredients 411: Yes, nutmeg may seem like an odd inclusion here, but it adds the slightest sweet-spicy note that complements the nuts and basil. Just don't go overboard! Use a kitchen grater to grate the nutmeg just a few times into the pesto.

Serving Suggestions: Use any leftover pesto to spread on pizza crusts, slather on crusty breads, dollop on soups, or mix with sandwich fillings!

Romesc-oat Sauce

MAKES ABOUT 1½ CUPS

wheat
(optionally) gluten **FREE**
soy

This is my version of the classic romesco sauce that originates from Spain, which can be thick enough to be called a dip or spread. There are plenty of variations on the recipe, though most include white bread to add structure. My adaptation uses healthier rolled oats that are lightly toasted until golden to give an earthier flavor to this sauce, along with just a hint of smoked paprika. It is versatile and delicious kept thick, or thinned as a sauce.

½ cup toasted oats (use GF-certified for gluten-free version; see note)

1¼ cups roasted red pepper (about 1½ medium-size to large red peppers; see note)

1 medium to large clove garlic

½ cup toasted almonds

½ teaspoon sea salt
Freshly ground black pepper

1½ tablespoons red wine vinegar (see note about peppers)

2 tablespoons extra-virgin olive oil (optional; you can reduce or omit)

⅛ teaspoon smoked paprika

2 to 4 tablespoons water, or more to thin as desired (see note)

In a food processor, combine all ingredients, starting with about 2 tablespoons of the water, and puree until smooth, adding more water to thin as desired.

Season to taste with additional salt and/or pepper (if using the sauce straight as a dip or spread or to top vegetables, and so forth, you probably won't need extra seasoning, but if tossing into pasta, you may want to add extra salt to the sauce or add it when mixing with the pasta).

If This Apron Could Talk: When thinning, add the water about a tablespoon at a time, until you achieve the desired consistency. Keep in mind that when using for pasta, you can thin later by adding some pasta cooking water, rather than dilute the sauce when first pureeing it.

If you chill the sauce, it will thicken more as it refrigerates, as the oats continue to absorb any moisture.

Ingredients 411: Place the oats on a baking sheet lined with parchment, and bake in a preheated 425°F oven for 7 to 10 minutes, until golden, tossing once or twice. Watch closely, as the oats can burn quickly.

You can use roasted red peppers from a jar, or roast them yourself; see "Plant-Powered Pantry," page xxxviii. If using jarred peppers, check the ingredients for vinegar. If they are marinated in vinegar, you may want to omit the vinegar altogether, or reduce, adjusting to taste.

Serving Suggestions: Kept thick, this sauce can be used as a spread or dip. It is like a roasted red pepper dip but with more texture and a deeper flavor profile. Try it as a base for your next pizza! It can also be thinned slightly to use as a sauce to kick up unseasoned tofu or beans, and of course, to toss with pasta.

Tomato Artichoke Pasta

SERVES 3 TO 4

wheat gluten soy **FREE**

I make a variation of this dish fairly often. One of the quickest and easiest things to do when you don't know what to cook is get some good olive oil, garlic, and herbs going in a pan, add a few other vegetables of interest, then toss with pasta. My go-to veggies are artichokes and tomatoes (unless sliced fennel gets its way). I love the simplicity of this dish, and rarely measure things when making it, but for the purpose of outlining a recipe, here you have measurement. Get to it!

3 to 4	tablespoons olive oil
6 to 7	large cloves garlic, minced or grated (I use a kitchen grater)
½	teaspoon dried oregano
1	teaspoon dried basil
½	teaspoon sea salt
2 to 3	cups frozen artichokes (see note)
¼	cup white wine (optional)
2½	cups roughly chopped tomatoes
¾ to 1	pound cut whole-grain pasta (e.g., rotini or penne; see "Plant-Powered Pantry," page xxxv)
	Handful of torn fresh basil leaves and/or pitted kalamata olives (optional)
	Coarse salt and freshly ground black pepper, for finishing (optional, but so good!)
1 to 2	tablespoons olive oil, for finishing (optional)

In a large skillet (I use cast iron, but you can use a pot if you don't have a large skillet; see note), combine the 3 to 4 tablespoons of olive oil, garlic, oregano, basil, ½ teaspoon of the salt, pepper, and artichokes. Cook covered over medium-low heat for 6 to 8 minutes to soften the garlic and start to cook the artichokes.

In the meantime, begin cooking the pasta according to the package directions. (Alternatively, this sauce can be partially or fully premade, and then reheated for when you are ready to cook your pasta).

Lower the heat beneath the first pot, if necessary—do not let garlic brown or burn. Add the wine (if using), turn the heat to high to bring to a boil and let bubble for a minute or two. Reduce the heat to medium-low again and add the tomatoes. Cook for 3 to 5 minutes to soften the tomatoes, or cook longer (10 minutes or more) if you don't care for raw tomatoes and prefer them cooked through.

Once the pasta is cooked, drain but leaving a little cooking water clinging to the pasta (do not rinse the pasta!). Add the pasta and basil (if using) into the artichoke mixture and toss. Add coarse salt and/or pepper to taste, if desired. Serve with a little drizzle of olive oil to finish the dish.

If This Apron Could Talk: Your cooking vessel, whether a skillet or pot, should be large enough to hold the cooked artichokes and tomatoes, and then also the cooked pasta, as you will be tossing the pasta with the artichoke mixture after cooking and draining.

Ingredients 411: I love frozen artichokes, and I really love how they encapsulate so much of the seasoning in this pasta dish. When I make this, I can use most of the full bag of artichokes, which is about 3 cups. I like to add them whole, straight from the bag, but my family doesn't feel the artichoke love quite as much as I do! They prefer a little less, and to have them chopped smaller (note that when you chop them smaller, 2 cups chopped equals about 3 cups unchopped). So, you can choose to roughly chop them before adding them to the pan, or add them whole, adjusting the quantity to your own level of artichoke love!

That said, frozen artichokes can be difficult (if not impossible!) to find. Feel free to use canned or marinated (well rinsed to remove their oil) in place of frozen.

Make It More-ish! Have fresh spinach or chard on hand? Chop or julienne, and throw in a couple of handfuls during the last few minutes of cooking (heat through until just wilted but still a vibrant green). You can even use more greens and replace some of the artichokes, if you like.

Protein Power: Adding ¾ to 1 cup of white beans to the sauté will bulk up the pasta, adding more nutrition and substance.

White Sauce

MAKES ABOUT 3½ CUPS

wheat gluten soy **FREE**

Using rice or millet flour as the base for the roux not only gives you a gluten-free white sauce, but also is less likely to clump and get gummy in the cooking process. The sauce is still thick and rich, and delicious tossed into pasta or layered in lasagna noodles.

¼ cup olive oil (reduce to 3 tablespoons, if desired)

5 tablespoons millet flour or rice flour (see note)

¼ cup white wine (optional; see note)

3 to 3½ cups plain unsweetened nondairy milk (almond or soy preferred; see "Plant-Powered Pantry," page xxxiii)

1 to 1¼ teaspoon sea salt (see note)
Freshly ground black pepper
About ⅛ teaspoon freshly grated nutmeg

1 to 2 large cloves garlic (or more, if you love garlic), grated (I use a kitchen grater)

In a medium-size saucepan, whisk the olive oil with the flour over medium heat. Cook, whisking, for a couple of minutes, but don't allow the mixture to burn (lower the heat, if necessary, and don't cook for more than a few minutes).

Lower the heat to low, and while whisking, gradually add the wine and about ½ cup of the milk, until the mixture is smooth and fully blended. Continue to add the milk gradually, about ½ cup at a time, increasing the heat to medium-high and continuing to whisk to keep mixture smooth

Add 1 teaspoon of the salt, and the pepper to taste, nutmeg, and garlic, and bring the mixture to a gentle boiling bubble. Once at a slow bubble, cook for a minute or two, then turn off the heat.

Add extra pepper or salt to taste, if desired. As the mixture cools, whisk occasionally to prevent a skin from forming on top—or cover the surface of the sauce with a piece of lightly oiled parchment paper.

Toss the white sauce into your pasta of choice or layer into lasagna noodles.

Ingredients 411: You can adjust the milk to the desired consistency, using additional milk to thin, if preferred. Add milk to the sauce if using it in a baked casserole, as it will thicken more with baking.

Start with just 1 teaspoon of salt, and then add more to taste, if desired. The amount of salt you might like will depend on the brand of milk used, how much sauce is used in proportion to the pasta, and also your personal taste and brand of salt.

Kid-Friendly: The alcohol in the wine will burn off with cooking, but if you want to make the sauce without the wine, you can do so and it will still be delicious. Simply follow the recipe, omitting the wine and gradually adding ½ to 1 cup of the milk, whisking to incorporate, followed by the remaining milk.

Savvy Subs and Adds: If using rice flour, you can use white or brown. Also, you can use all-purpose gluten-free flour (e.g., Bob's Red Mill) in part. A substitution of 2 to 3 tablespoons of gluten-free flour for 2 to 3 tablespoons of the rice flour is my choice. (Using much more of the gluten-free flour becomes noticeable in flavor.) I enjoy the millet flour version. Spelt flour also works well in this sauce, if gluten isn't a concern.

If you like nutritional yeast, add several tablespoons (or more, to taste) to this sauce—it makes a cheesier sauce that is also very tasty

"Fit-tuccine Alfredo" with Chanterelle Bread Crumb Topping

SERVES 4 TO 5

(optionally) wheat
(optionally) gluten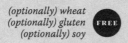
(optionally) soy

Go ahead and ladle on as much sauce as you want with this Alfredo sauce! While it isn't low fat, it is, of course, cholesterol free, and also low in saturated fat. Creamy, thick, luscious . . . ladle away!

SAUCE (SEE NOTE FOR
SOY-FREE VERSION):

½ cup raw cashews (see notes for soy-free version)
2 tablespoons raw pine nuts
2 to 3 tablespoons extra-virgin olive oil
1¼ to 1½ cups plain unsweetened nondairy milk (almond or soy preferred; see "Plant-Powered Pantry," page xxxiii)
1 cup Mori-Nu silken, firm, or extra-firm tofu (this is not one full package, please measure; see note for soy-free version)
½ tablespoon arrowroot powder (see note for soy-free version)
1 teaspoon sea salt
Freshly ground black pepper (generous is good)
1½ teaspoons onion powder
¼ teaspoon (generous) freshly grated nutmeg

FOR SAUTÉ:

1 tablespoon extra-virgin olive oil
4 large cloves garlic, minced or pressed
A few pinches of salt
½ to ¾ cup white wine (see note)

Start to heat the water for your pasta. Preheat the oven to 400°F, if you will be making the optional bread crumb topping.

Prepare the sauce: Place the sauce ingredients in a blender (start with 1¼ cups of the milk) and puree on high until very, very smooth, adding the remaining milk once smooth. Stop to scrape down the blender as needed and puree again until smooth.

Next, prepare the sauté: place the oil in a lidded deep skillet or large pot over medium or medium-low heat. Add the garlic and salt. Cook covered for a few minutes, lowering the heat, if necessary, to prevent the garlic from burning. After a few minutes, add the wine and turn heat to high.

Let the wine simmer for a few minutes, to burn off the alcohol. Then lower heat to medium and add sauce mixture. Whisk the sauce continuously as it heats. Let it come up to a gentle bubble but not a rolling boil; keep uncovered. After a few minutes, once the sauce has thickened, lower the heat to keep the sauce warm until the pasta is ready (alternatively, you can reheat the sauce when ready to cook the pasta). If you'd like a thinner consistency, whisk in the remaining ¼ cup of milk.

PASTA:

¾ to 1 pound dried fettuccine or other noodles (use wheat- or gluten-free versions for those options)

CHANTERELLE BREAD CRUMB TOPPING:

1½ cups dried whole-grain bread crumbs (or use wheat- or gluten-free alternative; see note)

1 (14-ounce) package dried chanterelle mushrooms (see note)

2 teaspoons truffle oil

1½ to 2 teaspoons olive oil

⅛ teaspoon sea salt

Prepare the topping, if using: In a food processor, combine the bread crumbs and dried mushrooms. Process until crumbly. Transfer to a baking sheet lined with parchment paper. Add the oils and salt, and mix well (using your hands is easiest). Bake for 5 minutes, toss, then bake for another 3 to 5 minutes or more, checking at the 3-minute mark to ensure the crumbs aren't burning. Bake until golden brown, checking frequently, as the crumbs will turn from golden brown to burnt quite quickly.

Once the pasta is cooked, drain (don't rinse). You can either serve the pasta in a bowl and top with the sauce, or toss it directly into the sauce in the pot.

Serve topped with extra freshly grated nutmeg and black pepper to taste, and sprinkled with Chanterelle Bread Crumb Topping, if desired. (You will likely have extra bread crumb topping left over; simply refrigerate in a sealed container for another meal.)

Adult-Minded: I like using the full ¾ cup of white wine in the sauce. The alcohol burns off, but you are left with great flavor. However, if you'd prefer less of a pronounced wine taste in the sauce, use just ¼ cup.

Allergy-Free or Bust! For soy-free adaptation of this recipe, omit the silken tofu and add these ingredients to the sauce mixture: another ⅓ cup of cashews (for ½ cup + ⅓ cup total), another 1 cup of milk (for 2¼ cups total), and another ½ tablespoon of arrowroot (for 1 tablespoon total).

Ingredients 411: See above notes to make a soy-free version of this sauce. With the soy (silken tofu) version, the sauce will be thicker and opaque . . . but the taste is fantastic, either way! If using the silken tofu, opt for the regular firm or extra-firm varieties, not the "lite."

I have tried different varieties of dried mushrooms and find chanterelles work the best. Dried oyster mushrooms are too tough and don't process well; dried portobellos process well but make bread crumbs that are quite dark and burn easily. But you can experiment with other mushrooms, if you like. Or you can omit the mushrooms and use the truffle and olive oils to add a beautiful aroma to your bread crumbs.

Make your own bread crumbs (and use up any heels of bread) by processing slices in a food processor until finely ground. Use your bread of choice—whole grain, wheat free, gluten free, and so on. If you want a really crunchy topping, use store-bought dried bread crumbs.

Mac-oh-geez!

SERVES 4

(optionally) wheat
(optionally) gluten
soy **FREE**

This is comfort food. A macaroni 'n' cheese type of casserole, this dish is made *without* tofu or cheese substitutes. The sauce is creamy, rich, and luscious, and has a crunchy bread crumb topping (like my mom used to make). Indeed, this is *gooood* comfort food.

3 to 3½ cups dried cut pasta (e.g., macaroni, penne; I use brown rice pasta; see "Plant-Powered Pantry," page xxxv; see note) (about 10 ounces dried)

SAUCE:
1½ cups plain unsweetened nondairy milk (almond or soy preferred; see "Plant-Powered Pantry," page xxxiii)
¾ cup raw cashews (see note for nut-free version)
½ cup raw Brazil nuts or raw almonds
3 tablespoons freshly squeezed lemon juice
1 medium clove garlic
2 teaspoons arrowroot powder
1 teaspoon sea salt
½ teaspoon onion powder
¼ teaspoon (rounded) dry mustard
1 cup water
2 tablespoons extra-virgin olive oil (you can reduce or omit, but it does add richness)

Preheat the oven to 375°F. Lightly oil an 8 by 12-inch baking dish

Start cooking the pasta.

Meanwhile, prepare the sauce: Starting with about ½ cup of the milk, blend all the sauce ingredients in a blender until very, very smooth (may take a few minutes in a standard blender). Add the remaining 1 cup of the milk and blend again.

Once the pasta is almost tender, fully drain (don't rinse). Mix the noodles with the sauce and immediately pour into the prepared baking dish. (It will look like there is a lot of runny sauce—it will thicken up, really; trust the pasta!)

BREAD CRUMB TOPPING (OPTIONAL):

½ to 1 cup dried whole-grain bread crumbs (or use wheat- or gluten-free alternative; see note)

½ to 1 tablespoon olive oil

A few pinches of sea salt

Prepare the topping: Mix the topping ingredients in a small bowl, then sprinkle over the top of the casserole.

Cover the casserole with foil and bake for 17 to 18 minutes. Then remove the foil and bake for another 5 to 7 minutes, or until the topping is golden brown and crisped. Don't over-bake, or the sauce will get thick, and will continue to thicken as it stands.

Remove from the oven and place the casserole on a hot plate (rather than on top of the oven, because the residual heat from the oven will continue to thicken the sauce). Serve!

Allergy-Free or Bust! When our baby was about a year old, I created a nut-free version of this dish, replacing the nuts with tahini, along with a few other changes. For this tahini version, substitute ½ cup of tahini for the nuts. Increase the arrowroot to 1 tablespoon and add 3 tablespoons of nutritional yeast, ¾ teaspoon of agave nectar, and 1 teaspoon of roughly chopped fresh rosemary.

If This Apron Could Talk: This may not seem like a lot of pasta . . . but once it cooks and soaks up some of the sauce, this dish makes enough to happily serve four. I usually stick to about a 3¼-cup measure (as I love the saucy stuff)! You can use up to 3½-cup measure, but I highly recommend stopping there! . . . You'll lose out on the sauce and instead will have a dry casserole.

This casserole can be made in advance. After combining the pasta and sauce and transferring to a baking dish, cover with foil. When ready to bake, sprinkle with the bread crumbs and re-cover with foil. When baking, allow another couple of minutes for the casserole to heat through.

If you have leftovers, place in a heatproof dish. Drizzle in a touch of nondairy milk to remoisten the mixture. Cover with foil and bake until heated through, then remove the foil for a couple of minutes to crisp up the topping again.

Ingredients 411: Make your own bread crumbs (and use up any heels of bread) by processing slices in a food processor until finely ground. Use your bread of choice—whole grain, wheat free, gluten free, and so on. If you want a really crunchy topping, use store-bought dried bread crumbs. If you like lots of that bread-y kind of topping, use the full 1 cup, but if you like more of the saucy stuff (like me), use just ½ to ¾ cup. Or divvy the bread crumbs over the top of the casserole to please family members—less on one side, more on the other!

Baked Macaroni with Broccolini in a Creamy Walnut Gravy

SERVES 4 TO 5

(optionally) wheat
(optionally) gluten **FREE**

This casserole makes broccolini (or broccoli) comfort food. Macaroni is baked with blanched broccolini in a creamy "gravy" made from toasted walnuts, and topped off with bread crumbs. Just make it!

1 to 1½	tablespoons olive oil
¾	cup chopped onions
3	medium to large cloves garlic, chopped roughly
¼	teaspoon (rounded) sea salt
	Freshly ground black pepper (fairly generous is good)
3	tablespoons millet flour (see note)
1	cup vegan vegetable stock (see "Plant-Powered Pantry," page xlii)
1¾	cups plain unsweetened nondairy milk (almond or soy preferred; see "Plant-Powered Pantry," page xxxiii)
1½	cups walnuts (toasted is good for flavor)
1	tablespoon tamari
1	teaspoon vegan Worcestershire sauce (omit or use gluten-free vegan Worcestershire for a wheat- or gluten-free version)
½	teaspoon dried sage
½	teaspoon Dijon mustard
2¾ to 3	cups dried brown rice macaroni (or other cut pasta of choice; see "Plant-Powered Pantry," page xxxv and note)
2½	cups broccolini or broccoli, tough stems trimmed, tender stems and florets cut into bite-size pieces

Preheat the oven to 375°F and lightly oil an 8 by 12-inch (or similar size) baking dish.

In a saucepan over medium or medium-low heat, combine the oil, onion, garlic, salt, and pepper. Lower the heat, if necessary, to prevent the garlic from burning. Cover and cook for 7 to 9 minutes, until the onion is softened and translucent. Remove the cover, add the flour, and stir. Cook for just 2 to 3 minutes to cook flour slightly (to remove the raw flour taste).

Add the stock, and whisk to incorporate. Add 1½ cups of the milk, still whisking, and then the walnuts, tamari, Worcestershire, sage, and mustard). Whisk again but turn off heat (so the mixture isn't too hot before blending).

Transfer the mixture to a blender and puree until very smooth, then transfer back to the saucepan. Use the remaining ¼ cup of milk to rinse all of the remaining sauce from the blender and add to the saucepan. Bring to a low boil over medium-high heat, stirring frequently, until thickened (3 to 5 minutes). Once thickened, remove from the heat and pour ¾ to 1 cup into the bottom of the prepared baking dish, reserving the rest of the gravy.

Meanwhile, in another pot, cook the macaroni, according to the package directions, until almost tender. Add the broccolini and cook for just 1 minute more. Remove the broccolini and drain (using a colander or sieve) and then set aside to top the casserole (see note). Then drain the pasta.

Transfer the macaroni to the baking dish. Toss the broccolini into the reserved gravy, and then top the pasta with the mixture, making sure to scrape out all that delectable sauce and get it into the dish (use another 1 to 2 tablespoons of milk, if needed, to loosen the sauce, seriously, get all the sauce)!

BREAD CRUMB TOPPING:

½ to ¾ cup whole-grain bread crumbs
(use wheat-free or gluten-free for
that option; see note)
A few pinches of sea salt

½ to 1 tablespoon olive oil

Prepare the topping: In a separate bowl, combine the bread crumbs with the salt and olive oil. Sprinkle over the macaroni. Cover the dish with aluminum foil and bake for 15 to 18 minutes, then remove the foil and bake for another 5 to 8 minutes, to crisp up the bread crumb topping.

Remove from the oven and let cool for about 5 minutes, then serve in portions.

If This Apron Could Talk: It is an attractive presentation to drain the broccolini separately from the pasta and then layer it on top of the pasta. However, for a shortcut, feel free to drain everything at once, and simply top the combined macaroni and broccolini with the gravy and bread crumbs.

This casserole is saucier with less pasta, so don't go past a 3-cup measure for best results.

Ingredients 411: Make your own bread crumbs (and use up any heels of bread) by processing slices in a food processor until finely ground. Use your bread of choice—whole grain, wheat free, gluten free, and so on. If you want a really crunchy topping, use store-bought dried bread crumbs.

Savvy Subs and Adds: I like the consistency of millet flour, but you can also use whole wheat pastry flour or spelt flour.

White Bean Sweet Potato Pasta Sauce

SERVES 3 TO 4

wheat gluten soy **FREE**

This sauce is thick and sumptuous without being too rich or oily, and it can be made with or without the wine.

2	tablespoons olive oil
3	large cloves garlic, chopped roughly
½	teaspoon dried oregano
½ to ¾	teaspoon sea salt
	Freshly ground black pepper
¼	cup white wine (optional; if not using wine, simply add extra water later)
1½	cups cooked yellow-flesh sweet potato (see note)
2	cups cooked navy or cannellini (white kidney) beans (drained and rinsed if using canned)
1	cup vegan vegetable stock (see "Plant-Powered Pantry," page xlii)
½ to ¾	cup water (to thin as desired, using extra if not using wine)
1½	teaspoon chopped fresh thyme
	A few pinches of freshly grated nutmeg
1 to 1½	tablespoons freshly squeezed lemon juice
¾ to 1	pound whole-grain pasta of choice (see "Plant-Powered Pantry," page xxxv)
	Extra olive oil, for finishing (optional)

In a pot, combine the 2 tablespoons of olive oil, garlic, oregano, ½ teaspoon of the salt, and the pepper to taste. Cook covered over low or medium-low heat for 4 to 6 minutes, to soften the garlic.

In the meantime, begin cooking the pasta according to the package directions. Alternatively, this sauce can be partially or fully premade, and then reheated when you are ready to cook your pasta.

Lower the heat, if necessary—do not let the garlic brown or burn. Remove the cover, add the wine (if using), turn heat to high to bring to a boil, and let bubble for a minute or two. Add the sweet potato, white beans, vegetable stock, and ½ cup of the water.

Turn off the heat, and with an immersion blender, puree the mixture in the pot until very smooth. Turn on the heat to medium again and cook for 7 to 10 minutes, or until heated through. Add the thyme, nutmeg, and lemon juice and stir. To finish, you can add another 1 to 2 tablespoons of olive oil (for a richer flavor; you can omit), allowing it to warm for several minutes. Add an extra ¼ teaspoon or more of salt to taste (note that the sauce may need more seasoning once tossed with the pasta), and thin out with additional water, if preferred. Alternatively, you can reserve about ½ cup of the pasta water to use to thin the sauce.

Serve over or tossed with the pasta.

Ingredients 411: I cook the sweet potato in advance by baking it whole in the oven. Simply scrub the potato, leaving the peel intact, and place on a baking sheet lined with parchment. Bake in a 400°F oven for 45 to 60 minutes, until tender throughout (the time depends on the size of the potato). You can substitute orange-fleshed sweet potato in this recipe, but I prefer it with the yellow-fleshed kind. Just don't substitute standard white potatoes.

Kid-Friendly: This sauce works well in a baked pasta casserole. Simply cook your pasta of choice (3 to 3½ cups dried) and then toss with the sauce. Top with bread crumbs and a sprinkle of vegan cheese, if you like. Also, it can be layered with lasagna noodles, with other fillings such as cashew cheese or roasted vegetables.

9 C Is for Cookie, That's Good Enough for Me

I love to create cookie recipes—so much that this book could well have been a cookie cookbook. My cookie journey started with one simple (now signature) recipe: my Homestyle Chocolate Chip Cookies from *Vive le Vegan!* I was intent on making a vegan cookie taste really freaking good—and good it was! Here, I've made them even better, using whole-grain flours that are wheat free and gluten free. (Look for the wheat-free and gluten-free designations.) And they are healthier, using alternative sweeteners—and for most cookies, less of these sweeteners—as well as less oil, than do other cookie recipes, vegan or otherwise.

Chocolate lovers can look forward to decadent treats such as Triple-Threat Chocolate Coconut Macaroons, Terry's Chocolate Orange Cookies, and Double Chocolate Chippers—and that's just a few of the drop cookies! To please nonchocolate cravings, there are Lemon Cranberry Cornmeal Cookies, Snifferdoodles, Kamut Hazelnut Cookies, and Matcha Green Tea Pistachio Biscotti—and more. When the holidays roll around, pull out your flours for Gingerbread Folks, Sugar Cutout Cookies, Almond Cardamom Toffee Cookies, and Gingery Cookies . . . not that you can't include some chocolaty offerings for your festive parties—by all means, do!

Cookie bars aren't left out: Cream Cheese Brownies with Salted Dark Chocolate Topping will knock your socks off! Or maybe you're a caramel-and-chocolate combo kind of girl like me . . . get to "Hello Vegan" Bars, and quick! Find a soft spot for goji berries with Chocolate Goji Macadamia Crispy Squares, and then sit your toosh back and relax in a berry patch . . . gather just enough of those berries to make Berry Patch Brownies and some Fresh Blueberry Oat Squares.

I've even added some raw options, and Award-Winning Frosted B-raw-nies might be your new favorite brownie recipe (ever!). But don't let them keep you from making Raw Banana Nut Squares with Coconut Cream Cheese Frosting, Raw Chocolate Truffles, and Raw Chai Bars.

Good enough for me. Good enough for you, too!

Note: If this is your first outing with vegan baked goods, don't panic! Check out the "Plant-Powered Baking Notes," which follow.

Plant-Powered Baking Notes

Vegan baking is one of the most misunderstood components of eating vegan. The perception is that one simply cannot bake without eggs—or butter! Well, yes you can! And not only is it healthier and cruelty free—it's often easier.

There are some tricks to the vegan baking trade, and others specific to my own style of baking, which is without white flour and usually wheat free . . . and, for most recipes, with only minimal added fat.

Baking Procedures

Ingredient Preparation: As with cooking, preparation is key for your baking. That is, read the recipe through first, and place your ingredients at your fingertips. Just as you are pulling out your flours and sweet-

eners, you might realize you are running low. Better to be prepared than a frustrated baker!

Pan Preparation: To make it even easier to remove your cakes from your pans, after wiping a little oil inside your pans, cut a piece of parchment to put in the bottom of each. If it's a round cake pan, insert a round piece to roughly fit the bottom of the pan, and placing it in after a light wipe of oil. It doesn't have to be perfectly round, or even the exact size, just a roughly cut circle placed in the bottom. For other pans, such as loaf and brownie pans, you can also place strips of parchment to cover the bottom and up one direction of the pan, for easier removal of your baked good after cooling.

Measuring and Mixing: When measuring dry ingredients, lightly scoop them into your measuring cup or spoon and then level off with your finger or a butter knife. I also measure wet ingredients in standard measuring cups (rather than glass). I find it easier to judge the measurement, rather than trying to get the eye-level line on a glass measuring cup. I have always baked this way, and find it more convenient.

Mix your dry ingredients separately from your wet ingredients, unless the recipe specifies otherwise. Then the wet mixture is typically blended into the dry mixture (again, unless otherwise stated). When adding wet to dry, it is important to mix until you have fully incorporated the ingredients, activating the leavening agents and any glutens in the flours. But it's also important not to overmix the batter as it can become tough, especially if using more gluten-rich flours such as spelt and barley—and especially wheat. Nongluten mixes are far more forgiving, and you may find them easier to work with than their gluten-based counterparts (this was very true for me when making the Gluten-Free Piecrust in the next chapter).

Egg Replacers: People are really perplexed by the idea of not using eggs in baking. And when I'm asked how to replace eggs, I'm sometimes perplexed to answer, because with most recipes it's really not that hard and I don't even need to think about having to make something work to replace the X number of eggs that should be in the recipe! In fact, for most recipes, a little baking powder and/or baking soda do the trick just fine for leavening. If binding is needed, sometimes the natural gluten in the flours do the job; other times, a little pureed fruit or xanthan gum step in.

Still, there are some recognized egg replacers in vegan baking, and here are a few:

Flax meal: Helps provide structure and tenderness to a recipe, particularly useful in muffins and quick breads, and some cookies. When combined with a liquid such as water or nondairy milk, flax meal becomes gelatinous, or "eggy." The general rule is to mix 1 tablespoon of flax meal with 3 tablespoons of liquid, to be the equivalent of one "egg." It is helpful to allow the mixture to sit for a few minutes to become "eggy" before using it. Whole flaxseeds can

be ground to make flax meal yourself, or you can buy it (I use Bob's Red Mill brand) in the refrigerated section of the grocery store. Whether store-bought or homemade, ensure that it is stored at home in the freezer. It does not need to be thawed before using.

Ground white chia Seeds: Ground chia (see "Plant-Powered Pantry," page xxvii) is very effective in giving that eggy structure to baked goods, similar to flax meal. It is denser and more absorbent than flax meal, and I have found that you can typically use less ground chia than the amount of ground flax meal that is called for. For instance, if a recipe lists 2 tablespoons of ground flax meal, 1 to 1½ tablespoons of ground chia will probably do just fine.

Nondairy yogurts: Once upon a time, only soy yogurts were available, and many weren't very good. Now we have coconut-, almond-, and rice-based yogurts in addition to soy varieties, and they have improved in taste and texture. (Also see the recipe for my cashew-based Vanilla Yogurt, which can be used in my recipes as an alternative to store-bought yogurts.) Nondairy yogurts offer moisture and tenderness to baked goods, and are especially useful in cake and cupcake recipes, and muffins and quick breads. Vanilla or plain varieties are usually the choice, and in general, ¼ cup of soy yogurt replaces one egg.

Silken tofu, pureed: I rarely use silken tofu as an egg replacer, though it is well known and used. I prefer to use pureed fruit or nondairy yogurt as a substitute. I find it tedious to puree a small amount of silken tofu for a recipe—plus sometimes the remainder is wasted. If you do wish to use it, as with soy yogurt, ¼ cup blended silken tofu replaces one egg.

Applesauce or pureed banana: These are two of my favorite egg replacers because they are easy, nonallergenic for most people, and add natural flavor and sweetness to baked goods. They do wonders to add moisture and stability, and also help reduce the amount of oil you need to add to a recipe. Typically, ¼ cup of applesauce or pureed bananas replaces one egg, but I usually add more for muffin or quick bread recipes for flavor and sweetness. I prefer to puree bananas (with an immersion blender and deep cup) over mashing. The texture is smoother and more consistent. But, for most recipes mashing the bananas with a fork will do the trick, too. Other fruit purees, such as pureed canned pumpkin or pumpkin pie mix, are also sometimes used.

Baking soda or baking powder, with an acid: Many vegan dessert and baking recipes use either baking soda, or a combination of baking soda and baking powder together with an acid such as citrus juice, vinegar, applesauce, or even molasses or regular unsweetened cocoa powder. These acidic elements react with the alkaline baking soda, creating air bubbles that leaven, or lighten and lift, the batter. The addition of baking powder, once it becomes wet in a batter and then heated, produces air bubbles, allowing the batter to rise better. Sometimes a recipe requires nothing more than a little extra baking powder for leavening. Be sure to use a nonaluminium baking powder.

Xanthan gum: Although xanthan gum is more obscure than the other egg replacers listed here, it's a marvelous ingredient for wheat-free and especially gluten-free baking. Xanthan gum is a natural vegan starch made from a fermentation process, and can be purchased in health food stores. In addition to help bind ingredients, it also works well in frostings and puddings to provide structure without adding other starches, or more important, without adding shortenings and/or extra sugar. It doesn't need heat to thicken, and a little goes a very long way.

Wheat- and Gluten-Free Baking

I bake wheat free because I like it. We don't have wheat or gluten intolerances intolerances in our family. But when I began baking with more healthful ingredients, moving away from white flour to whole wheat flour, I soon had people asking for wheat-free options. Once I began experimenting with other flours such as spelt and oat, I preferred their taste and texture, even if some extra testing was required.

For this book, I had more people asking for gluten-free recipes, so I have done my best to offer a balance of both wheat-free and gluten-free recipes.

The distinction between wheat free and gluten free is sometimes blurred, and can be confusing. And the idea of baking without wheat or gluten—along with no dairy or eggs—well, that just sounds ridiculous! But wheat-free baking is fairly uncomplicated with some relatively simple substitutions required for the more common all-purpose or whole wheat flours. Gluten-free baking becomes a little trickier, and can require more tweaking and testing to get the results "just right."

So, what's the difference between wheat free and gluten free? Flours (and grains) that are wheat free *but not gluten free* include:

- barley
- kamut
- oats (see note)
- rye
- spelt

While spelt and kamut are ancient grain relatives to wheat, they are a different grain and so are often tolerated by people that cannot eat common forms of wheat.

Gluten is a protein that is found in wheat and also the aforementioned grains. Gluten provides elasticity, and also offers binding to baked goods. Wheat-free, gluten-free grains and starches include:

- amaranth
- arrowroot
- buckwheat
- corn
- millet
- oats (see note)
- potato
- quinoa
- rice
- sorghum
- tapioca
- wild rice

Nut flours, including almond meal and coconut flour, can also be used in gluten-free baking.

The wheat-free flours I use most are spelt, oat, and barley, often in combination, but sometimes on their own. Spelt is one of my favorite flours as it usually substitutes well for wheat flours with just a few minor adjustments. In my experience, when substituting spelt flour, you will need slightly more than the wheat flour measurement. For instance, when 1 cup of all-purpose wheat flour is listed, I substitute 1 cup + 2 to 4 tablespoons of spelt (usually the full 1¼ cups for cookies; 1 cup + 2 tablespoons for cakes, but it varies from recipe to recipe). So, if you want to "de-wheat" your own recipes, keep this measurement conversion in mind. Oat flour is also one of my favorites because it has that naturally sweet "oaty" flavor, a delicate texture and creamy color.

You will notice that some of my recipes specify "light or sifted spelt flour," typically finer baked goods such as cookies and cakes where a lighter final product is desirable. I can purchase spelt flour presifted, which is helpful because it has a lighter and finer texture, and it helps to remove any coarse bits that might lurk in the flour. Look for light or sifted spelt flours in your stores, and if you are only able to find regular whole-grain spelt flour, sift it through a fine sieve and then discard the grainier remnants. Otherwise, if a recipe simply states "spelt flour" (usually heartier baked recipes such as muffins), you can use regular whole-grain spelt flour (e.g.: Bob's Red Mill) or use light or sifted flour, your choice.

I enjoy the ease spelt, barley, and oat flours offer when mixing batters (they don't get overworked as easily as wheat flour–based recipes) and prefer the taste and texture of the final product. While these flours are certainly more expensive than common wheat flour, if you need to make wheat-free changes in your diet, the reality is that most alternative flours are pricier than their mass-produced wheat counterpart.

Gluten-free baking is not quite as simple. Because no gluten is present to help bind the batters, help is needed from stabilizers and binders such as xanthan gum. Gluten-free baking requires a lot of trials and testing to get the right mix of flours (e.g., some combination of millet flour, rice flour, tapioca starch flour, and/or sorghum flour) and also stabilizers and other elements. If you don't feel like exploring the correct balance of gluten-free flours for your beloved recipes, you can instead experiment with commercial gluten-free flour mixes (e.g., Bob's Red Mill gluten-free all-purpose flour). Be sure to follow the guidelines for including xanthan gum or other stabilizers in the recipe, for best results.

Ingredients 411: Oats require clarification. There are certified gluten-free oat products available, such as rolled oats and oat flour. Most people with gluten-free allergies or intolerances can use these gluten-free oat products. Some cannot. In my recipes, I considered the majority and have designated recipes as having a gluten-free option if certified gluten-free oat products are used. Obviously, if you cannot eat gluten-free oats, these recipes will not be suitable for you.

Triple-Threat Chocolate Coconut Macaroons

MAKES 13 TO 15 SMALLISH MACAROONS

*wheat
gluten* **FREE**
soy

These cookies are out-of-this world good! They are chewy and moist, and rich and chocolaty. They are especially good just warm after baking, but if they do make it to your fridge, they'll still be fantastically delicious. Another bonus: As there is no flour in this recipe, these are naturally gluten free!

½   cup vegan dark chocolate chips
1   teaspoon organic extra-virgin coconut oil, at room temperature (see "Plant-Powered Pantry," page xxix)
1⅛ cups unsweetened fine- or medium-shred coconut (check label to ensure sulfite free; see note)
¼   cup unrefined sugar
⅛   teaspoon sea salt
¼   cup unsweetened cocoa powder
1¼ teaspoons baking powder
3   tablespoons vanilla nondairy yogurt (see note)
1   teaspoon pure vanilla extract
2   tablespoons vegan chocolate chips (small chips are great)

Preheat the oven to 350°F. Line a baking sheet with parchment paper.

Melt the ½ cup of dark chocolate chips with the coconut oil in a bowl fitted over a saucepan of simmering (not boiling) water. Stir until just melted and the coconut oil is incorporated into the chocolate. Remove the mixture from the heat and allow to cool.

Meanwhile, in a bowl, combine the coconut, sugar, and salt, sifting in the cocoa powder and baking powder. Then stir in the yogurt, vanilla, and melted chocolate. Mix well; the batter should be thick but moist. Add the ⅛ cup of chocolate chips and stir. Chill for 5 to 7 minutes.

Take about 1 rounded tablespoon of the batter and roll in your hands. Place on the prepared baking sheet (don't flatten). Repeat with the remaining batter. Bake for 11 minutes.

Remove from the oven, let cool on the pan for 3 to 4 minutes, then transfer to a cooling rack.

If This Apron Could Talk: These cookies are quite soft and almost fragile after baking. Be sure to let them cool for several minutes on the baking sheet before transferring to a cooling rack. The cookies will firm up after cooling—and particularly so after refrigeration.

Ingredients 411: I use either Bob's Red Mill medium-shred coconut or Let's Do . . . Organic finely shredded coconut. If the coconut has a larger shred, the macaroons will not hold together well. Also, if using a fine shred, you'll notice that the batter is much denser than when made with a medium shred. With a fine shred (e.g., Let's Do . . . Organic), you can measure a touch on the scant side; even 1 cup plus 1 tablespoon will do.

Berry- and fruit-flavored yogurts do not taste great in this recipe, vanilla yogurt works best. Use coconut- or almond-based yogurts for a soy-free option, or you can use my Vanilla Yogurt.

Terry's Chocolate Orange Cookies

MAKES 14 TO 16 COOKIES

wheat soy **FREE**

As a child, we would often get Terry's chocolate oranges for Christmas. That combination of chocolate with citrus has always been a favorite of mine—and it works equally well in a cookie. These are also just a little less sweet, so the chocolate and orange flavors really stand out. I like to make these cookies just a touch bigger than my other drop cookies—more deliciousness per cookie!

¼ cup organic extra-virgin coconut oil, at room temperature

¼ cup brown rice syrup

2 to 3 tablespoons freshly squeezed orange juice

¼ cup unrefined sugar

½ teaspoon pure vanilla extract

¼ teaspoon orange oil (optional; or use about ½ teaspoon additional orange zest)

1¼ cups light or sifted spelt flour, or barley flour

¼ cup unsweetened cocoa powder

1 teaspoon orange zest

1 teaspoon baking powder

¼ teaspoon baking soda

¼ teaspoon sea salt

3 to 4 tablespoons vegan chocolate chips

CHOCOLATE DRIZZLE TOPPING (OPTIONAL):

¼ cup vegan chocolate chips

Preheat the oven to 350°F. Line a baking sheet with parchment paper.

In a mixer fitted with the paddle attachment, beat the coconut oil and brown rice syrup on low speed for just a half minute or so until mixed, and then add 2 tablespoons of the orange juice and the sugar, vanilla, and orange oil. Mix well on low speed.

In a separate bowl, combine the flour, cocoa, orange zest, baking powder, baking soda, salt, and chips. Mix, then add half of the dry mixture. Mix on low speed to incorporate with the wet ingredients, then add the remaining dry mixture. Mix on low speed for just about a minute, until the dough comes together and is forming a ball on the paddle. (The batter should be moist with just 2 tablespoons of juice, but if it is dry and not coming together, add more of the orange juice, 1 teaspoon at a time, just until it comes together). Place the bowl in the refrigerator for about 20 minutes to chill.

Scoop large spoonfuls of the batter (about 1½ tablespoons each; a cookie scoop works very well, but isn't essential) and place on the prepared baking sheet. Bake for 11 minutes.

Remove from the oven, let cool on the pan for about a minute, then transfer to a cooling rack.

Prepare the optional chocolate drizzle: Melt the chocolate in a bowl fitted over a saucepan of simmering (not boiling) water. Once melted, use a spoon to drizzle the chocolate over the cooled cookies (it is helpful to place them back on the parchment-lined baking sheet, to catch the drips).

Chocolate Cornmeal Cookies

MAKES 12 TO 14
MEDIUM-SIZE COOKIES

wheat
gluten **FREE**
soy

Who says that gluten-free cookies can't be ridiculously tasty? The cornmeal gives these a nubbly crunch that makes these irresistible!

⅓ cup corn flour or finely stone-ground cornmeal (see "Plant-Powered Pantry," page xxix)

⅓ cup millet flour

¼ cup unrefined sugar

¼ teaspoon sea salt

3 tablespoons unsweetened cocoa powder

3 tablespoons tapioca starch flour

1 teaspoon baking powder

¼ teaspoon baking soda

¾ teaspoon xanthan gum

A few pinches of freshly grated nutmeg (see note)

¼ cup vegan chocolate chips (see note)

3 tablespoons pure maple syrup

2 tablespoons brown rice syrup

1 teaspoon pure vanilla extract

2½ to 3 tablespoons organic canola, almond, or avocado oil

Preheat the oven to 350°F. Line a baking sheet with parchment paper.

In a bowl, combine the dry ingredients (including the chips), sifting in the cocoa powder, tapioca starch flour, baking powder, baking soda, and xanthan gum, and stirring well.

In another bowl, combine the maple syrup, brown rice syrup, vanilla, and then the 2½ tablespoons of the oil, stirring well. Add the wet mixture to the dry, mixing to fully incorporate, working in the remaining ½ tablespoon of oil a little at a time, if needed. The batter should be thick and cohesive and not dry or powdery, but also not oily.

Place spoonfuls of the batter (1 to 1½ tablespoons each) on the prepared baking sheet. Bake for 11 minutes.

Remove from the oven, let cool on the pan for no longer than a minute, then transfer to a cooling rack.

Savvy Subs and Adds: The taste of nutmeg is faint in these cookies, but I enjoy the extra flavor element it contributes. Some other options include adding 1 to 1½ teaspoons of orange zest (or you can use an orange-flavored dark chocolate bar, broken up, instead of the plain chocolate chips), 1 teaspoon of lemon zest, or ½ teaspoon of almond extract for a light cherry flavor. You can also add some chopped nuts, such as almonds or walnuts.

Chocolate Cherry Pecan Cookies

MAKES 12 TO 14
MEDIUM-SIZE COOKIES

wheat
soy **FREE**

These cookies combine that classic homemade chocolate chip cookie flavor with chewy dried cherries and crunchy, buttery pecans! You will have a hard time believing that these tasty morsels have no dairy, eggs, or wheat.

1	cup + 3 tablespoons spelt flour (see note)
¼	cup unrefined sugar
¼	teaspoon sea salt
¼ to ⅓	cup vegan chocolate chips
¼	cup lightly crushed or chopped pecans
1	teaspoon baking powder
¼	teaspoon baking soda
⅓	cup pure maple syrup
1	teaspoon pure vanilla extract
¾ to 1	teaspoon almond extract (see note)
¼	cup neutral-flavored oil (see "Plant-Powered Pantry," page xxxii)
¼	cup dried unsulfured cherries, sliced in half

Preheat the oven to 350°F. Line a baking sheet with parchment paper.

In a bowl, combine the dry ingredients (including the chips and pecans), sifting in the baking powder and baking soda, mixing well.

In a separate bowl, combine the maple syrup with the vanilla and almond extracts, then mix in the oil and cherries. Add the wet mixture to the dry, and stir until just incorporated (do not overmix).

Place small scoops of the batter, 1 to 1½ tablespoons (a cookie scoop is easiest) on the prepared baking sheet and flatten a little. Bake for 11 minutes, until just golden (if you bake for much longer, they will dry out).

Remove from the oven, let cool on the pan for just a minute (again, to prevent drying), then transfer to a cooling rack.

Ingredients 411: Look for a sifted spelt flour, or sift yourself through a fine sieve to remove any grainy textures. You can use whole wheat pastry flour, if you prefer. You will need less flour, though, about 1 slightly scant cup (about 1 cup less ½ to 1 tablespoon).

The almond extract echoes the flavor of the dried cherries. If you aren't overly keen on almond extract, try these cookies with just ½ or ¾ teaspoon the first time round.

Make It More-ish! These make a great base for a really special dessert treat: ice-cream cookie sandwiches. Using two cookies that have been completely cooled in the refrigerator, spread some softened nondairy ice cream on the underside of one cookie, then place the other cookie on top. Wrap in plastic wrap and freeze until firm!

Double Chocolate Chippers

MAKES 14 TO 18 COOKIES

wheat
soy **FREE**

This is a standard wheat-free recipe for a double chocolate chip cookie that you can play with to embellish as you like. For instance, you can replace some or all of the dark chocolate chips with vegan white chips, add chunks of vegan chocolate instead of chips, and add toasted chopped nuts such as pecans, walnuts, or almonds.

1¼ cups light or sifted spelt flour
¼ cup unsweetened cocoa powder
3 tablespoons unrefined sugar
¼ to ⅓ cup vegan chocolate chips (use combination of dark and white chips, if you like)
¼ teaspoon salt
1 teaspoon baking powder
¼ teaspoon baking soda
¼ cup + 1 tablespoon pure maple syrup (scant ⅓ cup)
1½ teaspoons pure vanilla extract
¼ cup neutral-flavored oil (see "Plant-Powered Pantry," page xxxii)

Preheat the oven to 350°F. Line a baking sheet with parchment paper.

In a bowl, combine the dry ingredients (including the chips or your substitute of choice) in the baking powder and baking soda, and mix well.

In a separate bowl, combine the maple syrup with the vanilla, then stir in the oil until well mixed. Add the wet mixture to the dry, and stir until just incorporated.

Place spoonfuls of the batter (about 1 tablespoon) on the prepared baking sheet and flatten a little. Bake for 11 to 12 minutes (11 minutes if cookies are smaller, 12 if they are larger).

Remove from the oven, let cool on the pan for a minute (not much longer, to prevent drying), then transfer to a cooling rack.

If This Apron Could Talk: If cookie batter is dry when mixing, add another teaspoon of maple syrup plus 1 teaspoon of oil and incorporate. The batter should be thick and somewhat moist (but not too oily), so go easy with adding extra oil.

Troll Cookies

MAKES 11 TO 13 COOKIES

wheat soy

If you have kids, you know the challenge of nonvegan treats at school. This recipe originated when our daughter's class was doing a fairy tale–themed baking week. She brought the recipes home and we veganized them. This one's the best of the bunch. Watch out; these cookies will have you trolling back to the refrigerator for another sneaky nibble!

¼ cup spelt flour

1 cup rolled oats

3 tablespoons unrefined sugar

⅛ teaspoon (rounded) sea salt

2 tablespoons vegan chocolate chips

¾ teaspoon baking powder

¼ cup natural peanut butter (see note)

1 tablespoon organic extra-virgin coconut oil, at room temperature (see "Plant-Powered Pantry," page xxix)

2 tablespoons flax meal, or 1½ tablespoons ground white chia seeds

¼ cup mashed ripe banana (not too overripe, just yellow with some brown flecks)

2 to 2½ tablespoons pure maple syrup or agave nectar

1 teaspoon pure vanilla extract

Preheat the oven to 350°F. Line a baking sheet with parchment paper.

In a bowl, combine the dry ingredients (including the chips), sifting in the baking powder. Stir well.

In another bowl, first combine the peanut butter with the coconut oil, stirring to fully integrate the oil and mix well. Then add the flax meal, banana, 2 tablespoons of the maple syrup, and the vanilla and stir. Add the wet mixture to the dry, stirring until just incorporated. (The batter should come together with 2 tablespoons of sweetener, but if not, add the extra ½ tablespoon or more; see note).

Place spoonfuls of the batter (about 1 tablespoon each) on the prepared baking sheet. Bake for 11 to 12 minutes, until the cookies are set to the touch (they will firm more with cooling).

Remove from the oven, let cool on the pan for a minute or two, then transfer to a cooling rack.

Allergy-Free or Bust! Try a nut butter such as cashew or almond, if peanut allergies are present.

Ingredients 411: Sometimes the texture of peanut butter varies. You may have one that is thin and another that is thicker and drier. Also, the butter bottom of the jar tends to be much drier, even if you've stirred after opening the jar. If your peanut butter is dry, you may need a touch more maple syrup to help bring the batter together, and/or use a scant measure of the oats.

Savvy Subs and Adds: These cookies have a soft, slightly sticky texture, rather than being crispy-chewy. For additional crunch in the cookie, try using chunky peanut butter.

Krispie Chip Cookies

MAKES 13 TO 15 COOKIES

wheat soy **FREE**

Growing up, my sister Debbie made a wicked version of chocolate chip cookies with crisp rice cereal. My sweet-tooth had fond memories of those cookies, so I decided to do my own version based on my classic Homestyle Chocolate Chip Cookies but modified slightly. You'll enjoy the slight crunch and chew that the crisp rice offers up, plus the hint of cinnamon! Thanks for the inspiration, big sis.

1 cup + 3 tablespoons light or sifted spelt flour
1 teaspoon baking powder
¼ teaspoon (rounded) baking soda
¼ cup unrefined sugar (see note)
¼ teaspoon sea salt
  A few pinches of ground cinnamon
⅓ cup pure maple syrup
¼ teaspoon blackstrap molasses
1 teaspoon pure vanilla extract
¼ cup (slightly scant) neutral-flavored oil (see "Plant-Powered Pantry," page xxxii)
¼ to ⅓ cup vegan chocolate chips
¾ cup natural brown rice crisp cereal (not puffed rice, I use Nature's Path brand; see note)

Preheat the oven to 350°F. Line a baking sheet with parchment paper.

Place the flour in a bowl and sift in the baking powder and baking soda. Add the sugar, salt, and cinnamon, and stir until well mixed.

In a separate bowl, combine the maple syrup with the molasses and vanilla, then stir in the oil until well mixed. Add the wet mixture to the dry, along with the chocolate chips, and stir just until well incorporated (do not overmix. Refrigerate for about 10 minutes (see note). Then stir in the crispy cereal.

Place spoonfuls of the batter (about 1 rounded tablespoon each) on the prepared baking sheet and flatten a little. (The batter may seem a little crumbly. Do your best to form into scoops; the batter will do its thing while baking and the cookies will hold together nicely!) Bake for 11 to 12 minutes, until just golden (if you bake for much longer, they will dry out).

Remove from the oven, let cool on the pan for a minute (not much longer, to prevent drying), then transfer to a cooling rack.

If This Apron Could Talk: Refrigerating the batter helps keep the crispy cereal crisp once stirred in. Try to not let the batter sit long after mixing in the cereal, as the cereal will gradually absorb some of the moisture from the batter and begin to soften and lose its crunch. So, after mixing, try to get into the oven quickly. Also, don't refrigerate the batter much longer than 10 minutes as it will get too firm, making it difficult to work in the cereal.

Ingredients 411: I use the Nature's Path Crispy Rice Cereal, which is brown rice–based and not very sweet. If you use another variety that is sweetened more (such as a cocoa-flavored cereal), you can reduce the sugar to 3 tablespoons to cut down on the sweetness.

"Raisinet" Cookies

MAKES 15 TO 18 COOKIES

wheat
soy FREE

My buddy Vicki mentioned that she adapted one of my cookie recipes to include chocolate with the raisins. She went on about how good the two tasted together. Of course—chocolate-covered raisins! I got to work making a new cookie to capture the beauty of that chocolate and raisins combination. These "Raisinet" (or "Glosette" for my Canadian readers) cookies are now a personal fave.

1 cup barley or sifted spelt flour
⅓ to ½ cup rolled oats (see note)
¼ cup unsweetened cocoa powder
1 teaspoon baking powder
¼ teaspoon (rounded) baking soda
¼ cup raisins
¼ cup vegan chocolate chips (smaller-size chips are good, such as the Enjoy Life brand)
3 tablespoons unrefined sugar
¼ teaspoon sea salt
⅓ cup pure maple syrup
1 teaspoon blackstrap molasses
1½ teaspoons pure vanilla extract
¼ cup neutral-flavored oil (see "Plant-Powered Pantry," page xxxii)

Preheat the oven to 350°F. Line a baking sheet with parchment paper.

In a bowl, combine the flour, oats, and cocoa, sifting in the baking powder and baking soda. Add the raisins, chips, sugar, and salt, and stir well.

In a separate bowl, first combine the maple syrup with the molasses and vanilla, then stir in the oil until well mixed. Add the wet mixture to the dry, and stir until just incorporated.

Place spoonfuls of the batter (about 1 tablespoon each) on the prepared baking sheet and flatten a little. Bake for 11 minutes.

Remove from the oven, let cool on the pan for just a minute (not much longer, to prevent drying), then transfer to a cooling rack.

Ingredients 411: Using ⅓ cup of oats will give a slightly softer cookie that spreads a little more when baking. Using ½ cup will give a firmer cookie treat.

Almond Cardamom Toffee Cookies

MAKES 14 TO 15 COOKIES

wheat soy **FREE**

These cookies are crunchy, with a toffeelike flavor. Plus, with a simple change of the measurement of milk, you can have two versions of them. If you use the 1-tablespoon measurement, they are crunchy and toothsome; with the 2-tablespoon measurement, the cookies spread out more like a lace cookie.

1	cup raw almonds
½	cup unrefined sugar
¼	teaspoon (scant) sea salt
1¼	tablespoons organic extra-virgin coconut oil
1½	tablespoons light or sifted spelt flour
2	tablespoons pure maple syrup
¼	teaspoon ground cardamom
¼	teaspoon blackstrap or other molasses
1 or 2	tablespoons nondairy milk (use 2 tablespoons for thinner, lacier cookies)
½	teaspoon pure vanilla, or ¼ to ½ teaspoon almond extract

Preheat the oven to 350°F. Line a baking sheet with parchment paper.

Pulse the almonds and sugar in a food processor until very crumbly and fine. Add the remaining ingredients and process until the mixture has come together and somewhat formed a dough.

Place tablespoons of the batter (a small cookie scoop works well) on the prepared baking sheet. (I bake in two batches, because these cookies flatten and spread). Flatten cookies (not too flat, but so not in a mound) with the palm of your hand or the bottom of a glass. Bake for 12 minutes, until bubbly and golden.

Remove from the oven, let cool on the pan for a couple of minutes to set, then transfer to a cooling rack to cool. (The cookies are fragile when still warm, so transfer to rack carefully). Refrigerate the cooled cookies in an airtight container.

Serving Suggestions: These are elegant served as an ice-cream garnish. Try with Chai Peanut Butter Ice Cream, and don't forget a dollop of Lemon-Scented Whipped Cream.

Snifferdoodles

MAKES 15 TO 18
SNIFFERDOODLES

wheat
soy **FREE**

I had originally called these Maple Sugar Snickerdoodles. However, one day my middle daughter called them Snifferdoodles. I loved the name so much I had to go with it! They are delicious, and terrific for bringing to school or other parties, where allergies such as to peanuts, nuts, wheat, and even chocolate are always an issue.

¾ cup + 1 tablespoon sifted spelt flour

¼ cup + 2 tablespoons oat flour

⅓ cup unrefined sugar

¼ teaspoon ground cinnamon (see note for anise adaptation)

¼ teaspoon sea salt

1 teaspoon baking powder

¼ teaspoon (rounded) baking soda

¼ cup pure maple syrup

2 teaspoons pure vanilla extract

3 tablespoons neutral-flavored oil (see "Plant-Powered Pantry," page xxxii)

COATING:

2 teaspoons fine-textured unrefined sugar

1 teaspoon ground cinnamon

Preheat the oven to 350°F. Line a baking sheet with parchment paper.

In a bowl, combine the dry ingredients, sifting in the baking powder and baking soda, mixing well.

In a separate bowl, combine the maple syrup, vanilla, and oil. Add the wet mixture to the dry, and stir until just incorporated. Place the mixture in the fridge for about 5 minutes.

While the cookie mixture chills, mix the coating ingredients together in a separate small bowl.

Remove the cookie mixture from the fridge, and take small spoonfuls of the batter (about ½ tablespoon each; see note) of the batter and roll in your hands to form balls. Place on the prepared (you will still need to coat them, so just place randomly on the lined pan until ready to move to that step). Continue until you have used all the batter. Roll each ball in the coating mixture, and then place back on the lined pan, this time spacing out the cookies evenly. Do not flatten them! Bake for 10 minutes.

Remove from the oven (if you bake for much longer, they will dry out), let cool on the pan for no more than a minute (again, to prevent drying), then transfer to a cooling rack.

If This Apron Could Talk: I make these cookies a little smaller than most of the others. They are perfect for little hands when bite size. Because they are smaller, you should get a yield of between 18 to 25 cookies, and the baking time will be only 10 to 11 minutes. If you choose to make them a little larger, the yield should be 13 to 15 cookies; bake for 11 to 12 minutes.

You may have extra sugar mixture after coating the cookies. Don't throw it away! Use it to sprinkle on ice cream, bagels, toast, yogurt, or cereal!

Ingredients 411: Look for a sifted spelt flour, or sift it yourself through a fine sieve to remove any graininess.

If the batter is a touch dry when mixing, use another ½ to 1 teaspoon of oil and mix with another smidgen (about 1 teaspoon) of maple syrup. Depending on the brand of flour used and/or time of year, this is a good trick. Simply fold the oil and syrup into the batter, and repeat if needed. Just don't overdo it—the batter should be thick and not too wet or oily, or the cookies will spread out flat and join when baking.

Make It More-ish! After making these cookies, I learned about *biscochitos*, which are Mexican cookies flavored with anise and sprinkled with cinnamon sugar. To make a *biscochito* instead of a Snifferdoodle, omit the ¼ teaspoon cinnamon from the batter and replace it with ¾ to 1 teaspoon of aniseeds, crushed just slightly between your fingers before mixing in (if you love that licorice flavor, use the full 1 teaspoon, or more)!

You can also make different shapes with the batter, if you first refrigerate it for 20 or more minutes to get firmer. Roll out about ¼ inch thick and cut into shapes before dusting with the cinnamon sugar.

Kamut Hazelnut Cookies

MAKES 14 TO 16 COOKIES

wheat soy **FREE**

These cookies make a super snack cookie. They are made with wholesome ingredients, including kamut flour, flax meal, and nut butter, and they aren't overly sweet. They have a moist, soft texture that kids will enjoy.

2 tablespoons organic extra-virgin coconut oil, at room temperature (see "Plant-Powered Pantry," page xxix)
¼ cup pure maple syrup
2 tablespoons brown rice syrup
3 tablespoons hazelnut butter
¼ cup flax meal
1½ teaspoons pure vanilla extract
¾ cup kamut flour
½ cup almond meal
1 teaspoon baking powder
¼ teaspoon sea salt
1 teaspoon orange or lemon zest
2 to 3 tablespoons roughly chopped hazelnuts or almonds
3 to 4 tablespoons vegan chocolate or white chocolate chips (optional)

Preheat the oven to 350°F. Line a baking sheet with parchment paper.

In a mixer fitted with the paddle attachment, combine the coconut oil, maple syrup, brown rice syrup, nut butter, flax meal, and vanilla. Mix on low speed for about a minute to incorporate.

In a separate bowl, combine all the dry ingredients, including the nuts and chips (if using), and stir to mix. Add about half of the dry mixture to the wet mixture. Use the mixer briefly to partially incorporate the dry mixture, then add the remaining dry mixture. Continue to beat on low speed, just until the mixture comes together and forms a dough on the paddle.

Scoop spoonfuls of the batter (about 1 tablespoon each) and place on the prepared baking sheet. Bake for 12 minutes.

Remove from the oven, let cool on the pan for about a minute, then transfer to a cooling rack.

Make It More-ish! And when I say the chocolate chips are optional, I mean you can opt for 3 tablespoons—or the full 4!

Savvy Subs and Adds: Almond butter substitutes beautifully for hazelnut butter, and I use this variation often. If doing so, also sub ½ teaspoon of almond extract for ½ teaspoon of the vanilla.

Pecan Date Nibblers

**MAKES ABOUT
16 TO 20 NIBBLERS!**

*wheat
(optionally) gluten* **FREE**
soy

I'd been hankering for a baked cookie using dates as the primary sweetener; looking for a good pairing, I used pecans—perfect with their natural butteriness. The first batch was a winner, and these healthy, tasty little nibblers needed repeating!

1   cup whole pecans
1   cup pitted medjool dates
1   tablespoon organic extra-virgin coconut oil, or almond or other nut butter
1   teaspoon pure vanilla extract
3   tablespoons pure maple syrup
½   cup + 1 tablespoon light or sifted spelt flour (see note for gluten-free option)
1   teaspoon baking powder
¼   teaspoon (scant) sea salt
½   teaspoon ground cinnamon
1   teaspoon lemon or orange zest (optional)

Preheat the oven to 350°F. Line a baking sheet with parchment paper.

In a food processor, first pulse the pecans until just crumbly. Then add the dates, coconut oil, vanilla, and maple syrup. Pulse again until the dates are broken up into smaller pieces (but not fully processed, leave some chunkier pieces).

In a bowl, sift in the flour and baking powder, and then stir in the salt, cinnamon, and zest. Add the dry mixture to the processor and pulse until the mixture starts to come together. (It does not need to be fully formed into a dough, but should hold together when pressed or squeezed into a ball in your hand.) Once at this stage, stop processing.

Place spoonfuls of the dough (about a tablespoon each) on the prepared baking sheet. Bake for 11 to 12 minutes.

Remove from the oven, let cool on the pan for a minute, then transfer to a cooling rack.

Allergy-Free or Bust! For a gluten-free version, replace the spelt flour with ⅓ cup of rice flour, 1½ tablespoons of tapioca starch flour, and ½ teaspoon of xanthan gum. That easy!

Lemon Cranberry Cornmeal Cookies

MAKES 11 TO 13 SMALL
TO MEDIUM COOKIES

wheat
gluten **FREE**
soy

These cookies have a delightful lemony tang yet are still a cookie-sweet treat. They are ideal for people with wheat or gluten allergies—and you'll be surprised that gluten-free cookies can taste so lovely! If you're not super keen on cranberries, try other dried fruit (look for unsulfured), such as dried cherries or dried blueberries.

¼ cup dried cranberries

2½ tablespoons macadamia butter

1 tablespoon organic extra-virgin coconut oil

1 tablespoon agave nectar

1½ tablespoons pure maple syrup

1 tablespoon freshly squeezed lemon juice

½ cup corn flour

3 tablespoons millet flour

2 tablespoons tapioca starch flour

1 teaspoon baking powder

¼ teaspoon baking soda

½ teaspoon xanthan gum

2½ tablespoons unrefined sugar

¼ teaspoon sea salt

1½ teaspoons lemon zest

1 to 2 tablespoons unrefined sugar (for dusting cookies)

Preheat the oven to 325°F (see note). Line a baking sheet with parchment paper.

In a food processor, combine the cranberries, macadamia butter, coconut oil, agave nectar, maple syrup, and lemon juice, and pulse just to start to mix the ingredients.

In a separate bowl, combine the dry ingredients, except the dusting sugar. Add the dry ingredients to wet mixture, and pulse to break up the cranberries (the mixture will splatter some and you will need to scrape down the processor bowl once or twice). Process slightly until the mixture starts to come together. (It does not need to be fully formed into a dough, but should hold together when pressed or squeezed into a ball in your hand.) The cranberries will partially break up and create ruby flecks in the dough. Once the batter reaches this stage, stop processing. Refrigerate the batter for 15 to 20 minutes.

Take spoonfuls of the dough (about a tablespoon each), roll in the unrefined sugar, place on the prepared baking sheet, and flatten just slightly. Bake for 11 minutes, until just starting to turn a light golden on the very tippy edges.

Remove from the oven, let cool on the pan for a minute, then transfer to a cooling rack.

If This Apron Could Talk: Most cookie recipes bake at 350°F. These cookies tend to brown on the bottom too quickly at that temperature, so lower the heat to 325°F.

Make It More-ish! If you like white chocolate chips, add just a sprinkling to the batter, about 2 tablespoons.

Orange Almond Cranberry Chip Biscotti

MAKES 12 TO 18 BISCOTTI

wheat
soy **FREE**

Fresh orange zest with chopped almonds, cranberries, and chocolate chips make an irresistible combo in this wheat-free cookie.

⅓ cup organic extra-virgin coconut oil at room temperature, or neutral-flavored oil (see "Plant-Powered Pantry," page xxxii)

⅔ cup unrefined sugar

⅓ cup vanilla or plain nondairy milk

1 tablespoon pure maple syrup

1 teaspoon pure vanilla extract

¼ to ½ teaspoon pure almond extract, or ¼ teaspoon orange oil (or lemon oil if using lemon zest; see below)

2¼ cups light or sifted spelt flour

2½ teaspoons baking powder

½ teaspoon (scant) sea salt

1½ teaspoons orange zest (use kitchen grater to grate the zest; lemon zest is also delicious)

¼ cup roughly chopped whole almonds

3 to 4 tablespoons dried cranberries

2 to 3 tablespoons vegan dark chocolate chips

Preheat the oven to 350°F. Line a baking sheet with parchment paper.

In a mixer fitted with the paddle, blend the coconut oil and sugar together on low speed. Add the milk, maple syrup, and extracts, and blend again.

In a separate bowl, combine the flour, baking powder, salt, and zest. Mix well, then add to the mixer. Beat on low speed, and as mixture is just coming together, add the almonds, cranberries, and chips. Mix until the dough just comes together on the paddle.

Form into one large ball with your hands (don't overhandle), and then halve the mixture. Form each half into a log about 1 inch thick, 3 to 4 inches wide, and 8 to 9 inches long. Place on the prepared baking sheet, leaving space between the logs, and bake for 26 to 28 minutes, until golden around the edges.

Remove from the oven and let cool for 10 to 15 minutes (see note). Using a serrated knife, cut the biscotti logs on a slight diagonal into strips 1 to 1 1/2 inches thick. Place the cut biscotti, cut side down, back on the lined baking sheet, and bake at 350°F for another 11 to 16 minutes (less time for chewier cookies, longer for crispier ones), flipping the biscotti to the other side halfway through the baking time.

Remove from the oven and let cool on baking sheet for a minute or two, and then transfer to a cooling rack to cool completely.

If This Apron Could Talk: Leave the biscotti logs on the baking sheet set on top of a cooling rack, rather than try to move the semibaked logs back and forth to a cooling rack. You can also slice the logs directly on the baking sheet before baking again; just be sure to spread out and place cut side down for the second baking.

Make It More-ish! For additional decadence, dip the ends of the fully baked biscotti in good-quality melted vegan chocolate. then let cool on a baking sheet lined with parchment paper.

Savvy Subs and Adds: Another beautiful variation is a pistachio, white chip, and lime biscotti. Replace the almonds with raw pistachios, the dark chocolate chips with vegan white chips, and the orange zest with lime zest.

Matcha Green Tea Pistachio Biscotti with Sugar Dusting

MAKES 12 TO 18 BISCOTTI

Pistachios add a nutty sweetness to balance the earthy green tea in these biscotti. Dusted with a scattering of green tea sugar, these biscotti are as elegant as they are delicious.

wheat soy **FREE**

⅓ cup organic extra-virgin coconut oil at room temperature, or neutral-flavored oil (see "Plant-Powered Pantry," page xxxii)

½ cup+ 2 tablespoons unrefined sugar

⅓ cup plain nondairy milk

1 tablespoon pure maple syrup or agave nectar

1½ teaspoons pure vanilla extract

1¼ cups light or sifted spelt flour

1 cup oat flour

2½ teaspoons baking powder

1¼ teaspoons matcha green tea powder

½ teaspoon sea salt (little scant)

¼ cup raw pistachios

DUSTING SUGAR:

1 tablespoon unrefined sugar

¼ teaspoon matcha green tea powder

Preheat the oven to 350°F. Line a baking sheet with baking parchment.

In a mixer fitted with the paddle, blend the coconut oil and sugar together on low speed. Add the milk, maple syrup, and vanilla, and blend again.

In a separate bowl, combine the flours, baking powder, green tea powder, and salt. Mix, and then add to the wet mixture. Mix on low speed, and as mixture is just coming together, add the pistachios. Mix until the dough just comes together on the paddle.

Remove from the oven and let cool (see note) for 10 to 15 minutes. Using a serrated knife, cut the biscotti logs on a slight diagonal into strips 1 to 1½ inches thick. Form into one large ball with your hands (don't overhandle), and then halve mixture. Form each half into a log about 1 inch thick, 3 to 4 inches wide, and 8 to 9 inches long). Place on the prepared baking sheet, leaving space between the logs, and bake for 26 to 28 minutes, until golden around the edges.

Remove from the oven to let cool for 10 to 15 minutes (see note). Using a serrated knife, cut the biscotti logs on a slight diagonal into strips 1 to 1½ inches thick. Mix the dusting sugar ingredients on a plate, then spread out and coat each cookie in the mixture, mostly coating the cut sides. Return the biscotti cut side down to the lined baking sheet and bake for 11 to 16 minutes (less time for softer cookies, longer for crispier ones), flipping the biscotti halfway through the baking time.

Remove from the oven and let cool on baking sheet for a minute or two, and then transfer to a cooling rack to cool completely.

If This Apron Could Talk: Leave the biscotti logs on the baking tray to cool on top of a cooling rack rather than try to move the semibaked logs back and forth to a cooling rack. You can also slice the logs directly on the baking tray before baking again; just be sure to spread out and place cut side down for the second baking.

Gingery Cookies

MAKES 14 TO 17 COOKIES

wheat **FREE** *soy*

When I first made these, I had planned to make a pretty standard ginger cookie. But then I thought about how much I love ginger in chocolate bark, and decided to throw in a handful of chocolate chips. It's up to you to keep them more traditional, or perked up with chocolate—or double chocolate! Try all three versions, and you might have a hard time choosing a favorite!

1⅓ cups light or sifted spelt flour
¼ cup unrefined sugar
2 to 3 tablespoons chopped crystallized ginger (optional; see note)
¼ teaspoon sea salt
1 teaspoon ground ginger
½ teaspoon ground cinnamon
¼ teaspoon ground allspice
⅛ teaspoon ground cloves
½ teaspoon baking soda
¾ teaspoon baking powder
1 tablespoon blackstrap molasses
¼ cup pure maple syrup
1 to 1½ teaspoons pure vanilla extract
¼ cup neutral-flavored oil (see "Plant-Powered Pantry," page xxxii)
3 to 4 teaspoons fine-granule unrefined sugar, for coating

Preheat the oven to 350°F. Line a baking sheet with parchment paper.

In a bowl, combine the dry ingredients, including crystallized ginger, sifting in baking powder and baking soda, and stir well.

In another bowl, combine the molasses, maple syrup, and vanilla and stir to fully incorporate. Then add the oil, stir, and add the wet ingredients to the dry. Mix until just incorporated.

Take spoonfuls of the batter (1 to 1½ tablespoons each), and form into balls in your hand. Roll in the sugar and place on the cookie sheet. Very slightly press to lightly flatten the cookies. Bake for 11 minutes.

Remove from the oven, let cool on the pan for a minute, transfer to a cooling rack, and then nibble.

Make It More-ish! Need a double-chocolate gingery cookie? You've got it! Simply make these substitutions: Use just 1 cup + 2 tablespoons of spelt flour, add 3½ tablespoons of unsweetened cocoa powder, and either keep the crystallized ginger or replace it with 3 to 4 tablespoons of vegan chocolate chips. Gingery chocolaty goodness!

Savvy Subs and Adds: If you don't have crystallized ginger, you can skip it or add another pinch of ground ginger to the dry mixture. Or throw in a handful of chocolate chips for an unexpected ginger cookie twist!

Gingerbread Folks

MAKES 15 TO 20 CUTOUTS

wheat *soy* **FREE**

A variation on the holiday classic, these cookies have a slight chewiness and crunch, with a delicious, lightly spiced flavor.

1½ cups + 1 tablespoon light or sifted spelt flour
1 teaspoon baking powder
¾ teaspoon baking soda
¼ + ⅛ teaspoon sea salt
1 teaspoon ground cinnamon
⅛ teaspoon ground cloves
¾ teaspoon ground ginger
⅛ teaspoon ground allspice
⅓ cup organic extra-virgin coconut oil, at room temperature or use organic neutral-flavored oil (see "Plant-Powered Pantry," page xxxii and note)
½ cup unrefined sugar
2 tablespoons blackstrap molasses
2 tablespoons nondairy milk (see note)
2 tablespoons pure maple syrup

Preheat the oven to 350°F. Line a baking sheet with parchment paper.

In a large bowl, combine the flour, baking powder, baking soda, salt, cinnamon, cloves, ginger, and allspice.

Using a stand mixer fitted with the paddle attachment, combine the coconut oil, sugar, molasses, milk, and maple syrup, beating on medium speed for several minutes until creamy, and stopping to scrape the bowl as needed. Mixing at low speed, add the dry mixture about ½ cup at a time, over about a minute or so. Continue blending until the dough comes together in one or two balls on the paddle, separating cleanly from the inside of the mixing bowl.

Transfer to a clean, dry countertop. Roll out the dough to about ¼ inch thick. (If you are having trouble rolling the dough—if it is sticking—sandwich the dough between two sheets of parchment paper and roll your pin on top of the parchment, instead of directly on the dough.) If the dough has become too pliable (this may happen if your room is slightly warm), transfer to the fridge for 10 to 15 minutes to firm slightly. Once rolled fairly evenly to ¼ inch thick, use cookie cutters to cut the dough into shapes. A spatula (offset or regular) will help lift the cookies off your counter and to the prepared baking sheet. Space the cookies at least an inch or so apart. Bake for 10 to 11 minutes.

Remove from the oven and let cool on the pan for at least a couple of minutes. The cookies will firm more as they cool, and even more after they are chilled. Refrigerate the cookies in an airtight container. Decorate as desired, such as with the simple gingerbread icing.

SIMPLE GINGERBREAD ICING
(OPTIONAL):

1   cup natural powdered sugar
    (see "Plant-Powered Pantry,"
    page xxxvi)
1½ to 2   tablespoons vanilla nondairy
    milk

To prepare the icing: In a bowl, mix the sugar with 1½ tablespoons of the milk, until very smooth. Add the extra ½ tablespoon or so of milk, if needed, to thin mixture to a soft enough consistency that can be squeezed through a piping or resealable plastic bag (snip one corner if using a plastic bag).

After decorating the gingerbread, allow the icing to dry on the cookies before stacking.

If This Apron Could Talk: I like the size this batch of dough makes—enough for fifteen or more cookie cutouts. If, however, you prefer to bake in larger quantities, simply double this recipe and bake the cookies in batches. Finish cutting all of your cookies, and then refrigerate the shapes until ready to bake the next batch . . . or refrigerate the dough first and cut out only one batch's worth at a time as they bake. Note: If you are refrigerating the dough for more than 30 to 40 minutes, it will need to soften briefly at room temperature to roll out, as the coconut oil hardens when cooled.

Ingredients 411: Any nondairy milk can be used, though I like the hint of flavor a soy nog gives to the batter!

Sugar Cutout Cookies

MAKES 13 TO 15 CUTOUTS

wheat (optionally) gluten soy **FREE**

These cookies began as a spelt-based sugar cookie, but I just wasn't happy with the texture after several trials. Once I tinkered in a gluten-free direction, I scored a cookie with a crunchy bite and a slightly chewy texture. These are delicious with just a sugar sprinkle, but also are wonderful decorated with icing. If you go this route, omit the sugar sprinkle, so you can easily decorate after the cookies have cooled.

3	tablespoons organic extra-virgin coconut oil, at room temperature
½	cup unrefined sugar
2 to 2½	tablespoons nondairy milk
¼	teaspoon lemon extract (optional)
½	cup + 1 tablespoon millet flour
¼	cup + 1 tablespoon oat flour (use GF-certified oat flour for gluten-free version)
2	tablespoons rice flour (see "Plant-Powered Pantry," page xxxviii)
¼	cup tapioca starch flour
½	teaspoon baking powder
½	teaspoon agar powder
¼	teaspoon sea salt
1 to 2	teaspoons fine-granule unrefined sugar, for sprinkling

Preheat the oven to 350°F. Line a baking sheet with parchment paper.

Using a mixer fitted with the paddle attachment, combine the coconut oil, sugar, 2 tablespoons of the milk, and lemon extract (if using), beating on medium speed for several minutes until creamy, and stopping to scrape the bowl as needed.

In another bowl, combine the flours, baking powder, agar, and salt. Mixing on low speed, add the dry mixture about ½ cup at a time, for about a minute or so. Mix until the dough is coming together. This will take a couple of minutes, and you will see it become smooth and start to form together (though, not completely into a ball) and it will hold together when pressed. But if after a few minutes it isn't coming together, add the remaining ½ tablespoon of milk and mix again (if still not together, add another ½ to 1 teaspoon of milk, but avoid adding too much as the dough will become wet).

Roll out the dough to about ¼ inch thick. (If you are having trouble rolling the dough—if it is sticking—sandwich the dough between two sheets of parchment paper and roll your pin on top of the parchment, instead of directly on the dough.) If the dough has become too pliable (this may happen if your room is slightly warm), transfer to the fridge for 10 to 15 minutes to firm slightly. Once rolled fairly evenly to ¼ inch thick, use cookie cutters to cut the dough into shapes. A spatula (offset or regular) will help lift the cookies off your counter and to the prepared baking sheet. Space the cookies at least an inch or so apart. Once the cookies are all on the sheet, sprinkle the sugar over top. Place the baking sheet in the freezer for 5 to 10 minutes before baking. Then remove from freezer and transfer directly to the oven. Bake for 14 minutes (see note).

Remove from the oven and let cool for at least a couple of minutes on the pan for at least a couple of minutes. The cookies will be a little fragile while warm, but will firm more as they cool, and even more after they are chilled. Refrigerate in an airtight container.

If This Apron Could Talk: After baking for 14 minutes, the cookies will have firmness around the edges and into the center, once cooled, but will still maintain a slightly chewy bite. For a drier cookie, bake for another minute or two.

I like the size this batch of dough makes, but if you prefer to bake in larger quantities, simply double this recipe and bake the cookies in batches. Finish cutting all of your cookies, and then refrigerate (or briefly freeze) the shapes until ready to bake the next batch . . . or refrigerate the dough and cut only one batch's worth at a time as they bake. Note: If you are refrigerating the dough for more than 30 to 40 minutes, it will need to soften briefly at room temperature to roll out, as the coconut oil hardens when cooled.

Fresh Blueberry Oat Squares

MAKES 16 SQUARES

wheat
(optionally) gluten **FREE**
soy

These squares are similar to date squares, but made with blueberry and whole-grain goodness! Because you can use frozen blueberries, you can make these treats any time of the year.

FILLING:

- 3 cups fresh or frozen blueberries
- ⅛ teaspoon sea salt
- 3 tablespoons coconut sugar or other unrefined sugar
- 2 teaspoons freshly squeezed lemon juice
- 1 tablespoon arrowroot powder
- ½ teaspoon agar powder

BASE AND TOPPING:

- 2 cups rolled oats (see note; use GF-certified for gluten-free version)
- 1 cup spelt flour or oat flour (use GF-certified for gluten-free version)
- ½ teaspoon (scant) sea salt
- 1½ teaspoons lemon zest
- ½ cup pure maple syrup
- 1½ teaspoons pure vanilla extract
- 2 tablespoons neutral-flavored oil (see "Plant-Powered Pantry," page xxxii)

For the filling: in a saucepan over medium heat, combine the blueberries, salt, and sugar. Cover and let the berries soften until they release their juices, stirring occasionally, a few minutes for fresh berries, several more for frozen. Once the berries have broken down and the mixture is becoming more like a sauce, lower the heat and simmer for 7 to 8 minutes, covered.

In a small bowl, stir the lemon juice with the arrowroot and agar (it will be thick). Remove 2 to 3 tablespoons of the warmed blueberry juices and stir into the arrowroot slurry, 1 tablespoon at a time. This will help loosen that mixture and also tempers the arrowroot and agar, making it less likely to clump in the sauce. After the mixture has loosened, add it to the blueberry sauce, immediately stirring it. Increase the heat slightly to bring mixture back to a boil for just a minute or so. Then remove from the heat, transfer the mixture to a bowl, and let chill in refrigerator for 20 to 30 minutes, stirring occasionally to prevent a skin from forming on top of the mixture.

Meanwhile, prepare the base and topping: Preheat the oven to 350°F. Lightly oil or line an 8-inch square cake pan with parchment paper.

In a large bowl, combine the dry ingredients, including the zest.

In a small bowl, combine the maple syrup, vanilla, and oil. Add the wet mixture to the dry, and stir until well mixed; the consistency will be crumbly yet hold together somewhat when pressed. Transfer about two-thirds of the mixture to the prepared pan and press in evenly. Pour the chilled (can be warm, just not hot) blueberry mixture on top, then sprinkle with the remaining crust mixture. Bake for 25 minutes, until the blueberry filling is bubbly and the topping is golden in spots.

Transfer the pan to a rack to cool, and then to the fridge to cool completely before cutting into squares.

Savvy Subs and Adds: Quick oats can be substituted in whole or part for the rolled oats; however, the texture of the squares will be different. Using the rolled oats, the squares will have a chewier texture and a nuttier flavor, whereas the quick oats become softer and also absorb more of the moisture of the blueberry layer.

Berry Patch Brownies

MAKES 16 TO 20 BROWNIES

wheat soy **FREE**

Warning: These brownies are deep chocolaty, fudgy and sticky, and with bites of berry bursting flavor.

BROWNIE DOUGH:

½ cup vegan dark chocolate chips or chunks

¼ cup plain nondairy milk

1 cup + 1 tablespoon sifted or light spelt flour

¾ cup unrefined sugar

½ teaspoon sea salt

¼ cup unsweetened cocoa powder

1 teaspoon baking powder

1 tablespoon arrowroot powder

3 tablespoons pure maple syrup or agave nectar

1 teaspoon pure vanilla extract

¼ to ½ teaspoon almond or cherry extract (optional, if you want to enhance the berry flavor in the brownies)

3 tablespoons neutral-flavored oil (see "Plant-Powered Pantry," page xxxii)

BERRY LAYER:

3½ to 4 tablespoons raspberry jam

½ cup fresh or frozen blueberries

2 tablespoons vegan dark chocolate chips

Preheat the oven to 350°F. Line an 8-inch square cake pan with parchment paper.

First, prepare the brownie dough: Melt the chocolate with the milk in a bowl fitted over a saucepan with simmering (not boiling) water. Stir until melted together. Remove the mixture from the heat.

In a bowl, combine flour, sugar, and sea salt, and sift in the cocoa and baking powder.

In a small bowl, first combine the arrowroot with the maple syrup, stirring until smooth, then add the extracts and oil. Add the wet mixture into the melted chocolate mixture and stir. Add the chocolate mixture to the dry ingredients. Stir until the mixture becomes evenly mixed and thick.

Transfer the mixture to the prepared pan. Use a square of parchment to help press the mixture into pan evenly and spread it out. Next, spread raspberry jam over the top, and sprinkle with the blueberries and chocolate chips. Bake for 30 to 32 minutes.

Remove from the oven and let cool in the pan, running a spatula around the outer edge to loosen. (The brownies will not be set in the center, and will appear not fully cooked, but let cool and they will become fudgy!) Once completely cooled (refrigerating helps before cutting), cut into squares and dig in!

Make It More-ish! Ice-cream sundae anyone? You've already got the brownies combined with the berry sauce—why not just add some ice cream! Try Macadamia Ice Cream or Chocolate Lovers Ice Cream. Top with small pieces of the brownies. And if you need a little more berry sauce, try the Warm Strawberry Sauce.

Chocolate Goji Macadamia Crispy Squares

MAKES 12 TO 16 SQUARES

*wheat
gluten* FREE
soy

This recipe elevates a traditional crispy rice square, making it a little more sophisticated with dark chocolate, macadamia nuts, goji berries, and a hint of orange. If you are new to goji berries, this sure is a sweet way to get acquainted!

1¼ cup vegan dark chocolate chips (7½ to 8 ounces)

1½ tablespoons organic extra-virgin coconut oil, at room temperature (see "Plant-Powered Pantry," page xxix)

¼ teaspoon (scant) sea salt

1 to 1½ teaspoons orange zest

1 cup dried goji berries (see note)

½ cup roughly chopped and crushed macadamia nuts (can use other tender, sweet nuts, such as pecans or cashews)

¾ cup natural brown rice crisp cereal (not puffed rice; I use Nature's Path brand)

Line an 8-inch square cake pan with parchment paper.

First melt the chocolate with the coconut oil and salt in a bowl fitted over a saucepan with simmering (not boiling) water. Stir until just melted and the coconut oil is incorporated into the chocolate. Remove the mixture from the heat.

Add the orange zest, goji berries, nuts, and cereal and stir. Transfer the mixture to the prepared pan. Press the mixture evenly into the pan. Place in the refrigerator and chill until completely cool, then cut into squares.

If This Apron Could Talk: You can also drop these cookies onto a baking sheet lined with parchment to make simple drop cookies instead of squares, if you prefer.

Savvy Subs and Adds: If you prefer, you can switch the goji berry and rice cereal measurements, using ¾ cup of goji berries and 1 full cup of brown rice cereal. Also, you can substitute other dried fruit in place of some of the goji berries; for instance, using dried blueberries and cranberries for about half of the amount of the goji berries.

"Hello Vegan" Bars

MAKES 16 TO 20 BARS

wheat (optionally) gluten soy **FREE**

This is my adaptation of the classic Hello Dolly Bars. Beyond being free of animal products and refined flours and sugars, these bars have an extra-thick caramel layer that is positively sumptuous. Instead of a graham cracker base, they have a more satisfying and toothsome oat and coconut crust. Topped with pecans, coconut, and chocolate chips, these are a little piece of cookie bar heaven!

CARAMEL TOPPING:

- 1 cup full-fat coconut milk (refrigerate the can in advance, if possible; use only the thick cream (see "Plant-Powered Pantry," page xxviii)
- 2 tablespoons arrowroot powder
- ¾ cup unrefined sugar (see note)
- ⅛ teaspoon sea salt
- 1 teaspoon pure vanilla extract

BASE:

- 1½ cups oat flour (use GF-certified for gluten-free option)
- ½ cup unsweetened shredded coconut (look for unsulfured brand)
- ¼ teaspoon (rounded) sea salt
- 3 tablespoons brown rice syrup or agave nectar
- 2 tablespoons organic extra-virgin coconut oil, at room temperature

TOPPINGS:

- ⅓ to ½ cup vegan chocolate chips
- ⅓ cup broken or roughly chopped pecans
- ⅓ cup unsweetened shredded coconut
  A few pinches of sea salt

Preheat the oven to 350°F. Line an 8-inch square cake pan with parchment paper.

First, prepare the caramel topping: In a small saucepan, whisk about half of the milk with the arrowroot. Then add the remaining milk, whisking, and the remaining caramel ingredients. Heat the mixture over medium-high heat, whisking frequently, until it just reaches a boil. Then remove from the heat and transfer to a bowl to let cool slightly while preparing the base. (Continue to whisk or stir occasionally to prevent a skin from forming on the caramel. If a skin does start to form, you can whisk it into the mixture, or it fairly thick, simply remove and discard the skin, if you prefer.)

Prepare the base: In a bowl, combine the oat flour, coconut, and salt, then add the brown rice syrup and coconut oil. Mix with your fingers to help work in the syrup and oil. Once the mixture can hold together somewhat when pressed, transfer to the prepared pan. Press evenly into the bottom of the pan. When caramel has cooled slightly (can still be warm, just not hot), pour over the base. Then layer on each of the toppings, sprinkling over the caramel, followed by sprinkling on a couple of pinches of salt. Bake for 20 minutes.

Remove from the oven and place the pan on a cooling rack. Let cool slightly and then refrigerate to fully cool before slicing into bars.

If This Apron Could Talk: You can chill the coconut cream if you want, though it isn't necessary, but may help with some brands to separate the cream from the liquid. If refrigerating, after opening the can, scoop out 1 cup of the thick cream. If not refrigerating, carefully and slowly pour the cream to get your 1-cup measurement. As you pour, you will notice where the cream separates from the watery liquid, so don't include this liquid.

Ingredients 411: I use coconut sugar in this recipe, and it gives a beautiful caramel color to the cream. If you don't have coconut sugar, Sucanat is a good substitute. Or, if using a light-colored unrefined sugar, add a smidgen of molasses (¼ teaspoon or so, not too much as the flavor is strong) to your filling mixture while simmering, to help deepen the color.

Creamed Cheese Brownies with Salted Dark Chocolate Topping

MAKES 16 TO 20 BROWNIES

wheat
soy **FREE**

No faux cream cheese to be found in these deep, rich, fudgy brownies. Cashews stand in for a cream cheese–like layer, which takes these brownies to, "OMG these are freaking good!" 'Nuff said—go make them.

CREAM CHEESE LAYER:

1 cup soaked raw cashews
2 tablespoons freshly squeezed lemon juice
3 tablespoons water
1 tablespoon pure maple syrup
2 tablespoons vanilla nondairy yogurt (if using coconut yogurt instead of soy, add another 1 teaspoon lemon juice), can also use Vanilla Yogurt, page 235
1 teaspoon pure vanilla extract
⅛ teaspoon (rounded) sea salt

BROWNIE LAYER:

1 cup + 2 tablespoons sifted or light spelt flour
¾ cup unrefined sugar
½ teaspoon sea salt
⅓ cup unsweetened cocoa powder
1½ teaspoons baking powder
1 tablespoon arrowroot powder
3 tablespoons pure maple syrup
1 teaspoon pure vanilla extract
¼ cup + 1 tablespoon plain or vanilla nondairy milk
3½ tablespoons neutral-flavored oil (see "Plant-Powered Pantry," page xxxii)

Preheat the oven to 350°F. Line an 8-inch square cake pan with parchment paper.

Prepare cream cheese layer: Puree all those ingredients with an immersion or high-speed blender until very, very smooth (a mini food processor can also be used, but it usually doesn't produce as smooth a texture as does an immersion blender). Process for several minutes, if necessary, until very smoothed out.

Prepare the brownie layer: In a separate bowl, combine the flour, sugar, and salt, and sift in the cocoa and baking powder.

In a small bowl, first combine the arrowroot with the maple syrup, stirring until smooth, then add the vanilla, milk, and oil. Add the wet mixture to the dry. Stir until evenly mixed and thick. Transfer about two-thirds of the mixture to the prepared pan. Use a square of parchment to help the press mixture into the pan evenly and spread it out. Spread the cream cheese layer over the top. Then, as best as you can, spread the remaining brownie batter over the cheese layer. You can take pieces and lightly spread first with your fingers and place in patches over the cream cheese layer—and it doesn't have to fully cover; there can be spaces—most will fill in and come together while baking.

TOPPING:

⅓ to ½ cup vegan chocolate chunks (use a good-quality dark chocolate bar, broken or cut into small chunks)

A few pinches of coarse sea salt

Add the topping: Place the chocolate chunks on top, and then sprinkle with the salt. Bake for 28 to 30 minutes.

Remove from the oven and let cool in the pan, running a spatula around the outer edge to loosen. (The brownies will appear not fully cooked, but do not cook longer—I repeat, do not cook longer! Instead, let cool and they will become fudgy!) Once cooled, score the brownies with a sharp knife to ease cutting the chocolate before it completely hardens. Then refrigerate brownies to cool more, cut into squares and dig in!

If This Apron Could Talk: Trust the baking process! The amount of batter used for the base—and then topping— looks like it cannot possibly fill out to form a beautiful brownie. Lucky for us, the oven creates some magic in about half an hour!

Raw Banana Nut Squares with Coconut Cream Cheese Frosting

MAKES 16 TO 20 SQUARES

wheat gluten soy **FREE**

Years ago, I was obsessed with a sort of banana square—a homemade one with a banana filling sandwiched between graham crackers and topped with a powdered sugar frosting. This is my raw, vegan, and much healthier adaptation . . . and I like it even more!

BASE:
1 cup raw macadamia nuts
⅔ cup raw pecans
½ cup pitted medjool or honey dates
¾ cup dried unsulfured bananas (not crisp banana chips; dice or slice into small pieces; see note)
⅛ teaspoon (scant) sea salt
¼ teaspoon freshly grated nutmeg
Seeds from 1 vanilla bean (see "Plant-Powered Pantry," page xlii), or 1 teaspoon vanilla extract)

BANANA LAYER:
¾ to 1 cup thinly sliced fresh banana (about 1 medium-size to large banana)
1 to 2 teaspoons lemon juice

FROSTING:
½ cup (well packed) raw coconut butter (I use Artisana)
¼ cup + 1 tablespoon raw agave nectar
1 teaspoon apple cider vinegar or freshly squeezed lemon juice
A few pinches of ground cinnamon
A few pinches of sea salt

Line an 8-inch square cake pan with parchment paper.

Prepare the base: In a food processor, combine all ingredients for the base. Pulse until the mixture comes together, scraping down sides as needed. Process only until the nuts are well broken down and incorporated with the dried fruit. Avoid overprocessing, as it makes the nuts release their oils and the base becomes oily (but at the same time, be sure the mixture will hold together when pressed with your fingers).

Transfer the mixture to the prepared pan and press firmly and evenly into the pan (using a square of parchment to press with is easiest).

Next, in a small bowl, prepare the banana: Toss the sliced bananas with the lemon juice. Arrange these slices on top of the base, as evenly as possible, and very gently press the slices into the base, just to help them hold before layering on the frosting.

Prepare the frosting: Combine all the ingredients in a mini food processor, or mix very well by stirring in a bowl). Smooth the frosting over the base, covering the bananas and base as well as possible. Refrigerate for an hour or more until set. Cut into squares and serve!

Ingredients 411: Dried bananas are funny-looking specimens. They are just like a banana but shriveled and brown, and so, unfortunately, they don't look too a"peel"ing! But they taste so great in this recipe, try to get past the initial visual impression. Cutting them into small pieces will help with the processing.

Savvy Subs and Adds: If you want to substitute coconut oil for the coconut butter, you can do so, but you'll also need some cashew butter in the frosting. So, you can use ¼ cup + 1 tablespoon of cashew butter (preferably raw), and 3 tablespoons of coconut oil.

Raw Chai Bars

MAKES 14 TO 16 RECTANGULAR BARS OR 18 TO 21 SQUARES

wheat gluten soy **FREE**

These bars couple the warm, enchanting spices of chai tea with the sweetness of a dessert bar and the healthy goodness of a raw treat.

½ cup raw cashews
1 cup pitted medjool dates
⅓ cup raisins
¾ cup raw pecans
¼ teaspoon (scant) sea salt
½ teaspoon ground cinnamon
¼ teaspoon ground ginger
⅛ to ¼ teaspoon freshly grated nutmeg
A few pinches of ground cardamom
A few pinches of ground cloves (about ¹⁄₁₆ teaspoon)
¾ teaspoon pure vanilla extract, or seeds from 1 vanilla bean ("Plant-Powered Pantry," page xlii)
1½ teaspoon freshly squeezed lemon juice
½ teaspoon lemon zest

Line a loaf dish or similarly sized small pan with parchment paper.

Place the cashews, dates, and raisins in a food processor. Pulse until the nuts and fruits are crumbly, then add the pecans and the remaining ingredients and process again, scraping down the sides of the bowl a couple of times, until the mixture has come together and becomes sticky (don't overprocess, as pecans can make mixture too oily if overworked).

Transfer the mixture to the prepared loaf dish. Press the mixture firmly into the pan (using a small piece of parchment is easiest). Refrigerate for a couple of hours and then cut into bars or squares and serve!

Make It More-ish! If you want to frost these bars, use the frosting from Raw Banana Nut Squares with Cream Cheese Frosting.

Award-Winning Frosted B-raw-nies

MAKES 16 TO 20 B-RAW-NIES!

*wheat
gluten
soy* **FREE**

Let them eat brownies! You can feel good about munching on these raw brownies, made with nuts and dates. Don't pass on making the frosting; it's what makes these brownies especially delicious. I entered these brownies in a gluten-free recipe contest—and they took home first prize (for my first-ever contest)!

BASE:

- 1 cup raw almonds (see note)
- ¼ cup raw cashews
- ½ cup raw walnuts
- 2 cups (packed) pitted medjool dates (see note)
- ⅓ cup raw cocoa or regular unsweetened cocoa powder
- ¼ teaspoon sea salt
- 1 to 1½ teaspoons pure vanilla extract, or seeds from 1 vanilla bean (see "Plant-Powered Pantry," page xlii)

FROSTING:

- ½ cup coconut butter (not coconut oil; see "Plant-Powered Pantry," page xxviii)
- ¼ cup raw agave nectar (see note)
- 2 tablespoons raw cocoa or regular unsweetened powder
  Pinch of sea salt

Line an 8-inch square cake pan with parchment paper.

Prepare the base: In a food processor, process the almonds and cashews until very fine (the almonds are the harder of the two, and need to be worked until crumbly), 1 to 2 minutes. Add the walnuts and dates, and pulse until the mixture is quite crumbly but not yet coming together. Then add the cocoa powder, salt, and vanilla and pulse. Process until the mixture comes together. (It should be sticky and hold together when pressed with your fingers.) You don't want to overmix (to prevent the nuts from releasing their oils; see note), but the mixture does need to hold and be sticky. If it's not doing so, add a few drops of water, as your dates might be dry.

Once you have a good, sticky mixture that will hold together, press into the prepared pan. Use a small piece of the parchment to help press and flatten the mixture evenly into the pan. Press it firmly to ensure the mixture holds.

Prepare the frosting: In a mini food processor, first combine the coconut butter and agave nectar until smooth. Then add the cocoa powder and salt, and pulse again until just incorporated. Do not overprocess, or the frosting will begin to separate with the heat of the churning and become oily. (If you don't have a mini food processor, you can follow the same steps stirring by hand in a bowl.)

Smooth the frosting over the base, and refrigerate for an hour or more until set. Cut into squares and serve! You can also freeze the squares after cutting, and enjoy them out of the freezer!

Ingredients 411: If your dates are on the dry side, add a few teaspoons of water, one at a time, to the mixture while processing, to help it come together.

If This Apron Could Talk: If you process the mixture too long, the heat generated by the food processor will bring the oils out of the nuts. If this happens, the brownies won't be ruined necessarily, but they will have an oily appearance and be oily to the touch.

Make It More-ish! For a Chocolate Cherry B-rawn-ie variation, substitute ¼ cup of dried organic pitted cherries for ¼ cup of the dates, and add ½ teaspoon of pure almond extract to the base mixture.

Savvy Subs and Adds:
- A combination of ¾ cup of almonds and ½ cup of cashews also works well.
- Although it isn't technically a raw ingredient, pure maple syrup can be substituted for the agave nectar.

Raw Chocolate Truffles

MAKES ABOUT 12 TRUFFLES

wheat gluten soy FREE

These raw chocolate truffles are virtually a guiltless chocolate indulgence, and they are easier to make than traditional truffles! There are two versions here, one using coconut oil, and the other using coconut butter.

COCONUT OIL VERSION:

¼ cup (scant) organic extra-virgin coconut oil

3 tablespoons cashew butter

1 teaspoon orange zest (optional)
A few pinches of sea salt

3 to 3½ tablespoons raw agave nectar (adjust sweetness to taste; see note)

¼ teaspoon orange oil or almond extract

½ cup + 2 tablespoons unsweetened cocoa powder

1 to 2 tablespoons raw sugar (I use raw coconut sugar) or raw unsweetened cocoa powder, for dusting (optional)

COCONUT BUTTER VERSION:

¼ cup (packed) coconut butter, (I use Artisana brand; see note if substituting coconut oil)

1½ tablespoons raw cashew or other nut butter (see note if substituting coconut oil)

1 teaspoon orange zest (optional)
A few pinches of sea salt

3 to 3½ tablespoons raw agave nectar (adjust sweetness to taste; see note)

¼ teaspoon orange oil or almond extract

½ cup raw cocoa or regular unsweetened cocoa powder (see note if substituting coconut oil)

1 to 2 tablespoons raw sugar (I use raw coconut sugar) or raw unsweetened cocoa powder, for dusting (optional)

In a mini food processor, combine all the ingredients except the cocoa powder and optional sugar or cocoa powder for dusting. Pulse to mix well. Then add the cocoa powder and pulse again, until the ingredients are fully combined and the mixture starts to stick together. (Be careful not to overprocess, as the mixture can become oily.)

Refrigerate the mixture for 30 to 45 minutes, until it becomes firm enough to scoop and roll lightly in your hands. Take small scoops (about a tablespoon or less each) and gently roll into balls. Place the sugar and/or cocoa powder (can use either or both) in a bowl and toss each truffle in the topping to coat. Refrigerate the truffles to firm up again, then enjoy!

Ingredients 411: You need at least 3 to 3½ tablespoons of liquid sweetener such as agave to get a good consistency for these truffles. I typically use about 3½ tablespoons, but you can use a little less or a little more, as desired. Note that if you use close to 4 tablespoons, the truffles get a touch softer.

Protein Power: If you'd like to add some hemp seeds to the truffles, pulse them in at the end. About 2 tablespoons is nice; if your truffle mixture is at all dry or stiff, add another ½ tablespoon or so of agave nectar.

Savvy Subs and Adds: The orange note in these truffles is really flavorful; however, you can omit the orange rind and substitute another extract such as almond or vanilla.

Hazelnut butter is also tasty in these truffles, though I haven't found raw hazelnut butter and have only used the roasted variety.

While not technically raw, pure maple syrup can be substituted for the agave nectar.

Raw Carob Goji Truffles

MAKES 12 TO 14 TRUFFLES

wheat
gluten **FREE**
soy

Carob can be an acquired taste, and is not necessarily a given substitute for chocolate (there isn't any true substitute for chocolate, in my opinion)! Still, carob can be enjoyed for its own unique flavor profile. Here, I've paired it with nutty, mellow cashew butter; fruity, earthy goji berries, and a touch of almond extract, for a delicious, easy, and healthful truffle! If you don't have, or don't care for, goji berries, try substituting dried blueberries or cranberries for an equally tasty treat.

3	tablespoons organic extra-virgin coconut oil
2½ to 3	tablespoons raw cashew butter (see note)
3	tablespoons goji berries (see note)
	A few pinches of sea salt
3	tablespoons raw agave nectar (see note)
¼ to ½	teaspoon pure almond extract (optional; I use ½ teaspoon)
½	cup (not packed) raw carob powder
1 to 2	tablespoons unrefined sugar, for dusting

In a mini food processor, combine the coconut oil, 2½ tablespoons of the cashew butter (see note), goji berries, salt, agave, and almond extract and puree until fairly smooth (don't process too long, just until it smoothes out). Add the carob powder and pulse for another few moments, until the mixture just comes together (do not overwork by pureeing for too long, or it will become oily; see note).

Refrigerate the mixture for 5 to 10 minutes, and then roll small scoops of the mixture (about ½ tablespoon each) into a ball in your hands (see note). Once all the balls are formed, place the unrefined sugar in a bowl and toss the truffles in the sugar. Nibble immediately, or place in a covered container and refrigerate.

If This Apron Could Talk: You can refrigerate for longer if that's more convenient, and then let the mixture sit at room temperature for 5 to 10 minutes or more, long enough to make it soft enough to scoop and form into balls.

If you are finding the mixture dry and crumbly when you have started to process it, rather than process further and overwork the mixture, try adding the remaining cashew butter, about 1 teaspoon at a time, and process again. Then check the consistency by pressing a small amount of the mixture together with your fingers. If it holds together well when pressed, you will be able to form truffles, so no need to process more.

Savvy Subs and Adds: While not technically raw, pure maple syrup can be substituted for the agave nectar. Similarly, regular (roasted) cashew butter can be substituted for raw.

10 Let Them Eat Cake, Pies, and Pudding

Ever watch kids eat cupcakes at parties? Most of them lick the frosting and leave the cake. I get them. I was one of those kids. I love frosting, too. But those neon-colored, sickly sweet frostings are not where it's at. I've come up with frostings that are made with much less sweetener and that are far lighter and more delicious—Fluffy Macadamia Mallow Frosting, Cooked Vanilla Frosting, or Sugar-Free Cashew Glaze, anyone? You'll also find frostings that have no margarine and no soy (No-Butter Cream Frosting, Double-Trouble Chocolate Ganache, Coconutty Frosting)—creamy, luscious, thick, mallowy, delicious. Yep, you will love these alternative frostings, and you'll want to just eat them straight from the mixing bowl.

But really, what's frosting without cake? From Pumpkin Cake, Sugar-Free Chocolate Cake, Banana-Scented Vanilla Cake,

Fresh Orange Cake, and Blueberry Coffee Cake with Cinnamon Walnut Crumble Topping, they're fabulous, and they're wheat or gluten free.

Don't worry—pie's fully represented here, too—with more wheat- and gluten-free options. Try Apple-of-My-Eye Pie, Three's Company Pie, To-Live-For Pecan Pie, or Banana Butter Pie to get going . . . and if you are up for making your piecrust from scratch, there's a Rustic Piecrust or a scrumptious (and hard to believe it's gluten free!) Gluten-Free Piecrust. This chapter also covers some raw treats, as well as all sorts of finger-licking toppings and sauces for desserts, and a couple of puddings, to boot.

As with all my desserts, I have worked hard and recipe-tested myself silly to give you cakes, pies, and puddings that find a way to make healthy (or healthier) meet delicious—using alternative flours for allergy modifications and less refined sweeteners, and not using any processed products such as soy cream cheeses, sour creams, or margarines. This I do for the love of baking, and for the joy of bringing healthier desserts into your life. So do something for me and get your plant-powered baking apron on. (And, if you want to let me know how much you love the goodies, I'm all ears!)

Pumpkin Cake

MAKES 2 ROUND CAKE LAYERS

wheat
soy **FREE**

This cake is a new family favorite. Moist and just lightly spiced with traditional pumpkin pie spices, it is absolutely ideal for an autumnal party or birthday, or as part of a Thanksgiving menu. But it is so delicious, you may want to make it other times of the year!

2¼ cups sifted or light spelt flour (see note)

½ cup + 2 to 4 tablespoons unrefined sugar (see note)

½ teaspoon sea salt

1 teaspoon ground cinnamon

¼ teaspoon freshly grated nutmeg

⅛ teaspoon ground allspice
A few pinches of ground cloves (about ¹⁄₁₆ teaspoon)

2 teaspoons baking powder

½ teaspoon baking soda

¾ cup pure pumpkin puree (not pumpkin pie mix; I use Farmer's Market organic brand)

1 cup plain or vanilla nondairy milk

¼ cup pure maple syrup

2 teaspoons pure vanilla extract

1 tablespoon freshly squeezed lemon juice

¼ cup neutral-flavored oil (see "Plant-Powered Pantry," page xxxii)

Preheat the oven to 350°F. Lightly oil two 8-inch round cake pans, and line the bottom of each with parchment paper, if desired.

In a large bowl, combine the flour, sugar, salt, cinnamon, nutmeg, allspice, and cloves, sifting in the baking powder and baking soda. Mix well.

In a separate bowl, whisk the pumpkin puree with the milk, maple syrup, vanilla, and lemon juice. Add the wet mixture to the dry, along with the oil, and mix until just incorporated.

Pour the batter evenly into the prepared pans. Bake for 24 to 27 minutes, or until a toothpick inserted in the center of each comes out clean.

Remove from the oven and let cool in pans on a cooling rack.

If This Apron Could Talk: To adapt this cake to cupcakes, line about 20 compartments of a muffin tin and fill about halfway with the batter. Bake in a preheated 350°F oven for 16 to 18 minutes (test with a toothpick). Also, because this batter is quite healthful, the cupcakes can double as muffins. You can add chopped walnuts or pecans to the batter to make the muffins a little heartier, and fill the liners a little fuller, if you like, than you would for cupcakes (in this case, bake a minute or two longer).

Savvy Subs and Adds: If you'd like to use wheat flour in this recipe, you can substitute 2 cups (with a light hand measuring that second cup) of whole wheat pastry flour.

I like this batter with the ½ cup + 2 tablespoons of sugar. But if you want it just a touch sweeter, add the extra 2 tablespoons of sugar.

If frosting this cake with the Fluffy Macadamia Mallow Frosting, try topping with a sprinkling of chopped, toasted macadamia nuts. As this cake is slightly reminiscent of a carrot cake, you might opt to use another frosting (such as the No-Butter Cream Frosting, and add a few tablespoons of raisins and/or chopped toasted walnuts to the batter.

Sugar-Free Chocolate Cake

MAKES 2 ROUND CAKES

wheat *soy* FREE

This cake is made without any granulated sugar . . . and, it's also made without wheat flour! Despite these very wholesome adaptations, this chocolate cake is surprisingly moist and delicious, just as cake should be! (Don't dismiss it, really—don't!)

½ cup raisins (see note)
  Boiling water (to soak raisins)
2¼ cups sifted or light spelt flour
½ cup unsweetened cocoa powder
1½ teaspoons baking powder
1½ teaspoons baking soda
½ teaspoon sea salt
½ cup prunes (unsulfured)
½ cup unsweetened applesauce
½ cup pure maple syrup
2 tablespoons balsamic vinegar
2 teaspoons pure vanilla extract
1 cup cold water
⅓ cup + 1 tablespoon extra-virgin olive oil (see note)

Preheat the oven to 350°F. Lightly oil two 8-inch round cake pans, and line the bottom of each with parchment paper, if desired.

First combine the raisins with the boiling water in a bowl and let soak while preparing the other ingredients.

In a large bowl, sift together flour, cocoa powder, baking powder, and baking soda, then add the salt and mix well.

In a blender, combine the prunes, applesauce, maple syrup, vinegar, and vanilla. Once the raisins have soaked for 5 or more minutes, drain and discard the water and add the raisins to the blender. Blend until the prunes and raisins are pulverized (but not too long, so the blended mixture doesn't become heated). Add the cup of cold water and blend again (again, try not to blend too long, so the mixture doesn't become too warm).

Add the blended mixture to the dry, along with the olive oil, and stir until incorporated.

Pour the batter evenly into the prepared pans. Bake for 23 to 25 minutes, or until a toothpick inserted in the center of each comes out clean.

Remove from the oven and let cool in pans on a cooling rack.

If This Apron Could Talk: I soak the raisins in enough boiled water just to cover them, about ½ cup of water. Normally I don't soak the prunes, because they are often softer and blend easier than the raisins. However, if the prunes you are using are a little on the tough side, go ahead and soak them with the raisins, using ¾ to 1 cup of boiled water. Just be sure to fully drain before using, and then blend with cold water, per the directions.

To adapt this cake to cupcakes, line about two dozen compartments of a muffin tin and fill about halfway to two-thirds full with the batter. Bake in a preheated 350°F oven for 16 to 18 minutes (test with a toothpick).

Ingredients 411: Normally I don't use olive oil in cakes because the taste can be prominent, especially the fruitiness of extra-virgin olive oil. But this cake is an exception, and I think the taste of the olive oil actually improves the overall taste, helping to balance the flavors of the pureed raisins and prunes. Resist the temptation to pass it up for another, neutral-flavored, oil!

Fresh Orange Cake

MAKES 2 ROUND CAKE LAYERS

wheat soy **FREE**

Fresh orange juice and orange zest bring life to your standard vanilla cake (which also happens to be wheat free). A small touch of cinnamon accents the orange very nicely, too!

2 cups + 2 tablespoons sifted or light spelt flour

1 cup unrefined sugar (a fine granule works best)

½ teaspoon (scant) sea salt

¼ teaspoon ground cinnamon (optional, but lovely)

1½ to 2 teaspoons orange zest

2 teaspoons baking powder

½ teaspoon baking soda

⅓ cup freshly squeezed orange juice

½ cup plain or vanilla nondairy yogurt (use soy-free yogurt or Vanilla Yogurt for a soy-free option; see "Plant-Powered Pantry," page xxxiii)

½ cup + 2 tablespoons plain unsweetened nondairy milk (almond or soy preferred; see "Plant-Powered Pantry," page xxxiii)

1 teaspoon pure vanilla extract

⅓ cup neutral-flavored oil (see "Plant-Powered Pantry," page xxxii)

Preheat the oven to 350°F. Lightly oil two 8-inch round cake pans and line the bottom of each with parchment paper, if you desire.

In a large bowl, combine the dry ingredients, including zest, sifting in the baking powder and baking soda, and stir well.

In a separate bowl, combine the orange juice, yogurt, milk, vanilla, and oil, and stir.

Add the wet mixture to the dry, and stir until just well combined.

Pour the batter evenly into the prepared pans. Bake for 23 to 25 minutes, or until a toothpick inserted in the center comes out clean.

Remove from the oven and let cool in the pans on a cooling rack before frosting. Once cool, frost as desired.

If This Apron Could Talk: To adapt this cake to cupcakes, line about two dozen compartments of a muffin tin and fill about halfway to two-thirds full with the batter. Bake in a preheated 350°F oven for 17 to 19 minutes (test with a toothpick).

Banana-Scented Vanilla Cake

MAKES 2 ROUND CAKE LAYERS

wheat
gluten **FREE**
soy

This cake has just a light banana flavor combined with fragrant vanilla. The banana helps add stability and moistness, so don't leave it out to make a vanilla-only cake. It is such a subtle flavor that is most lovely, and the cake is fluffy and moist, perfect for any special occasion.

1 cup millet flour
¾ cup rice flour (see note)
¼ cup arrowroot powder or tapioca starch flour
½ teaspoon xanthan gum
½ teaspoon agar powder
½ teaspoon baking soda
2 teaspoons baking powder
1 cup unrefined sugar
½ teaspoon (scant) sea salt
1 cup + 2 tablespoons plain unsweetened nondairy milk (almond or soy preferred; see "Plant-Powered Pantry," page xxxiii)
¾ cup pureed ripe banana (1½ to 2 small bananas, or 1½ medium-to large)
1 tablespoon apple cider vinegar
1½ teaspoons pure vanilla extract
⅓ cup neutral-flavored oil (see "Plant-Powered Pantry," page xxxii)

Preheat the oven to 350°F. Lightly oil two 8-inch round cake pans and line the bottom of each with parchment paper, if you desire.

In a large bowl, combine the flours, xanthan gum, and agar; sift in the baking powder and baking soda; then add the sugar and salt. Mix well.

In another bowl, stir the nondairy milk and banana together, and then add the vinegar, extract, and oil. Add the wet mixture to the dry, and stir until incorporated.

Pour the batter evenly into the prepared pans. Bake for 27 to 30 minutes, or until a toothpick inserted in the center of each comes out clean.

Remove from the oven and let cool in the pans on a cooling rack.

If This Apron Could Talk: Use an immersion blender or mini processor to puree the banana.

This cake take a little longer to set up than some of my other cake recipes. Just have patience, and watch until the layers become lightly golden around the edges and the centers are no longer dull and sticky looking (and test with a toothpick)!

To adapt this cake to cupcakes, line twenty to twenty-two compartments of a muffin tin and fill about halfway with the batter. Bake in a preheated 350°F oven for 22 to 24 minutes (test with a toothpick).

Ingredients 411: You can use white rice flour, brown rice flour, or a combination of both. Note that white rice flour gives a slightly lighter cake texture, and brown rice flour can impart a subtle aftertaste. For taste and texture, using all or some of white rice flour is preferred.

Chocolate Yogurt Cake

MAKES 2 ROUND CAKE LAYERS

Gluten-free cakes are dry and pasty right? Not this one! No sir, it's moist and tender, and quite irresistible!

*wheat
gluten* **FREE**
soy

½ cup rice flour (see "Plant-Powered Pantry," page xxxviii)

½ cup millet flour

½ cup sorghum flour

½ cup unsweetened cocoa powder

⅓ cup tapioca starch flour

½ + ⅛ teaspoon xanthan gum

½ teaspoon agar powder

1 teaspoon baking soda

1½ teaspoons baking powder

1 cup unrefined sugar

½ teaspoon (scant) sea salt

½ cup vanilla nondairy yogurt (use soy-free yogurt or Vanilla Yogurt for a soy-free option; see "Plant-Powered Pantry," page xxxiii)

1⅓ cups water

1 tablespoon apple cider vinegar

2 teaspoons pure vanilla extract (see note)

1½ teaspoons blackstrap or other molasses

¼ cup + 1 tablespoon neutral flavored oil (see "Plant-Powered Pantry," page xxxii)

Preheat the oven to 350°F. Lightly oil two 8-inch round cake pans and line the bottom of each with parchment paper, if desired.

In a large bowl, combine the dry ingredients, sifting in the cocoa, baking powder, and baking soda.

In another bowl, combine the yogurt, water, vinegar, vanilla, and molasses, stirring well. Add the oil and mix again. Add the wet mixture to the dry, and stir until incorporated.

Pour the batter evenly into the prepared pans. Bake for 28 to 32 minutes, or until a toothpick inserted in the center of each comes out clean.

Remove from the oven and let cool in the pans on a cooling rack.

If This Apron Could Talk: To adapt this cake to cupcakes, line twenty to twenty-two compartments of a muffin tin and fill about halfway with the batter. Bake in a preheated 350°F oven for 22 to 24 minutes (test with a toothpick).

Savvy Subs and Adds: If you like the flavor of almond extract, try replacing ½ teaspoon of the vanilla extract with ½ teaspoon of almond.

Blueberry Coffee Cake with Cinnamon Walnut Crumble Topping

SERVES 6 TO 8

wheat soy **FREE**

This cake almost melts in your mouth, with a soft, tender batter laced with blueberries and topped off with a crunchy, buttery-tasting cinnamon-walnut topping.

CINNAMON WALNUT CRUMBLE TOPPING:

- ¾ cup lightly chopped or crushed walnuts
- 3 tablespoons unrefined sugar
- 1¾ teaspoons ground cinnamon
  A few pinches of sea salt
- 1 tablespoon neutral-flavored oil (see "Plant-Powered Pantry," page xxxii)

CAKE:

- 1½ cups + 1 tablespoon sifted or regular spelt flour (see note)
- ¾ cup oat flour
- ¼ cup unrefined sugar
- ½ teaspoon ground cinnamon
- ⅛ teaspoon ground allspice
- ½ teaspoon sea salt
- 2 teaspoons baking powder
- ½ teaspoon baking soda
- ¼ cup pure maple syrup
- 2 tablespoons agave nectar (or more maple syrup)
- ⅔ cup plain or vanilla nondairy milk
- 2 teaspoon freshly squeezed lemon juice
- 1½ teaspoons vanilla
- ¼ cup neutral-flavored oil (see "Plant-Powered Pantry," page xxxii)
- 1 cup fresh or frozen blueberries (see note)

Preheat the oven to 350°F. Lightly oil an 8-inch square baking dish.

In a small bowl, combine the topping ingredients with a spoon or your fingers.

In a large bowl, combine the dry ingredients, sifting in the baking powder and baking soda.

In another small bowl, combine the maple syrup, agave nectar, milk, lemon juice, vanilla, and oil. Add the wet ingredients to the dry, mixing until just incorporated.

Transfer about two-thirds of the batter to the prepared pan. Distribute the blueberries over the batter (distribute more berries around the perimeter rather than in the center; see note), then top with the remaining batter, scraping out everything from your mixing bowl (simply dollop the topping in spots over the blueberries— you do not need to fully cover the berries). Sprinkle the topping mixture over top, and bake for 36 to 40 minutes, until the center of the cake has just set.

Remove from the oven and let cool in the pan on a cooling rack before serving.

If This Apron Could Talk: When distributing the blueberries, particularly if using frozen berries, it helps not to crowd the berries in the center of your cake. When too many berries sit in the center of the cake, the middle of the cake does not set well. So be sure to distribute generously around the edges of your cake, and then sprinkle just a little less into the center area.

Ingredients 411: You can use sifted spelt flour or regular whole-grain spelt flour. Sifted spelt flour will give a slightly lighter texture.

Lemony Luscious Almond Cake with Almond Maple Sauce

MAKES 1 CAKE,
WITH 1½ CUPS OF SAUCE

wheat soy FREE

I was intrigued while watching an episode of the British show *How to Cook Yourself Thin*, that whole boiled lemons were pureed into the batter of a cake! Such an inventive idea! I thought I must try a vegan version of this recipe myself. Although my cake is quite different, and isn't exactly intended to cook yourself thin . . . it *is* intended to bake your vegan self happy—and that it does! The Almond Maple Sauce is sweet but not overly rich. If you're looking for a creamier, richer sauce, try Rich Coconut Caramel Sauce. Or if you'd like a fruity sauce, try Fresh Strawberry Sauce or Warm Strawberry Sauce.

2	small organic lemons, left whole and unpeeled (see note)
1⅛	cups sifted or light spelt flour
1	cup almond meal
¾	cup unrefined sugar
1½	teaspoons baking powder
½	teaspoon baking soda
½	teaspoon (scant) salt
¼	cup organic extra-virgin coconut oil, at room temperature (see "Plant-Powered Pantry," page xxix)
½	cup plain nondairy milk (almond or soy preferred; see "Plant-Powered Pantry," page xxxiii)
¼	cup agave nectar
1½	teaspoons pure vanilla extract

First place the whole lemons (do not cut, prick, or peel) in a small saucepan and cover with water. Bring to a boil, then lower the heat and simmer partially covered for about 30 minutes. Remove the lemons from the pan and let cool enough to handle. While preparing the lemons, preheat the oven to 350°F. Lightly oil a 9-inch nonstick springform pan and line the bottom with parchment paper.

Meanwhile, in a bowl, combine the dry ingredients.

Holding the cooled lemons over a small bowl (to catch any juices), cut the lemons in half. Remove all seeds from the lemon and discard; also, trim the ends of each lemon (where the stems are) and discard. Place the remaining lemon with pulp (and reserved juices) in the blender, along with the coconut oil, milk, agave nectar, and vanilla. Puree until very smooth. Add the wet mixture to the dry, and stir until just incorporated.

Pour into the prepared pan. Bake for 30 to 33 minutes, or until a toothpick inserted in the center comes out clean.

Remove from the oven and let cool in the pan on a cooling rack.

ALMOND MAPLE SAUCE:

1 cup almond milk (unsweetened or vanilla)

⅓ to ½ cup pure maple syrup

½ teaspoon pure vanilla extract

¼ teaspoon sea salt

½ teaspoon almond extract

1 tablespoon (scant) arrowroot powder (see note)

⅛ teaspoon freshly grated nutmeg

Make the sauce: In a small saucepan, combine all the sauce ingredients, except the nutmeg, and whisk. Bring to a boil over medium-high heat, let boil just briefly (less than a minute), then remove from the heat. The sauce will not be thick at this point, but will thicken slightly after cooling. Let the sauce cool to warm (or cooled further) and drizzle over portions of the cake.

Ingredients 411: Try to use organic lemons in this cake, because the entire lemon (peel included) will be worked into the batter. Chemi-cake is not all too appetizing! Most organic lemons are quite small, but if by chance you have a larger lemon, use just one. Also, I'd recommend not substituting limes; I have tried this recipe with limes and the taste was too bitter.

You need arrowroot to thicken this sauce, but too much will make the sauce very thick and sticky. Use just a scant tablespoon of arrowroot (about 2½ teaspoons), and note that as the sauce cools, it will thicken more than when hot.

Fluffy Macadamia Mallow Frosting

MAKES 1¼ TO 1½ CUPS

wheat
gluten **FREE**
soy

This frosting has become one of my all-time favorites. It becomes thick and mallowy, and just slightly sweet. Really, I can eat it with a spoon. Truth be told, I usually stow enough away in the fridge so I can do just that! This recipe makes enough to frost one single-layer cake, so be sure to double the recipe for a double-layer cake or for twenty-four cupcakes.

1   (14-ounce) can regular (not "lite") coconut milk (refrigerate ahead of time; see "Plant-Powered Pantry," page xxviii and note)

⅛   teaspoon sea salt

½ to ¾   cup natural powdered sugar (see "Plant-Powered Pantry," page xxxvi)

    Seeds from 1 vanilla bean (see "Plant-Powered Pantry," page xlii)

2½ to 3   tablespoons macadamia nut butter (see note)

¼ to ½   teaspoon xanthan gum (see note)

Open the chilled can of coconut milk, without shaking or otherwise tipping much. You want to keep the cream solids as separate from the watery liquid as possible. Use a spoon to scoop out the thick cream into the bowl of a stand mixer (see note). You will get about ½ cup plus 2 to 4 tablespoons (see note). Get as much thick cream as you can without diluting it with the watery liquid sitting underneath. With the wire whip attachment, whip the cream at high speed for a minute or two, until it thickens and becomes fluffy. Then add the salt, sugar, vanilla seeds, and macadamia butter, and slowly bring the mixer to a high speed again to incorporate.

Stop the mixer, add the xanthan gum, and mix slowly to incorporate. Then whisk again at high speed for 30 seconds or so, until thickened (this will thicken more with chilling).

Transfer to an airtight container and refrigerate until ready to use. This frosting keeps for several days without deflating.

If This Apron Could Talk: You really need a mixer for this recipe. Don't try whisking by hand; the speed of the mixer is essential for whipping the thick, separated coconut milk.

Ingredients 411: Depending on how much thick cream you extracted from the can of coconut milk (without using any of the liquid), you may need more or less xanthan to help keep it firm for frosting. Usually about ¼ teaspoon will do, but feel free to use a little more, up to ½ teaspoon. The frosting will also firm more after refrigerating.

I like this frosting with ½ cup of sugar, or sometimes up to ¾ cup. If you like a sweeter frosting, add another few tablespoons of powdered sugar to taste, but not too much. The beauty of this frosting is its creamy-mallowy texture that is not overly sweet.

Savvy Subs and Adds: This frosting can be made without powdered sugar (substituting raw agave nectar, brown rice syrup, or pure maple syrup), but with some changes. Using maple syrup or agave, use ¼ to ⅓ cup; and for brown rice syrup, ⅓ to ½ cup. Then, if you want it sweeter, consider using a pinch of stevia to heighten the sweetness, as using much more liquid sweetener will thin out the frosting. You will need more xanthan gum to keep the frosting stable. Use close to ¾ teaspoon (don't go overboard, the frosting will firm more with chilling).

Vanilla seeds are really pretty in this frosting! But if you don't have a vanilla bean, feel free to substitute ½ to 1 teaspoon of pure vanilla extract.

Double-Trouble Chocolate Ganache

GANACHE #1 MAKES 2½ CUPS;
GANACHE #2 MAKES
ABOUT 2 CUPS

wheat
gluten **FREE**
soy

I can be indecisive—and this applies to recipes as much as anything else I do! So, when working with chocolate ganache, I've done it two ways, one that's a little sweeter using brown rice syrup, and another that is a little more "pure," in the sense that it uses just coconut milk and chocolate. The first option also makes a larger batch of ganache; the second, a little smaller yield which might better suit your use. Either way, it's delicious . . . so, I'll let *you* choose!

GANACHE #1:

1¾ cups vegan dark chocolate chips (10½ to 11 ounces)

⅔ cup regular coconut milk, or a thicker nondairy milk (such as almond or soy; see note)

¼ cup brown rice syrup

½ tablespoon organic extra-virgin coconut oil (or omit if using coconut milk rather than soy or almond; see "Plant-Powered Pantry" page xxix)

⅛ teaspoon sea salt

1 teaspoon pure vanilla extract (optional)

In a double boiler (or fit a metal or heatproof glass bowl over a saucepan filled with several inches of water) over medium-low heat, combine all the ingredients and gently stir until it's all melted and thoroughly incorporated.

Transfer to the refrigerator and chill until completely cool, then use to frost your cake (or use a mixer to quickly aerate and cool the frosting; see note). If you like, you can gently reheat to pour over the cake as a glaze (but don't heat too much; just warm enough to pour).

Ingredients 411: With ⅔ cup of milk, this ganache is thick enough to spread as a frosting. For a thinner consistency, add another couple tablespoons of milk. Also, it can be thinned to glaze by gently warming (as noted in directions).

GANACHE #2:

7 to 8 ounces vegan dark chocolate, roughly chopped, or about 1¼ cups vegan dark chocolate chips

1 cup regular (not "lite") coconut milk (use the creamy milk and discard the watery liquid; it's okay if the cup is a little scant)
A few pinches of salt

In a double boiler (or fit a metal or heatproof glass bowl over a saucepan filled with several inches of water) over medium-low heat, combine the chocolate, coconut milk, and salt and gently stir until it's all melted and thoroughly incorporated.

Transfer to the refrigerator and chill until it is cool enough to frost your cake (or use a mixer to quickly aerate and cool the frosting; see note). If you like, you can gently reheat to pour over the cake as a glaze (but don't heat too much; just warm enough to pour).

If This Apron Could Talk: To fluff up either ganache for a lighter, airier frosting, you can whisk it in a mixer. After heating through, transfer to a stand mixer fitted with the wire whisk attachment. Mix at high speed until cooled to room temperature, then transfer to the fridge to chill. Once chilled, whisk again at high speed, stopping to scrape down the sides of the bowl. You'll see the ganache lighten in color and become more fluffy.

I like the sweetness of this ganache as is, but if you want to fluff up the frosting and sweeten more for topping cupcakes and cakes, follow the directions to fluff with a mixer, and then add ¼ cup or more of powdered sugar while whisking.

No-Butter Cream Frosting

MAKES ENOUGH FROSTING FOR ONE 2-LAYER CAKE

wheat gluten soy **FREE**

This frosting has a light coconut flavor and is like a traditional buttercream—but without the use of butter or margarine.

⅓ cup organic extra-virgin coconut oil, at room temperature (see "Plant-Powered Pantry," page xxix)

¼ cup coconut butter, at room temperature (not coconut oil, I use Artisana brand; see "Plant-Powered Pantry," page xxviii)

3 to 3¼ cups (not packed) powdered sugar, sifted if lumpy (see "Plant-Powered Pantry," page xxxvi)

¼ + ⅛ teaspoon sea salt

2 teaspoons pure vanilla or other extract (optional; see note)

¼ to ⅓ cup regular (not "lite") coconut milk

In a stand mixer using a paddle attachment, cream the coconut oil and coconut butter at medium speed for a couple of minutes until creamy. Add 3 cups of the powdered sugar and mix on low speed until combined.

Increase the speed to medium-high and beat for a couple of minutes, then add the salt, vanilla, and ¼ cup of the coconut milk (add the remaining tablespoon, if desired, for desired consistency) and mix for another few minutes, until the mixture is smooth and creamy. Add the remaining ¼ cup of powdered sugar if you'd like a thicker buttercream.

Frost the cupcakes or cakes, or chill slightly before using (see note).

If This Apron Could Talk: This frosting will firm up considerably after chilling. Depending on the temperature in your kitchen, you may find it best to chill the freshly made frosting for 30 minutes or longer before frosting. If you make the frosting a day or two in advance, remove it from the fridge and let stand at room temperature for about an hour before frosting, or whip in the mixer to fluff up again.

Savvy Subs and Adds: Other extracts can be added to this frosting instead of vanilla, such as almond, anise, lemon, orange, or maple. Adjust amounts of other flavorings to taste. Note that the frosting will take on a slight caramel color with the addition of vanilla.

No-Butter Cream Chocolate Frosting

MAKES ENOUGH FROSTING FOR ONE 2-LAYER CAKE

wheat gluten soy **FREE**

Forget those tubs of prepared frostings full of junk. This frosting is thick and rich, and deeply chocolaty!

¼ cup organic extra-virgin coconut oil, at room temperature (see "Plant-Powered Pantry," page xxix)

¼ cup coconut butter, at room temperature (I use Artisana; (see "Plant-Powered Pantry," page xxviii)

1¾ cups (not packed) powdered sugar, sifted if lumpy (see "Plant-Powered Pantry," page xxxvi), plus 2 to 3 tablespoons (optional)

½ cup unsweetened cocoa powder, sifted if lumpy

¼ teaspoon sea salt

½ cup regular (not "lite") coconut milk

In a stand mixer using paddle attachment, cream the coconut oil with the coconut butter at medium speed for 2 to 3 minutes until creamy. Add the 1¾ cups of powdered sugar and the cocoa powder and mix on low speed until incorporated.

Increase the speed to medium-high and beat for a couple of minutes, then add the salt and coconut milk and beat for another few minutes, until the mixture is smooth and creamy. Add the extra powdered sugar, if necessary, to thicken.

Frost your cake or cupcakes (see note).

If This Apron Could Talk: This frosting will firm up considerably after chilling. Depending on the temperature in your kitchen, you may find it best to chill the freshly made frosting for 30 minutes or longer before frosting. If you make the frosting a day or two in advance, remove it from the fridge and let stand at room temperature for about an hour before frosting, or whip in the mixer to fluff up again.

Ingredients 411: This frosting will have a subtle coconut flavor from the coconut butter, as well as from the coconut milk. To lighten this coconut flavor, use soy creamer instead of coconut milk.

Cooked Vanilla Frosting

MAKES ENOUGH FROSTING
FOR ONE 2-LAYER CAKE

wheat
gluten **FREE**
soy

This frosting is made without margarine, and can be made without soy as well! It is not gritty sweet, but instead is mallowy and creamy delicious. It is made in the method of some traditional cooked frostings, but is vegan, gluten free, and a little healthier!

---

5 tablespoons millet (for gluten-free), barley, or spelt flour (see note)

1¼ cups natural powdered sugar, sifted if lumpy (see "Plant-Powered Pantry," page xxxvi)

½ teaspoon sea salt

¼ or ½ teaspoon agar powder (use ¼ teaspoon for barley or spelt flour, ½ teaspoon for millet)

1 cup + 2 tablespoons vanilla or plain unsweetened nondairy milk (almond or soy preferred; see "Plant-Powered Pantry," page xlii)

½ teaspoon pure vanilla extract, or seeds from 1 vanilla bean (see "Plant-Powered Pantry," page xlii)

½ cup organic extra-virgin coconut oil, at room temperature (see "Plant-Powered Pantry," page xxix)

In a saucepan over medium heat, whisk the flour with the sugar, salt, and agar. Gradually whisk in the milk. Cook, stirring frequently with a whisk at first, and then whisking almost constantly as the mixture thickens (take care that the mixture doesn't thicken on the bottom of the pan and clump; lower the heat to medium-low, if necessary). Add the vanilla, and keep heating and whisking the mixture until very thick and bubbling slowly.

Transfer to a stand mixer fitted with the paddle attachment. Mix on high speed for about 5 minutes, until the mixture has started to cool down. Add the coconut oil and beat for another few minutes, until the mixture is cool and creamy. At this point, you can either frost the cake or chill the frosting to whip up even fluffier.

To do so, refrigerate the mixer bowl of frosting until chilled (1 to 1½ hours). Then, instead of using the paddle attachment, affix the wire whisk attachment. Begin mixing slowly and then bring up to the fastest speed for a minute or two, until the frosting becomes lighter in color and fluffier. (If it doesn't, the frosting might need more chilling. Return the bowl to the fridge for another 30 minutes to an hour. Then whip at high speed again.)

Frost the cake or refrigerate the whipped mixture.

Ingredients 411: When using millet flour, because it is gluten-free, it is helpful to use extra agar to help stabilize the frosting, so use the full ½ teaspoon.

Savvy Subs and Adds: Cooked frosting traditionally uses all-purpose flour and butter. Coconut butter steps in for the dairy butter, and barley, spelt, or millet flour can be used in place of all-purpose. I like using millet flour. Because it is gluten free, it is easier to whisk and more forgiving, with less tendency to clump, than a gluten-based flour.

Coconutty Frosting

MAKES ABOUT 1 CUP OF FROSTING, ENOUGH TO GENEROUSLY FROST 12 CUPCAKES OR FROST TOPS OF A TWO-LAYER CAKE

wheat gluten soy **FREE**

Frosting does not need to be sugary, sickly sweet. Here, coconut oil combines with mellow (and naturally sweet) raw cashew butter or macadamia butter, and much less sugar than traditional frosting. It is thick and rich and buttery, and sweet enough to please big and little cake-hungry folk!

½ cup organic extra-virgin coconut oil, at room temperature (see "Plant-Powered Pantry," page xxix)

¼ to ⅓ cup raw cashew butter or macadamia butter (see note)

⅛ teaspoon sea salt

1½ tablespoons pure maple syrup

3 to 4 tablespoons natural powdered sugar (or more if desired; see "Plant-Powered Pantry," page xxxvi)

⅓ cup shredded coconut (optional; see note)

In a mixer fitted with the paddle attachment, cream together the coconut oil and nut butter. Then add the salt, maple syrup, 3 tablespoons of the sugar, and coconut (if using). Cream together again, and once smooth, taste. If you'd like to add extra sugar, go ahead. Note that the frosting will firm considerably once chilled.

Ingredients 411: If you cannot find raw cashew butter or macadamia butter, try regular cashew butter. It has a darker color, but the flavor and texture work well.

I like this frosting more buttery and creamy than sugary-sweet, so I use just few tablespoons of powdered sugar. You can add more powdered sugar to your preference. Keep in mind that the extra sugar will yield a stiffer frosting, and it will also thicken with refrigeration (as the coconut oil will harden). If the frosting becomes too thick or stiff with refrigeration, simply let sit at room temperature until it softens enough to spread or pipe.

Shredded coconut adds flavor, texture, and also stability to the frosting, but it is optional. Also, you can lightly toast the coconut in advance before adding it to the frosting, and/or add a sprinkle of toasted coconut to the finished frosted cake or cupcakes.

For a chocolate version, add 2 tablespoons of unsweetened cocoa powder when adding the powdered sugar, and either keep or omit the shredded coconut.

Cooked Chocolate Frosting

MAKES ENOUGH FROSTING
FOR ONE 2-LAYER CAKE

wheat
gluten **FREE**
soy

This chocolate frosting is an adaptation of the cooked vanilla frosting, and rivals my other chocolate frostings as my all-time favorite. Yep, I think it's won me over!

5 tablespoons millet (for gluten-free), barley, or spelt flour (see note)

1¼ cups natural powdered sugar, sifted if lumpy (see "Plant-Powered Pantry," page xxxvi)

3 tablespoons unsweetened cocoa powder

½ teaspoon sea salt

¼ or ½ teaspoon agar powder (use ¼ teaspoon for barley or spelt flour, ½ teaspoon for millet)

1 cup + 2 tablespoons chocolate nondairy milk (see note)

½ cup organic extra-virgin coconut oil, at room temperature (see "Plant-Powered Pantry," page xxix)

In a saucepan over medium heat, whisk the flour with the sugar, cocoa, salt, and agar. Gradually whisk in the milk. Cook, stirring frequently with a whisk at first, and then whisk almost constantly as the mixture thickens (take care that the mixture doesn't thicken on the bottom of the pan and clump; lower the heat to medium-low, if necessary).

Transfer to a stand mixer fitted with the paddle attachment. Mix on high speed for about 5 minutes, until the mixture has started to cool down. Add the coconut oil and beat for another few minutes, until the mixture is cool and creamy. At this point, you can either frost your cake or chill the frosting to whip up even fluffier.

To do so, refrigerate the mixer bowl of frosting until chilled (1 to 1½ hours). Then, instead of using the paddle attachment, affix the wire whisk attachment. Begin mixing slowly and then bring up to the fastest speed for a minute or two, until the frosting becomes lighter in color and fluffier. (If it doesn't, the frosting might need more chilling. Return the bowl to fridge for another 30 minutes to an hour. Then whip at high speed again.)

Frost the cake or refrigerate the whipped mixture.

Ingredients 411: When using millet flour, because it is gluten free, it is helpful to use extra agar to help stabilize the frosting.

Kid-Friendly: If making this for a children's party, you can add a touch more powdered sugar to the frosting. After whipping, taste, and if you think the cocoa flavor might be bitter for their taste buds, add another 3 to 4 tablespoons of powdered sugar. When adding the powdered sugar, be sure to turn off the mixer, and work it in slowly and then up to high speed (so as not to get a sugar dusting yourself)!

Make It More-ish! If you're feeling energetic, whip up this chocolate frosting and also the Cooked Vanilla Frosting, for a "black and white" cake. Choose a vanilla or chocolate cake batter, and simply frost half of each layer with the vanilla and chocolate frostings. Like a "black and white cookie" in cake form!

Savvy Subs and Adds: Cooked frosting traditionally uses all-purpose flour and butter. Coconut butter steps in for the dairy butter, and barley, spelt, or millet flour can be used in place of all-purpose. I like using millet flour. Because it is gluten free, it is easier to whisk and more forgiving, with less tendency to clump, than a gluten-based flour

A plain or vanilla almond milk can be substituted for chocolate. If so, you can add another 1 to 2 teaspoons of unsweetened cocoa powder to the whisking mixture.

Sugar-Free Cashew Glaze

MAKES ABOUT 1 CUP, ENOUGH
TO GLAZE 12 CUPCAKES OR THE
TOPS OF ONE 2-LAYER CAKE

This frosting uses only maple syrup or agave as the sweetener, and works best as a thick glaze. It is deeply satisfying and delicious, and worth a try as an alternative to a more traditional sugary frosting.

wheat
gluten **FREE**
soy

½ cup (packed) raw or roasted cashew butter (see note)

3 tablespoons raw coconut butter or organic extra-virgin coconut oil, at room temperature (see "Plant-Powered Pantry," page xxviii)

¼ teaspoon sea salt

⅓ cup pure maple syrup or agave nectar

1½ teaspoons pure vanilla extract

In a stand mixer using a paddle attachment, cream the cashew butter with the coconut butter or oil at medium speed for 2 to 3 minutes, until creamy (see note for chocolate version). Add the salt, maple syrup, and vanilla. Increase the speed to medium-high and beat for a couple of minutes, until the mixture is just smooth and creamy. Do not overwork.

Because it is dense, it helps to slightly warm this frosting by setting its bowl in a hot water bath. Glaze your cake or cupcakes and refrigerate, or first refrigerate the frosting and use to gently smooth onto your cake.

Ingredients 411: I use the Artisana brand of raw cashew butter. The flavor is mild and creamy, with a light nutty cashew flavor and also a creamy color. Roasted cashew butter will give the frosting a nuttier flavor and darker color, but is still delicious.

Make It More-ish! For a chocolate version, add 2 tablespoons of unsweetened cocoa powder after creaming the cashew and coconut butters; the vanilla extract can be omitted, if desired.

Lemon-Scented Whipped Cream

MAKES ⅔ TO ¾ CUP

wheat gluten soy **FREE**

Why whip dairy when you can whip coconut?! This cream is airy, fluffy, luscious, and has just a hint of lemon zest to lift the flavor. Xanthan gum helps add stability to the cream; I recommend using it.

1 (14-ounce) can regular (not "lite") coconut milk (refrigerated ahead of time; see "Plant-Powered Pantry," page xxviii)

1 to 2 tablespoons agave nectar (or can use maple syrup or natural powdered sugar; adjust sweetness to taste)

½ teaspoon lemon zest
Seeds from 1 vanilla bean (see "Plant-Powered Pantry," page xlii)

¼ teaspoon xanthan gum (optional but helpful; see note)

Open the can of coconut milk, without shaking or otherwise tipping much. You want to keep the cream solids as separate as possible from the watery liquid. Use a spoon to scoop out the thick cream into the bowl of a stand mixer. You will get about ½ cup + 2 to 4 tablespoons (see note). Add the other ingredients, and with the wire whip attachment, whip the cream at high speed for a minute or two, until it thickens and becomes fluffy.

Once thickened, transfer to an airtight container and refrigerate until ready to use. It keeps for several days without deflating.

If This Apron Could Talk: If you are having trouble getting the cream whipped (e.g., too much liquid got included with the cream), you can help firm up the cream with the addition of xanthan gum. Usually, if just 1 tablespoon of agave is used, no xanthan gum is needed. But if you use 2 tablespoons of agave (or more), it liquefies the cream and stability is needed. Typically ¼ teaspoon of xanthan gum will do the job, but you may need a pinch or two extra, depending on the mixture. I like adding the xanthan gum regardless, as it helps stabilize the cream.

I have experimented freezing this cream, and it thaws just perfectly, with the same texture and ready to use.

Savvy Subs and Adds: The vanilla seeds are really exceptional in this whipped cream, but feel free to use just a touch of vanilla extract, no more than ½ teaspoon.

Fresh Strawberry Sauce

MAKES 2 TO 2¼ CUPS

wheat gluten soy **FREE**

Sometimes, simple is best—such as when local, ripe strawberries are bursting with flavor, juicy and sweet, and need very little to transform them into a fresh sauce for topping desserts.

3 cups fresh or frozen strawberries or other berries of choice

1 to 1½ teaspoons freshly squeezed lemon juice

3 to 4 tablespoons pure maple syrup or agave nectar

3 to 4 tablespoons water (or more for frozen berries; see note)
Pinch of sea salt

Combine all the ingredients in a blender (starting with 3 tablespoons of water). Process until smooth. If more water is needed to thin the mixture, add a couple of teaspoons at a time until you reach desired texture (see note).

Store in an airtight jar for 2 to 3 days.

Ingredients 411: Frozen berries will require a little more water to blend; however, don't add too much, as the sauce will thin as it thaws. Add only as much as needed to be able to blend. With frozen berries you can expect to have a thick, slushy mixture after blending, which will thin out for serving after refrigerating for a couple of hours.

Because the sweetness of berries varies greatly, depending on the time of season (and also variety), taste the sauce. If additional maple syrup or another sweetener is needed, add a tablespoon or two, to taste.

Warm Strawberry Sauce

MAKES 1½ TO 1¾ CUPS

wheat gluten soy FREE

One strawberry sauce is just not enough! Sometimes you want a warm sauce to drizzle over ice cream or top pancakes and waffles. This sauce is so very simple, with just a few ingredients that won't overtake the beauty of the strawberries themselves.

1 pound fresh strawberries or other berries, sliced if large or left whole if small (about 3 cups)

2 to 4 tablespoons pure maple syrup or agave nectar (sweeten to taste, based on personal preference and also sweetness of berries)

A few pinches of sea salt

Place the berries, a few tablespoons of the maple syrup, and the salt in a saucepan over medium heat (add a splash of water, if needed, especially for other berries that are not as moist, such as blueberries). Let mixture come up to a bubble, then lower the heat to medium-low and cook at a slow bubble for 15 to 20 minutes, or until the fruit has broken down and the sauce has thickened slightly. Taste, and add additional sweetener, if desired.

Serve the sauce warm or cool (it will thicken more after cooling). If you'd like a smoother consistency, puree the sauce in a blender (after cooling slightly), and then strain to catch any seedy bits. Store in an airtight jar in the fridge for up to a week.

Rich Coconut Caramel Sauce

MAKES ABOUT 1½ CUPS

wheat gluten soy **FREE**

This is a marvelously simple caramel sauce that is naturally thick and rich, thanks to the coconut milk. After simmering to reduce, it becomes luscious and thick, almost like a *dulce de leche*.

1 cup regular (not "lite") coconut milk (use only the thick cream and discard the watery portion; you can refrigerate ahead of time to help separate, but this is not essential)

¾ cup + 1 tablespoon coconut sugar (see note)

⅛ teaspoon (rounded) sea salt

1 teaspoon pure vanilla extract

In a saucepan over medium heat, combine the coconut milk, sugar, and salt. Stir and bring to a boil (keep a close watch; it may boil over quickly). Once at a boil, lower the heat to low and simmer for 12 to 18 minutes, to reduce. Then stir in the vanilla and let cool. (The longer you simmer and reduce the sauce, the thicker it will become after cooling.)

This sauce refrigerates well and thickens more with chilling.

Ingredients 411: Coconut sugar has a deep caramel color and a beautiful flavor. Do not substitute a light-colored unrefined sugar in this recipe, as you won't get the rich color needed for a caramel sauce. Coconut sugar has become more available in grocery stores, but if you can't find it, substitute with another darker unrefined sugar such as Sucanat.

Vanilla Yogurt

MAKES ABOUT 1¼ CUPS

wheat
gluten **FREE**
soy

While this cashew-based "yogurt" doesn't contain any of those beneficial probiotics, it is an excellent substitute for commercially prepared soy, coconut, and other nondairy yogurts in recipes. Plus, it's tasty straight off a spoon!

  1 cup soaked raw cashews
  ⅓ cup unsweetened applesauce (preferably organic)
1½ to 2 tablespoons freshly squeezed lemon juice (see note)
  1 tablespoon pure maple syrup
  ⅓ cup nondairy milk (or more to thin if desired, but keep to ⅓ cup for use in recipes; use soy free for that option)
  ½ teaspoon pure vanilla extract
    Pinch of salt

In a high-powered blender, puree all the ingredients until very smooth. If using a standard blender, this may take a few minutes, scraping down the sides a few times.

Serve, or store in an airtight container.

If This Apron Could Talk: Use 1½ tablespoon of lemon juice for use in recipes, and if you'd like it tangier for eating straight, add the extra lemon juice to taste.

Kid-Friendly: I created this yogurt primarily as a substitute for premade yogurts in my recipes (e.g., BF Blueberry Muffins or Fresh Orange Cake). As such, it isn't overly sweet. Feel free to make it a little more fun for your little ones by stirring in extra maple syrup, or try a few spoonfuls of a berry, peach, or other fruit jam. Warm Strawberry Sauce would be especially delicious. Also note that this yogurt is nutritious for little ones that might not otherwise eat nuts or nut butters because of textural issues—nuts being too hard, and nut butters too sticky! This recipe brings cashews into a puddinglike form that *you* can customize with extra flavor and sweetness!

Tapioca Pudding

MAKES 2 CUPS

wheat gluten soy FREE

This pudding got me through many evening cravings during my third pregnancy! You see, as a kid and teen I always loved those small containers of rice and tapioca puddings. I already had recipes for rice pudding, and it was time to sort out tapioca!

¼ cup small pearl tapioca (I use Let's Do . . . Organic brand)
1 cup vanilla or plain nondairy milk
1½ cups water
1 teaspoon pure vanilla extract
3 to 4 tablespoons agave nectar or other liquid sweetener (or less or more to taste; see note)
¼ teaspoon sea salt
A few pinches of freshly grated nutmeg (optional)

In a saucepan over medium-high heat, combine the tapioca, milk, and water and stir. Bring to a boil, stirring frequently. Then lower the heat to low or medium-low and cook, uncovered, for 14 to 15 minutes, stirring occasionally, until the tapioca is cooked through and translucent. Add the vanilla, agave, salt, and nutmeg (if using), stir, and cook for another minute or two. (For a thicker consistency, continue to cook for another few minutes; however, do note that the pudding will thicken considerably once cooled.)

Remove from the heat and let cool some in the pan, then transfer to a heatproof dish or bowl and refrigerate until chilled.

If This Apron Could Talk: Trust the pudding! When you make this, it will appear too runny and that there aren't enough tapioca pearls for a finished pudding. But, I promise, this pudding will thicken up as it cools, the pearls will swell more, and you will have a thick, yummy pudding!

Ingredients 411: Adjust the sweetener according to the milk used. If using vanilla milk, you may want less sweetener, but with an unflavored nondairy milk, you may prefer the full 4 tablespoons of agave—or more to taste. Also, other sweeteners can be substituted (e.g., maple syrup or Sucanat, though they add a darker color than agave nectar).

Raw Orange Chocolate Pudding

MAKES ABOUT 2½ CUPS

wheat gluten soy **FREE**

This mousse (or pudding, depending on your opinion), is incredibly healthful, with a foundation of avocado and dates to create a smooth, sweet consistency and *no* added sweeteners. Kids will love it, and will have no idea how good it is for them!

Seeds from 1 vanilla bean (see "Plant-Powered Pantry," page xlii), or 1½ teaspoons pure vanilla extract

1 cup peeled, pitted, and roughly chopped ripe avocado (about 1 large or 1½ small to medium-size avocados)

1 cup pitted dates

⅓ cup raw or regular unsweetened cocoa powder

1 teaspoon orange zest (zest orange first and then juice)

½ cup fresh squeezed orange juice

⅛ teaspoon sea salt

In a food processor, puree all the ingredients. Puree until very, very smooth, stopping the processor to scrape down the sides several times while processing. This pudding is very thick. If you'd like to thin it, you can do so with more orange juice, or a splash of nut milk or water.

Serve or store in the refrigerator.

Pumpkin Pie Custard

MAKES 5 OR 6 CUSTARDS

wheat gluten soy **FREE**

These custards are magical—creamy, luscious, and like having a mini pumpkin pie (without the crust!) all to yourself! These are on our annual Thanksgiving and Christmas menus, definitely make them for your holiday celebrations—and with the brûlée topping!

- ⅔ cup (packed) pumpkin puree (not pumpkin pie filling) (I use Farmer's Market organic brand)
- ½ cup raw cashews
- 1¼ cups plain unsweetened nondairy milk (almond or soy preferred; see "Plant-Powered Pantry," page xxxiii)
- ½ cup unrefined sugar
- ¼ cup pure maple syrup
- 1 tablespoon freshly squeezed lemon juice
- 1¼ teaspoons agar powder
- 1 teaspoon arrowroot powder
- 1 teaspoon ground cinnamon
  A few pinches of freshly ground nutmeg
  Pinch or two of ground allspice
  Pinch or two of ground cloves
- 1 teaspoon pure vanilla extract
- ¼ teaspoon sea salt
  A few teaspoons unrefined sugar for caramelized topping (optional, see note)

Preheat the oven to 375°F. Place 5 or 6 ramekins (standard size) in an 8 by 11-inch glass baking dish. Bring roughly 3 cups of water to a boil in a kettle.

Meanwhile, in a blender, combine all the ingredients (except the sugar for topping) and puree until very, very smooth. (I use a Blendtec; if you don't have a high-powered blender, you will need to blend for a longer time, and scrape down the sides of the bowl a couple of times.)

Pour the boiled water into the baking dish to surround the ramekins (but don't get any water in the ramekins). Then pour the pureed pumpkin mixture evenly into each ramekin. If using six ramekins (mine are 3 inches in diameter—from the inside—and almost 2 inches deep), they will be about two-thirds full; if using five, they will be just about completely full. Carefully place the baking dish into the oven. Bake for 32 to 34 minutes, until the custards are set around the edges but a touch looser in the center.

Carefully remove the baking dish from the oven and let cool slightly until you can safely remove and transfer each custard to a cooling rack. Let cool a little more. The custards are best still a little warm, but can also be served chilled.

Make It More-ish! Turn these custards into Pumpkin Brûlée! Sprinkle ½ to 1 teaspoon of unrefined sugar over the top, and then use either a small butane torch or oven broiler to caramelize it. If using the oven broiler: Set the oven to BROIL, and then place the individual ramekins under the broiler for 3 to 5 minutes. Check after 3 minutes, and then again at the 4-minute mark. If not done, broil for another minute or so. If doing this brûlée finish, do it soon before serving, as the crunchy topping will soften if prepared too long in advance.

Making Vegan Piecrusts

Here are a few things to keep in mind when making vegan piecrusts.

- First of all, if you are new to pie baking, don't stress. These piecrusts are more forgiving than are many conventional pastry recipes.
- While it is useful to have the coconut oil at room temperature for effortless measuring (it is soft and scoopable when soft), do not melt the oil. It will result in different measurements, and it is also preferable to have the oil more solidified for distributing the fats through the crust. If your oil is melted at room temperature, refrigerate it until it firms up slightly but is still soft.
- Do your best to roll out the dough evenly and into a circle, but don't sweat it. Even if your pie dough is not rolled out into an even circle, you can place in a pie dish and patch with longer pieces if needed.
- If rolling out the dough gives you grief, you can take a shortcut. Flatten the dough and transfer to the pie plate, then use your hands to press the dough around the bottom and up the sides of the pie plate, much like you would do for a cookie- or nut-based crust. Because these crusts contain no or little gluten, handling them won't toughen them up.
- For easier nonstick rolling, place your dough between two pieces of parchment paper. Roll gently from the center out, turning your dough between rollings as you go, to make an evenly distributed disk 2 to 2½ inches larger than the diameter of your pan. You can estimate, or it might be useful to trace the circumference of the pan onto the underside of the bottom sheet, as a guide.
- Use a glass pie plate for best results, and lightly grease the bottom and sides of the plate, for the easier removal of your pie slices. Use the edge of a paper towel to lightly coat the inside of the plate.
- These crusts can be made in advance, shaped into a thick disk, wrapped in plastic wrap and refrigerated. When ready to use, remove from the fridge for 10 to 15 minutes or longer to make more pliable, and follow the directions to roll out.
- If there is any excess dough around the edge, simply trim it with a sharp knife or kitchen shears. For double crusts, you can crimp or press the two layers together after trimming (you may need to moisten with water for the Rustic Piecrust, but that's not necessary for the Gluten-Free Piecrust). This is where you can get fancy—if you like. Me, I either do a simple pinch with my fingers or press with the tines of a fork—but I'm not particular about it. You can lose patience trying to make it look "just right," so keep it simple; rustic folds or tucks are fine. Your family and friends won't care; they'll be too busy asking for seconds!

- Once your piecrust is fitted into your pie plate, place in the refrigerator or freezer to chill before baking (about 15 minutes in the freezer or 30 minutes in the fridge).
- For double-crust pies, be sure to cut steam vents into the top crust— simple slits with a sharp knife, or fancier, using mini cookie cutters!
- Before baking a double-crust pie, brush the top with a little nondairy milk and then sprinkle with just a little coarse, unrefined sugar. This brings a sparkly, pretty finish to your pie.
- If the crust edges are browning too much while baking, you can loosely wrap some aluminum foil just around the perimeter of the pie until it finishes baking.
- To prebake a single crust for an uncooked filling, prick the bottom with a fork and bake in a preheated 375°F oven for 20 to 25 minutes, or until the crust has become a little golden but not too brown, and isn't moist or sticky.
- Let's face it, there's not always time or enough patience to bake a crust from scratch! When you need a shortcut, look for the Wholly Wholesome brand of piecrusts and shells. They are good quality, and have always worked well in my testing.
- For precooked pie fillings that do not require a baked crust, also consider using the raw crusts in Raw Lemon-Lime Cheesecake with Coconut Nut Crust, Raw Chocolate Dream Mousse Pie, or Raw Strawberry Pie.

Rustic Piecrust

wheat
soy **FREE**

This is much like a traditional pastry crust, but with a mellow, naturally sweet "oaty" flavor. It also omits margarine and instead uses coconut oil. Use it anywhere you might use a standard pastry crust!

SINGLE CRUST:

½ cup light or sifted spelt flour

½ cup oat flour

½ cup corn flour or fine stone-ground cornmeal (see note)

1½ tablespoons unrefined sugar (or ½ tablespoon, if using for a savory filling)

¼ teaspoon sea salt

⅓ cup organic extra-virgin coconut oil, at room temperature (see "Plant-Powered Pantry," page xxix)

5½ to 6 tablespoons ice-cold plain nondairy milk

DOUBLE CRUST:

1 cup light or sifted spelt flour

1 cup oat flour

1 cup corn flour or fine stone-ground cornmeal (see note)

3 tablespoons unrefined sugar (or 1 tablespoon, if using for a savory filling)

½ teaspoon sea salt

⅔ cup organic extra-virgin coconut oil, at room temperature

11 to 12 tablespoons ice-cold nondairy milk (add ice cubes to milk)

In a food processor, combine the flours, sugar, and salt. Process for a few seconds to mix. Add the coconut oil, and pulse briefly to begin to break up and incorporate. Then add a few tablespoons of the milk for the double crust, 1 tablespoon at a time for single, pulsing, and then continue to add milk 1 tablespoon at a time after that, pulsing until the dough has just come together and has started to form a ball. (It doesn't have to be one unified ball; pulse just until some of the dough has started to come together.)

Remove the dough from the processor and shape into a ball. For the double crust, divide the dough in two (you can weigh each half for precision, if you like, but it's not necessary). If the dough has become warm, shape into a flattened disk, wrap in plastic wrap, and refrigerate for 20 to 30 minutes. (You can also refrigerate this dough for a few days before using, and remove from fridge for an hour or two before rolling, long enough for the coconut oil to soften again in the dough.)

When ready to use, place a flattened disk between two sheets of parchment for easiest rolling. Roll out the dough to 2 to 2½ inches larger than your pie plate. Place the bottom crust in a greased pie plate. Place this crust in the freezer for 15 to 20 minutes while preparing your filling, or prebake the crust if you will be using a no-bake filling in the pie.

For a double crust, roll out the second half of dough to a little larger than the diameter of your pan, place on top of the filling, and crimp the edges (don't trim; the baked crust is too tasty, and even if thicker in spots, is still fabulous, so keep things rustic).

Follow the directions for baking the specific pie filling, and if using a double crust, it's a nice idea to brush the top with a little nondairy milk and sprinkle a little sugar over the top.

If This Apron Could Talk: See "Making Vegan Piecrusts," page 239, for tips on making and rolling out dough.

This crust isn't very sweet, but if you want to use it for a savory pie or tart, use just ½ tablespoon of sugar in the single crust, and 1 tablespoon in the double.

Ingredients 411: Very finely ground cornmeal is similar to corn flour in texture. However, if it is a medium grind, the cornmeal will be too granular for this crust. Look for an organic corn flour or fine stone-ground cornmeal, Bob's Red Mill brand is a good choice.

Gluten-Free Piecrust

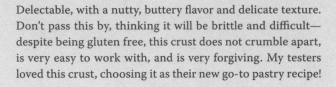

Delectable, with a nutty, buttery flavor and delicate texture. Don't pass this by, thinking it will be brittle and difficult—despite being gluten free, this crust does not crumble apart, is very easy to work with, and is very forgiving. My testers loved this crust, choosing it as their new go-to pastry recipe!

wheat gluten soy **FREE**

SINGLE CRUST:

- ¾ cup almond meal (see note)
- ¼ cup + 2 tablespoons rice flour or sorghum flour
- ¼ cup tapioca starch flour
- 2 tablespoons arrowroot powder
- 2 tablespoons unrefined sugar
- ¼ teaspoon sea salt
- 1 teaspoon xanthan gum
- 7 tablespoons organic extra-virgin coconut oil, at room temperature (see "Plant-Powered Pantry," page xxix)
- 3½ to 4 tablespoons ice-cold plain nondairy milk

In a food processor, combine the almond meal, rice flour, tapioca starch flour, arrowroot, sugar, salt, and xanthan gum. Process for a few seconds to mix these ingredients. Add the coconut oil, and pulse briefly to begin to break up and incorporate. Then add a few tablespoons of the milk for the double crust, 1 tablespoon at a time for single, pulsing, and then continue to add milk 1 tablespoon at a time after that, pulsing until the dough has just come together and has started to form a ball. (It doesn't have to be one unified ball; pulse just until some of the dough has started to come together.)

Remove the dough from the processor and shape into a ball. For the double crust, divide the dough in two (you can weigh each half for precision, if you like, but it's not necessary). If the dough has become warm, shape into a flattened disk, wrap in plastic wrap, and refrigerate for 20 to 30 minutes. (You can also refrigerate this dough for a few days before using, and remove from fridge for an hour or two before rolling, long enough for the coconut oil to soften again in the dough.)

When ready to use, place a flattened disk between two sheets of parchment for easiest rolling. Roll out the dough to 2 to 2½ inches larger than your pie plate. Place the bottom crust in a greased pie plate. Place this crust in the freezer for 15 to 20 minutes while preparing your filling (e.g., Apple-of-My-Eye Pie), or prebake the crust, if you will be using a no-bake filling in the pie.

DOUBLE CRUST:

- 1½ cups almond meal (see note)
- ¾ cup rice flour or sorghum flour
- ½ cup tapioca starch flour
- ¼ cup arrowroot powder
- ¼ cup unrefined sugar
- ½ teaspoon sea salt
- 2 teaspoons xanthan gum
- ¾ cup + 2 tablespoons organic extra-virgin coconut oil, at room temperature
- 7½ to 8 tablespoons ice-cold plain nondairy milk

For a double crust, roll out the second half of dough to a little larger than the diameter of your pan, place on top of the filling, and crimp the edges (don't trim; the baked crust is too tasty, and even if thicker in spots, is still fabulous, so keep things rustic).

Follow the directions for baking the specific pie filling, and if using a double crust, it's a nice idea to brush the top with a little nondairy milk and sprinkle a little sugar over the top.

If This Apron Could Talk: See "Making Vegan Piecrusts," page 239, for tips on making and rolling out dough.

Ingredients 411: I use an almond meal that has been processed from natural, unblanched almonds (skins still intact). As a result, the crust has flecks of a nutty brown color, which is quite pretty in the finished pie. If you can buy this almond meal (or make it yourself), go for it!

Apple-of-My-Eye Pie

wheat gluten soy **FREE**

This is your stop for apple pie filling. The apples are sliced thinly and bake up tender in a fragrant, juicy sauce. You can choose your favorite apples for this pie, as there will always be varying opinions about the "best" apples for apple pie! I like to use more than one variety, such as a combination of Fuji and Spartan, or a tart apple combined with a sweeter, crunchier variety such as Gala. Regardless of the type of apple, this is heavenly with the Gluten-Free Piecrust.

2 teaspoons freshly squeezed lemon juice
3 tablespoons pure maple syrup
3 tablespoons tapioca starch flour
¼ cup unrefined sugar
1¼ teaspoons ground cinnamon
⅛ to ¼ teaspoons freshly grated nutmeg
⅛ teaspoon ground allspice
⅛ teaspoon sea salt
6 cups peeled, cored, and thinly sliced apples (see note)
1 double piecrust (e.g., Gluten-Free Piecrust, page 242, or Rustic Piecrust, page 241), or use 2 prepared vegan pastry crusts
  Splash of nondairy milk, to brush pastry
1 to 2 teaspoons unrefined sugar, for sprinkling

Preheat the oven to 400°F.

In bowl large enough to hold the sliced apples, combine the lemon juice with the maple syrup and tapioca starch flour, stirring well to incorporate fully. Stir in the sugar, cinnamon, nutmeg, allspice, and salt. Add the apple slices to the mixture, and toss to coat.

Transfer the filling to the bottom piecrust (you can prebake this crust for 10 to 15 minutes, if you like, but this is not necessary).

Moisten the edge of the crust with water (you can skip this step if using the Gluten-Free Piecrust, as it easily holds to bottom crust), and place the top crust over the filling. Cut a few slits in the top crust to allow steam to exit while baking (alternatively, you can use cutout pastry shapes to form the top crust, or a lattice-top crust). Brush the top crust with the milk and sprinkle a teaspoon or two of sugar over the top.

Place the pie in the oven (with a baking sheet on the rack underneath to catch any drippings) and bake for 20 minutes. Then lower heat to 350°F and bake for another 30 to 35 minutes, until the top is lightly browned and the juices are thickened and bubbling, watching that the outer edges aren't browning too fast (see "Making Vegan Piecrusts," page 239). To check for doneness, pierce through the pie (where open or vented) with a skewer or sharp knife. If the apples are not tender when pierced, allow to cook for another 5 minutes.

Remove from the oven, transfer to a cooling rack, and let cool for an hour or more before serving. This pie is delicious served with vanilla nondairy ice cream, or Lemon-Scented Whipped Cream.

Raw Chocolate Dream Mousse Pie

SERVES 6 TO 8

wheat gluten soy **FREE**

Creamy, chocolaty, luscious. Yet no sugar, no flour, no oil. Yes, chocolate dreams do come true. The filling is adaptable and can be accented with other flavors, such as orange zest (or orange oil), almond extract, or mint (leaves or extract).

CRUST:

- 1 cup unsoaked raw almonds
- ¾ cup unsoaked raw pecans
- 1 cup (lightly packed) pitted dates
- 2 tablespoons raw unsweetened cocoa powder
- ¼ teaspoon (scant) sea salt
- ¼ teaspoon freshly ground nutmeg
- ½ teaspoon pure vanilla extract (see note)

FILLING:

- 1 cup peeled, pitted, and sliced or chopped ripe avocado (about 1 large or 1 to ½ medium-size avocados)
- ½ cup soaked raw cashews (about ⅓ cup unsoaked)
- ½ cup nut milk (or other nondairy milk if preparing nonraw)
- ½ cup pitted dates
- ¼ cup pure maple syrup
- ⅓ cup raw unsweetened cocoa powder
- ½ to 1 teaspoon pure vanilla extract (see note)
- ⅛ teaspoon sea salt

Lightly oil a pie plate with coconut or another oil.

Prepare the crust: Place the almonds in a food processor and pulse briefly until fine and crumbly. Add the crust remaining ingredients and process until the mixture becomes sticky. Stop to scrape down the bowl, if needed. The mixture should hold together when pressed with your fingers. If it's still a little dry or not sticking, pulse again, add another date (or two, if small honey dates) and process again. Use ½ to 1 teaspoon of water, as well, if not using vanilla extract.

Transfer the mixture to the prepared pie plate. Press the mixture evenly into the pan.

To prepare the filling: Place all the filling ingredients in a high-powered blender and puree for a minute or so on at medium-high speed, until completely smooth and no texture of the cashews remains. Stop to scrape down the blender and redistribute the ingredients. Puree again until very, very smooth—like a velvety pudding. This will take a few starts and stops for scraping down—even with a high-powered blender. Once the mixture is readily churning and smooth, it's ready.

Pour the filling into the crust, and tilt and smooth with a spatula to evenly distribute. Refrigerate for a couple of hours to set. (Optionally, you can also freeze the pie and serve at a later time, thawing most of the way before slicing.) Slice and serve.

Savvy Subs and Adds: If you'd prefer not to use vanilla extract, use the seeds from one vanilla bean (see "Plant-Powered Pantry," page xlii), using half for the crust and half for the filling.

Serving Suggestion: Serve as is, or topped with fresh strawberries, blueberries, or raspberries, or a ladleful of Fresh Strawberry Sauce.

Raw Lemon-Lime Cheesecake with Coconut Nut Crust and Fresh Mango Sauce

SERVES 6 TO 8

wheat gluten soy **FREE**

Raw cheesecakes trump any tofu or soy cream cheese version (at least for me)! I wanted to come up with my own signature raw cheesecake. This one combines the tang and flavor of both lemon and lime juice, and has a tropical twist with coconut in the crust and a fresh mango sauce for serving. The recipe makes a fairly large batch of mango sauce. You can halve the batch or save the extra to top other foods, such as yogurt or waffles. You can also try the Fresh Strawberry Sauce as a switch from the mango puree. Regardless of the sauce you choose, this dessert is heavenly.

CRUST:

1 cup soaked raw almonds (soak first, then measure; this is about ¾ cup unsoaked; see note)

1 cup unsoaked raw pecans

¾ cup pitted medjool dates

¼ cup unsweetened shredded coconut

1 teaspoon pure vanilla extract

⅛ teaspoon sea salt

Lightly oil the bottom and sides of a 9-inch springform pan (do not use tube liner).

Prepare the crust: Place the almonds and pecans in a food processor. Pulse until very crumbly, then add the remaining ingredients and process until the mixture will hold together when pressed.

Transfer the mixture to the prepared springform pan.

FILLING:

3¼ cups soaked raw cashews (soak first, then measure—this is about 2½ cups unsoaked; see "Plant-Powered Pantry," page xxxiv)

¼ cup freshly squeezed lemon juice

¼ cup freshly squeezed lime juice

1 teaspoon lemon zest

¼ teaspoon sea salt

½ cup + 1 tablespoon raw agave nectar
Seeds from 1 vanilla bean (see "Plant-Powered Pantry," page xlii)

½ cup (packed) coconut butter, at room temperature (I use Artisana; see "Plant-Powered Pantry," page xviii)

MANGO SAUCE:

1½ cups frozen mango chunks

½ cup water

2 tablespoons freshly squeezed orange juice

¼ cup raw agave nectar or pure maple syrup

½ teaspoon orange zest
Pinch of sea salt

To prepare the filling, place all the filling ingredients in a high-powered blender (see note). Puree until very, very smooth and lightened in color.

Pour the mixture over the crust and tip the pan back and forth to distribute evenly. Cover the pan with foil and pop into the freezer to set (you can freeze overnight, if you like, but freeze at least 3 to 4 hours so it can become firmer).

To prepare the mango sauce: Combine all the sauce ingredients in a blender and puree until smooth; refrigerate in a covered container until ready to serve.

To serve, remove the cake from the freezer for 30 minutes to 1 hour to soften slightly before slicing. Serve with the sauce.

If This Apron Could Talk: It's helpful to make the crust a day ahead if you have the time; it spreads out the preparation work and makes for easier cleanup!

Ingredients 411: If your measurement of almonds is a bit shy or generous, simply make up the difference with the pecans.

Raw Strawberry Pie

SERVES 6 TO 8

wheat gluten soy **FREE**

One summer after picking buckets full of local ripe strawberries, I wanted to make a pie deserving of their glorious, fresh flavor. I created this pie, and it did the strawberries proud!

CRUST:

1 raw pecans
¾ cup raw walnuts
1 cup (packed) pitted dates
¼ teaspoon (scant) sea salt
¼ teaspoon ground cinnamon

FILLING:

3 cups fresh strawberries (whole if small, or cut in half if large)
¾ cup unsoaked raw cashews (see note)
3 to 4 tablespoons raw agave nectar (adjust to taste)
1 teaspoon freshly squeezed lemon juice
A few pinches of sea salt
1 teaspoon lemon zest

Lightly oil a pie plate with coconut or another oil.

Prepare the crust: Place all the crust ingredients in a food processor and pulse briefly until crumbly and the mixture will hold together when pressed with your fingers.

Transfer the mixture to the prepared pie plate, pressing it evenly into the pan.

Prepare the filling: Place all the filling ingredients, except the lemon zest (and starting with 3 tablespoons of the agave nectar), in a high-powered blender (see note). Puree for a minute or so at medium-high speed until completely smooth and no texture of the cashews remains. Taste, and add the remaining tablespoon of agave, if needed, to sweeten, and puree again. Once smooth, stir in the lemon zest.

Pour the filling into the crust, then cover with aluminum foil or plastic wrap and place the pie in the freezer for at least 5 to 6 hours to set. After this time, the pie will be partially set, but can be sliced. You can freeze it longer, and remove the pie about 20 minutes before serving, to slice easily.

Ingredients 411: It is preferable to use unsoaked cashews because they have less moisture, and then can absorb some of the moisture from the strawberries as the pie sets. If using local seasonal berries, they tend to be softer and juicier than imported. Opt for another 2 tablespoons of cashews to help absorb the extra juices.

Serving Suggestion: Serve as is, or with Lemon-Scented Whipped Cream.

"Chocolate-Dipped Strawberries" Pie

SERVES 7 TO 8

wheat gluten soy **FREE**

I made this pie for my husband on Valentine's Day, inspired by the idea of chocolate-dipped strawberries. I had fresh strawberries on hand, but didn't want to simply dip them in chocolate . . . and I had this notion to include fresh strawberries in a chocolate truffle sort of pie. Although this pie is somewhat unconventional (what with folding the fresh strawberries into the chocolate filling), it is exceptionally tasty!

1   (160 ml) can regular (not "lite") coconut milk (see note)

3   tablespoons brown rice syrup

¾   teaspoon agar powder

1½ cups chopped vegan dark chocolate (about 8½ ounces)

1½ cups fresh strawberries, sliced (and cut in half if very large)

1   prepared vegan chocolate cookie piecrust (I use Wholly Wholesome brand), or Rustic Piecrust (page 241) or Gluten-Free Piecrust (page 242)

In a saucepan over medium heat, combine the coconut milk, brown rice syrup, and agar powder, stirring until the brown rice syrup and agar are dissolved and the coconut milk is hot but not boiling.

Remove from the heat, and pour the hot milk mixture over the chocolate (in a heatproof glass or metal bowl). Fold until the chocolate is melted.

Place in fridge to cool slightly (15 to 20 minutes). Remove from the fridge and fold in strawberries, taking care not to overmix (to not mush berries). Pour the mixture into the chocolate pie shell, and refrigerate until completely cool and set.

If This Apron Could Talk: This pie is best served the same day you make the pie. Make it earlier in the day for a dinner party, or in the morning for an afternoon dessert. The strawberries begin to break down the next day, and although the taste is still fine, the appearance of the pie is not quite as pretty.

Ingredients 411: I use Earth's Choice organic coconut milk, and this brand is available in 160 ml cans. If you cannot find this brand/size, 160 ml is the equivalent of about ⅔ cup, so simply measure this out from a 14-ounce can.

If using a pastry piecrust, be sure to prebake the piecrust before filling it (see "Making Vegan Piecrusts," page 239).

Savvy Subs and Adds: If you'd like to enhance the berry flavor of this pie, you can try adding ¼ to ½ teaspoon of cherry or almond extract when warming the milk mixture.

Three's Company Pie

SERVES 6 TO 8

All combinations here are winners—chocolate and peanut butter, banana and peanut butter, and chocolate and banana. Together, three's company, not a crowd!

(optionally) wheat
(optionally) gluten
soy **FREE**

1 cup vegan chocolate chips
⅔ cup natural organic peanut butter or nut butter such as cashew or almond (see note)
1 cup sliced ripe banana (not overripe as for banana bread, just lightly flecked)
1 tablespoon unsweetened cocoa powder
2 tablespoons pure maple syrup
1½ teaspoons pure vanilla extract
¼ teaspoon (scant) sea salt (see note)
¾ cup plain or vanilla nondairy milk
1 prepared piecrust of choice (I use Wholly Wholesome brand) or Rustic Piecrust (page 241) or Gluten-Free Piecrust (page 242)

TOPPINGS:
1 to 2 medium-size to large ripe banana, sliced
½ to 1 teaspoon freshly squeezed orange or lemon juice (use full teaspoon, if using 2 bananas)
½ tablespoon unsweetened cocoa powder
¼ cup chopped peanuts or your choice of nuts

Preheat the oven to 375°F.

Prepare the filling: Fit a metal or glass bowl over a saucepan on medium-low heat and filled with several inches of water, not touching the base of the bowl (or use a double-boiler). Place the chocolate chips in the bowl and stir occasionally as the water simmers (do not boil), letting the chocolate melt.

While the chocolate is melting, in a food processor, combine the peanut butter with the banana, process, and then add the cocoa, maple syrup, vanilla, and salt. Puree, scraping down the sides and base as needed to incorporate the sticky peanut butter. Then add the milk and puree again, until fully incorporated (again scraping the sides and base to work in the stickier parts of the mixture). Once the chocolate is melted, add to mixture in the food processor and puree, scraping down the sides of bowl as needed.

Pour the mixture into the piecrust (scraping out all filling from the bowl) and tip the pie back and forth gently to evenly distribute it.

Bake for 20 minutes. The pie will be firmer around the edges and a little looser in the center, but it will set further as it cools.

Carefully remove from the oven and place on a cooling rack. Let cool completely (refrigerate if needed) before adding the toppings.

Prepare the toppings: In a small bowl, toss the banana slices with the juice. Then layer the bananas (very random/rustic) on the pie, use a fine sieve to dust the cocoa over the top, then sprinkle the peanuts over everything. Slice and serve!

If This Apron Could Talk: This pie freezes very well, if you have leftovers. Slice into portions, pop into an airtight container, and then freeze. Take out sometime later when you need a fix!

Another pretty way to decorate this cake is to dust it lightly with some powdered sugar. Simply use about 1 tablespoon of powdered sugar, place in a fine sieve, and tap it lightly over the pie to dust and decorate.

Ingredients 411: Some natural peanut butters contain salt. Try to find a brand without salt. If the brand you have is salted, reduce the salt from ¼ teaspoon to just a pinch.

To-Live-For Pecan Pie

SERVES 6 TO 8

Pecan pie was always a favorite of mine in my pre-vegan days. My version is luscious and delicious, without having any eggs, butter, or cream—truly a pie to live for!

(optionally) wheat
(optionally) gluten
soy
FREE

FILLING:

1½ tablespoons arrowroot powder
½ + ⅛ teaspoon agar powder
1 (14-ounce) can regular (not "lite") coconut milk (using mostly the thick cream and not the watery portion; you will have about 1 cup + 2 to 3 tablespoons of cream)
¼ cup plain unsweetened nondairy milk (almond or soy preferred, see "Plant-Powered Pantry," page xxxiii)
½ cup brown rice syrup
⅓ cup agave nectar (or substitute pure maple syrup, which will have a darker color)
1½ tablespoons flax meal
¼ teaspoon freshly grated nutmeg
¼ teaspoon (rounded) sea salt
2 teaspoons pure vanilla extract

TOPPING:

1¼ to 1¾ cups whole or broken raw pecans (see note)
1½ to 2 tablespoons unrefined sugar, for topping
1 to 2 teaspoons neutral-flavored oil or organic extra-virgin coconut oil, at room temperature (see "Plant-Powered Pantry," page xxxii and xxix)
A pinch of sea salt
1 prepared vegan pastry piecrust (I use Wholly Wholesome brand), or use Rustic Piecrust (page 241) or Gluten-Free Piecrust (page 242)

Prepare the filling: In a saucepan, first whisk together the arrowroot and agar with about ¼ cup of the coconut milk or nondairy milk. Once it is incorporated, whisk in the remainder of the milks, as well as the brown rice syrup, agave nectar, flax meal, nutmeg, and salt. Bring the mixture to a low boil over medium-high heat, whisking frequently. Once at a boil, remove from the heat and whisk in the vanilla.

Transfer the mixture to a bowl and let cool in the refrigerator (can still be fairly warm), stirring occasionally.

Meanwhile, prepare the topping. Toss the chopped pecans with the sugar, oil, and salt. Set aside and preheat the oven to 375°F.

Once the filling is cooled somewhat, pour the filling into the pie shell (scraping out the bowl as best you can!) Bake for 15 minutes without pecan topping. Then lower the heat to 350°F and sprinkle the pie with the pecan mixture, ever so gently patting it into the surface of the filling. Bake for another 15 minutes.

Remove carefully from the oven (the filling will not be set) and let cool on a cooling rack. Once the pie is fully cooled, it will also be set (refrigerate, if desired). Slice and serve.

If This Apron Could Talk: Unlike with traditional pecan pies, I have kept the pecan topping more distinct from the custard filling. I prefer that the pecans maintain their crunch, rather than plumping and getting softer from absorbing some of the filling during the baking.

Ingredients 411: If using whole pecans, it's helpful to chop them roughly before using in the recipe. It's easier to cut the pie if the pecan pieces are broken up rather than kept whole. I prefer this pie with just 1¼ cups of pecans, but if you really love plenty of pecans in your pecan pie, use the full 1¾ cups. If using the greater amount of pecans, then also use the greater amount of sugar and oil to toss with the pecans.

Serving Suggestion: Serve with Lemon-Scented Whipped Cream, or a scoop of vanilla nondairy ice cream, or even a drizzle of a vanilla nondairy yogurt.

Raspberry Almond Torte

SERVES 6 TO 7

wheat
gluten **FREE**
soy

This gluten-free torte has a densely sweet and satisfying almond meal base, and is covered with a thickened raspberry sauce topping. It is tart yet sweet, indulgent yet light, sticky but a civilized bit of gluten-free vegan deliciousness!

RASPBERRY TOPPING:

- ½ tablespoon arrowroot powder
- 1½ tablespoons freshly squeezed lemon juice (zest first for base, then squeeze)
- 1⅓ to 1½ cups frozen or fresh raspberries
- 3 tablespoons unrefined sugar
  A few pinches of sea salt

TORTE BASE:

- 1½ cups almond meal (see "Plant-Powered Pantry," page xxiv)
- ⅓ cup millet flour or rice flour
- 1 tablespoon ground white chia seeds
- 1½ teaspoons lemon zest
- ¼ teaspoon sea salt (rounded)
- ⅓ cup unrefined sugar
- 1 tablespoon arrowroot powder
- ½ teaspoon xanthan gum
- 2½ tablespoons nondairy milk
- ¼ cup pure maple syrup
- 1 teaspoon pure vanilla extract
- ½ teaspoon pure almond extract

Preheat the oven to 350°F. Lightly oil an 8-inch round cake pan or small pie plate and line with parchment paper on the bottom and sides (cut a circle for the bottom and a separate strip to cover the sides).

Prepare the raspberry topping: In a small bowl, stir together the arrowroot and lemon juice until well blended. In a small saucepan over medium heat, combine the raspberries, arrowroot mixture, sugar, and salt. Cook until the mixture starts to slowly bubble and thicken, stirring frequently. Once thickened, turn off the heat.

Prepare the torte base: In a bowl, combine the almond meal, millet flour, chia seeds, lemon zest, salt, and sugar.

In a separate bowl, first stir the arrowroot and xanthan gum with the milk until smooth, then add the remaining wet ingredients and stir. Add the wet mixture to the dry, and stir until incorporated.

Transfer the base mixture to the prepared pan, lightly pressing it in and evening it out. Pour the raspberry mixture on top. Bake for 25 minutes.

Remove from the oven and transfer to a cooling rack to let cool completely. Slice into wedges, and serve.

Serving Suggestion: Serve with a dollop of Lemon-Scented Whipped Cream, or a scoop of nondairy vanilla ice cream.

Banana Butter Pie

SERVES 6 TO 8

(optionally) wheat
(optionally) gluten
(optionally) soy

FREE

Our daughters love bananas sliced with a thick slather of almond butter. One day, driving them to school, I thought, "Why not combine that in a pie?" With the sweetness of the bananas and nondairy yogurt, minimal sweetener is added.

2 cups (somewhat packed) sliced ripe bananas (freckled, but not too overripe; about 2½ large bananas)

½ cup + 1 tablespoon almond butter

¼ cup + 2 tablespoons vanilla nondairy yogurt (see note)

2 to 3 tablespoons coconut sugar or other unrefined sugar (adjust to taste)

1 tablespoon pure maple syrup

1 teaspoon pure vanilla extract

½ teaspoon agar powder

¼ teaspoon sea salt

¼ teaspoon ground cinnamon or freshly grated nutmeg
Pinch of ground cardamom (optional)

1 prepared vegan pastry piecrust (I use Wholly Wholesome brand) or use Rustic Piecrust (page 241) or Gluten-Free Piecrust (page 242)

Preheat the oven to 425°F.

In a food processor, combine all the filling ingredients (starting with 2 tablespoons of the sugar) until liquidy smooth, scraping down the sides and base of the bowl as needed, to incorporate the almond butter. Taste, and if it needs a little extra sweetness (depending on the sweetness of bananas and yogurt), add the extra tablespoon of sugar.

Pour the mixture into the piecrust (scraping out all filling from the bowl) and tip the pie back and forth gently to evenly distribute the filling. Bake for 10 minutes at 425°F, then lower heat to 350°F and bake for another 12 to 14 minutes. The pie will be firmer around the edges and a little looser in the center, but it will set further as it cools.

Carefully remove from the oven and place on a cooling rack. Let cool completely (refrigerate, if needed) before slicing to serve.

Ingredients 411: If the bananas aren't as ripe as you like, you may want to add the additional tablespoon of sugar, or more to taste.

Soy yogurt typically has more of a tangy flavor than does coconut yogurt. If using coconut yogurt, add 2 teaspoons of freshly squeezed lemon juice to the blended mixture.

Serving Suggestion: Try decorating with a light layer or piped edging of Lemon-Scented Whipped Cream, and then arrange slices of bananas around the edges of the pie (toss the slices first in lemon juice to prevent browning). A small amount of finely chopped almonds would also be a pretty finish on top of the cream and bananas.

Chocolate Raspberry Truffle Tart with Coconut Crust

SERVES 8

wheat
(optionally) gluten **FREE**
soy

A deeply rich, decadent chocolate truffle mixture covers a sweet, lightly crunchy and chewy coconut crust base coated with a thin raspberry layer. This tart is perfect for special-occasion desserts, but easy enough to make any day of the week.

CHOCOLATE TRUFFLE FILLING:

½ cup + 3 tablespoons regular (not "lite") coconut milk (refrigerate in advance; use the thick cream only; see "Plant-Powered Pantry," page xxviii)

3½ tablespoons organic extra-virgin coconut oil, at room temperature (see "Plant-Powered Pantry," page xxix)

½ teaspoon pure almond or vanilla extract

2 cups vegan chocolate chips or vegan chocolate bars broken into chunks (about 12 ounces)
Pinch of sea salt

Preheat the oven to 350°F. Lightly oil a 9-inch springform pan or a pie plate, using a small piece of paper towel to wipe the oil over the surface and up the sides.

In a double boiler (or fit a metal or heatproof glass bowl over a saucepan filled with several inches of water) over medium-low heat, combine the coconut milk, oil, and extract, stirring occasionally for several minutes until melted. Add the chocolate chips (reserving a small portion, about ¼ cup), and stir until the chocolate chips are just about melted. Then turn off the heat, add the remaining chocolate chips, and gently stir. Once just melted (do not overwork the chocolate), remove the saucepan from the heat and place on the counter to cool slightly while preparing the crust.

CRUST:

1 cup + 2 tablespoons oat flour (use GF-certified oat flour for gluten-free option; see note)

1 cup unsweetened shredded coconut

¼ teaspoon (rounded) sea salt

¼ cup pure maple syrup

2½ to 3 tablespoons organic extra-virgin coconut oil, at room temperature

RASPBERRY LAYER:

⅓ cup raspberry jam of choice

Prepare the crust: Combine the oat flour, coconut, and salt in a bowl. Stir well and add the maple syrup and 2½ tablespoons of the coconut oil. Mix well, using your fingers to incorporate, until the mixture will hold together easily when pressed. If it is still crumbly, add the remaining ½ tablespoon of oil.

Transfer the mixture to the prepared crust, pressing into the bottom. Bake for 13 to 14 minutes, until slightly golden on very edges.

Remove the pan from the oven and transfer to a cooling rack. Place in the fridge to let cool somewhat for 10 to 15 minutes. Once the crust is cooled to just warm, spread the layer of raspberry layer over the crust base, distributing as evenly as possible. Pour the truffle mixture into the crust and tip back and forth gently to distribute evenly over the crust. Refrigerate until completely cool (several hours). Before serving, let the pie sit at room temperature for 30 minutes or longer, to let the chocolate layer soften for slicing. Then cut into slices and serve.

Savvy Subs and Adds: If you'd like to use a prepared piecrust for this pie, go ahead and do so. Simply prebake the pie shell until lightly golden, let cool some, and then fill with the truffle layer per the directions.

Serving Suggestions: If you'd like to make this pie without the raspberry layer, try instead serving this pie with a simple fresh berry sauce that gives a bright, slightly tart contrast to the richness of the chocolate filling. Try Fresh Strawberry Sauce.

Orange Spice Cream Pie

SERVES 6 TO 8

(optionally) wheat
(optionally) gluten **FREE**

I toyed with this pie one year for Christmas dessert, and our guests loved it. If you enjoy the taste of warm spices such as cinnamon, cardamom, and ginger, give this pie a go—almost like chai in flavor, but lighter with the spices and with a hint of orange!

1 prepared piecrust of choice (I use Wholly Wholesome) or can use Rustic Piecrust (page 241) or Gluten-Free Piecrust (page 242)

FILLING:
1 (12.3-ounce) package extra-firm silken tofu
1 (14-ounce) can regular (not "lite") coconut milk (use the thick cream only and discard the watery liquid; you can refrigerate ahead of time to help separate, but it's not essential)
¼ teaspoon sea salt
2 tablespoons arrowroot powder
1 teaspoon agar powder
½ cup unrefined sugar (lighter color granules are best, so as not to darken filling)
¼ cup agave nectar (pure maple syrup can be substituted but will darken the filling)
½ teaspoon ground cinnamon
¼ to ½ teaspoon ground ginger
¼ teaspoon freshly grated nutmeg
⅛ teaspoon (scant) ground cardamom
⅛ teaspoon orange oil, or ½ to 1 teaspoon orange zest

Preheat the oven to 350°F. First, prebake the piecrust.

Bake the piecrust for about 10 minutes (a little longer for pastry crust, 12 to 14 minutes), then remove from the oven and let cool.

Prepare the filling: In a saucepan, combine all the ingredients, (except the orange zest, if using). Using an immersion blender, puree the ingredients until smooth. Then place over medium heat and bring the mixture to a low boil, whisking frequently (don't leave the stove for long, as the mixture can settle on the bottom of the saucepan and brown or burn). Once at a low boil, remove from the heat and let cool for about an hour. Once it has cooled somewhat, use the immersion blender to puree the mixture in the pot again (to smooth it out), and then stir in the orange zest, if using.

Pour the mixture into the pie shell and refrigerate for a couple of hours to set. Remove from the fridge and cut into wedges, and serve.

11 Dreena Dazs

I've made it no secret that my favorite sweet treat is ice cream (I've also never shown photos of my personal freezer stash). But if there is any food worthy of stocking as a treat, in my opinion it is ice cream (challenged heartily by chocolate)! Ice cream offers so many variations in flavors and textures, extra toppings, or add-ins, the options are really endless. If you love ice cream as I do, make a small investment in an ice-cream maker. It'll show you more love than any pair of new shoes.

While the flavor combos are endless, there are a couple of basics. These recipes use canned coconut milk as the creamy base, sometimes in conjunction with other nondairy milks and nuts such as cashews. Be sure to use the regular, not "lite" coconut milk. Ice cream needs the richness of the higher-fat coconut milk, otherwise it will be like an ice or sherbet, and not have the luscious, velvety smooth texture that

you are looking for in ice cream. My favorite brands of coconut milk are Thai Kitchen (organic) and Earth's Best (organic), but other brands will also work fine, see "Plant-Powered Pantry," page xxviii, for more on coconut milk.

Where another nondairy milk is specified in the recipe, I prefer to use almond, soy, or coconut milk (refrigerated, not canned). Obviously almond or coconut are better choices if you need a soy-free version, and vice versa if looking for an ice cream free of tree nut products. I typically don't use rice or hemp milks because the texture of rice milk is sometimes watery, and hemp milks can have a noticeable flavor that I prefer not to come through a finished ice cream. The choice is entirely yours, however, if you prefer rice or hemp milks to other nondairy milks.

The recipes include a small amount of guar gum. This isn't a common ingredient, but is very useful in homemade ice-cream mixtures. It contributes a mallowy thickness to the ice cream. If you buy a small packet, it will last you a while and is worth the purchase. My fellow ice-cream lovers understand this importance.

You'll see I remind you to check the sweetness after blending and adjust as needed. The room-temperature mix will seem sweeter to the taste buds than when the mixture is actually frozen. So you may want to make your blended mixture just a touch sweeter so the final ice-cream product has just the right level of sweetness!

Now, let's talk about some flavors! I cover all the basics—vanilla, chocolate, and strawberry, but with twists. You'll also find some different flavors and spice combinations: Pumpkin Pie, Macadamia, Eggnog, a lighter Banana Pear Soft-Serve, and Chai Peanut Butter! Be sure to try some of the "Make It More-ish!" suggestions, to really elevate your ice creams to the "Dreena Dazs" level they deserve!

I can't think of a better way to finish off my recipes than with ice cream. (And, if you read this chapter before all the others, I like your style!) Happy scooping.

Chai Peanut Butter Ice Cream

MAKES 4 TO 4¼ CUPS

Velvety, luscious, nutty, with a bouquet of chai spices. This is a unique flavor combination that really works—don't move on just yet, get to churning!

wheat gluten soy **FREE**

1 (14-ounce) can coconut milk (regular, not "lite")

½ cup natural peanut butter

1 cup plain or vanilla nondairy milk (see chapter introduction)

¾ cup coconut sugar or other unrefined sugar (see note)

2 tablespoons pure maple syrup

1 teaspoon pure vanilla extract

1 teaspoon ground cinnamon

½ teaspoon ground cardamom

¼ teaspoon ground allspice (see note)

¼ teaspoon ground ginger (see note)

¼ teaspoon freshly grated nutmeg

⅛ teaspoon sea salt
A pinch or two ground cloves (see note)

¼ teaspoon (rounded) guar gum

In a blender, combine all the ingredients and blend until thoroughly mixed, stopping to scrape down the blender bowl once or twice, if needed. Transfer the mixture immediately (see note) to an ice-cream maker (follow the directions of the specific model), and churn until the mixture is of soft-serve consistency.

Adult-Minded: If you generally like more spices in such sweets as gingerbread, pumpkin pie, spice cookies, and cakes, you can round the measures of the spices cinnamon, cardamom, allspice, and ginger, and add a pinch more of cloves.

Ingredients 411: If using vanilla nondairy milk, you might want to adjust the ¾ cup measure of sugar, starting with a little less, because vanilla milks are sweeter than plain. Keep in mind that the room-temperature ice-cream mixture will taste sweeter than when frozen.

Savvy Subs and Adds: Coconut sugar has a caramel flavor, and likewise a caramel-type flavor with undertones of coconut. It is a delicious and lovely sugar; however, if you cannot find it, try Sucanat or another unrefined sugar in its place.

Eggnog Ice Cream

MAKES ABOUT 4½ CUPS

wheat gluten **FREE**

If you're one of those that hoards packaged holiday nogs, this ice cream will be right up your alley. (And for those of you that stocked up on a carton or four too many of the shelf-stable nogs over the holidays, this ice-cream recipe will help you make very good use of it!)

2½ cups nondairy eggnog (I use So Nice brand; see note)
¾ cup + 2 tablespoons canned coconut milk regular (not "lite") (use the cream on top)
½ cup raw cashews
⅔ cup unrefined sugar (see note)
⅛ teaspoon sea salt
⅛ teaspoon freshly grated nutmeg
¼ teaspoon (rounded) guar gum
½ teaspoon pure vanilla extract

In a blender, combine all the ingredients and puree until very, very smooth, scraping down the sides of the blender as needed (see note). Transfer the mixture to an ice-cream maker (follow the directions of the specific model), and churn until the mixture is of soft-serve consistency.

Allergy-Free or Bust! If you make your own version of dairy-free eggnog using an alternative to soy milk (e.g., coconut, almond, or rice milk), this can be made soy free. Another alternative is to opt for a vanilla almond or coconut milk, increase the nutmeg to ¼ teaspoon, and add a pinch of cinnamon and the teensiest pinch of cloves, to mimic a commercial eggnog. I have yet to find a nondairy eggnog that is also soy free, but crossing fingers!

If This Apron Could Talk: I use my Blendtec to puree this mixture, and it really does wonders in smoothing out ice-cream purees before churning. If you don't have a high-powered blender, start pureeing the cashews with about half of the eggnog, to get them pulverized. Once they are smoothing out, add the remaining liquid and ingredients.

Ingredients 411: This amount of sugar makes the ice cream sweet enough for my taste, but feel free to increase or decrease slightly to your own preference. The sweetness will also be affected slightly by the brand of nondairy eggnog used in the mix. You may want to start with ½ cup of sugar, and add several additional tablespoons to taste after blending. Keep in mind that the room-temperature ice-cream mixture will taste sweeter than when frozen.

Make It More-ish! You must try this with a generous drizzle of Rich Coconut Caramel Sauce. Must, I say!

Pumpkin Pie Ice Cream

MAKES 3¾ TO 4 CUPS

wheat gluten soy **FREE**

In my world, every good dessert can take on a new form as ice cream. So here, I reconstruct pumpkin pie into a scoop of creamy, cold bliss!

¾ cup canned pumpkin pie mix (not pumpkin puree; I use Farmer's Market organic brand)

1 (14-ounce) can coconut milk (regular, not "lite")

⅓ cup raw cashews

½ cup plain or vanilla nondairy milk (see chapter introduction)

⅔ to ¾ cup unrefined sugar (see note)

⅛ teaspoon sea salt

¼ teaspoon ground cinnamon (optional)

¼ teaspoon (rounded) guar gum

½ teaspoon pure vanilla extract
Add-ins (optional): ½ to ¾ cup vegan ginger snaps, ginger cookies, or graham crackers, crumbled

In a blender, combine all the ingredients, except the add-ins, and puree until very, very smooth, scraping down the sides of the blender as needed. Transfer the mixture to an ice-cream maker (follow the directions of the specific model), and churn until the mixture is of soft-serve consistency. If using add-ins, add during last couple of minutes of churning. Serve, or freeze to firm more.

Ingredients 411: You can start with ⅔ cup of sugar, and then after blending the mixture (before churning), taste for sweetness. If you think you'd like the ice cream sweeter, add the additional sugar. Keep in mind that the room-temperature ice-cream mixture will taste sweeter than when frozen. I usually use close to the ¾ cup measure of sugar.

Macadamia Ice Cream

MAKES 4 TO 4½ CUPS

This ice cream is uncomplicated in process, and also in flavors. The ingredients are fairly simple, allowing the delicate flavor of the macadamia nuts to shine through.

wheat gluten soy **FREE**

1 (14-ounce) can coconut milk (regular, not "lite")
1 cup raw macadamia nuts, or ½ cup macadamia nut butter; see note)
1 cup plain or vanilla nondairy milk (see chapter introduction)
½ cup unrefined sugar (see note)
1 to 3 tablespoons agave nectar (see note)
⅛ teaspoon sea salt
1 to 1½ teaspoons pure vanilla extract
¼ teaspoon (rounded) guar gum

In a high-powered blender (see note), puree all the ingredients (starting with 1 tablespoon of the agave nectar) until very smooth, stopping to scrape down the blender bowl once or twice as needed. Taste, and add additional agave nectar to sweeten, if you like (see note). Transfer the mixture to an ice-cream maker (follow the directions of the specific model), and churn until the mixture is of soft-serve consistency. Serve, or freeze to firm more.

If This Apron Could Talk: A high-powered blender really works best to pulverize the macadamia nuts. If you don't have a Terminator blender, then use ½ cup of macadamia nut butter in place of the raw nuts.

Ingredients 411: Coconut sugar adds a beautiful flavor to this ice cream, but a lighter color sugar helps retain a light creamy color. Choose whichever you like. Note that a vanilla nondairy milk will be sweeter than plain. After blending, you can adjust sweetness with agave nectar, if desired or pure maple syrup (this will also make the ice cream darker, if used). Keep in mind that the room-temperature ice-cream mixture will taste sweeter than when frozen.

Savvy Subs and Adds: This is one of my favorite recipes, even though it looks fairly simplistic in concept and ingredients. But macadamia nuts are rich and yet have a delicate flavor, and so less is more in this ice cream.

Vanilla Bean Coconut Banana Ice Cream

MAKES 3¾ TO 4 CUPS

Coconut and banana simply make sense together—and an infusion of sensuous vanilla makes for creamy, dreamy proof!

wheat gluten soy **FREE**

1 (14-ounce) can coconut milk (regular, not "lite")

¼ cup coconut butter (see "Plant-Powered Pantry," page xxviii)

1 cup plain or vanilla nondairy milk (see chapter introduction)

1 cup frozen overripe bananas (cut into chunks before freezing)

½ cup coconut sugar or other unrefined sugar (see note)
Seeds from 1 vanilla bean (see "Plant-Powered Pantry," page xxix)

⅛ teaspoon sea salt

¼ teaspoon (rounded) guar gum

In a blender, first combine the coconut milk and coconut butter and puree (it helps to first blend the coconut butter with the milk to break down the solids and smooth the mixture before adding the frozen bananas, which can chill and solidify small particles of the coconut butter). Then add the milk, bananas, sugar, vanilla seeds, sea salt, and guar gum, and blend. Puree until very smooth, stopping to scrape down the blender bowl once or twice, as needed. Transfer the mixture to an ice-cream maker (follow the directions of the specific model), and churn until the mixture is of soft-serve consistency. Transfer the mixture to a container and place in the freezer to firm more.

Ingredients 411: Coconut sugar has a caramel flavor, and likewise a caramel-type flavor with undertones of coconut flavor. It is a delicious and lovely sugar; however, if you cannot find it, substitute another unrefined sugar in its place. Start with ⅓ cup, then adjust the sweetness with additional sugar to taste. This will depend on the brand and type of nondairy milk you use (whether it contributes much sweetness). Keep in mind that the room-temperature ice-cream mixture will taste sweeter than when frozen.

Make It More-ish! For extra coconut flavor, add ⅓ to ½ cup of dried coconut to the ice cream just before you finish churning. Also, a tiny amount (¼ to ½ teaspoon) of coconut extract could be added to the blended mixture—but not too much, or it will overwhelm the other flavors. Also try adding a ribbon of Rich Coconut Caramel Sauce just in last few seconds of churning—or, small cubes of Raw Banana Nut Squares with Coconut Cream Cheese Frosting.

Savvy Subs and Adds: You can also try substituting raw cashew butter or macadamia butter for the coconut butter.

You can substitute 1 to 1½ teaspoons of pure vanilla extract for the vanilla bean, if you like (though the flavor of the vanilla seeds is truly extraordinary, worth trying)!

Vanilla Hazelnut Ice Cream

MAKES ABOUT 3¼ CUPS

wheat gluten soy **FREE**

After creating my Chocolate Hazelnut Ice Cream (recipe follows), I loved it so much I wanted a vanilla version. For the vanilla, I also added some frozen bananas, as I like the flavor profiles together. More churning ahead . . .

1 (14-ounce) can coconut milk (regular, not "lite")
¼ cup hazelnut butter
1 cup plain or vanilla nondairy milk (see chapter introduction)
½ cup frozen overripe sliced banana (optional; if not using, you may need to add the extra amount of sugar)
⅓ cup pure maple syrup or agave nectar
1 to 3 tablespoons unrefined sugar (see note)
2 teaspoons vanilla
⅛ teaspoon sea salt
¼ teaspoon (rounded) guar gum

In a blender, combine all the ingredients (starting with 1 tablespoon of sugar; see note) and blend until smooth. Transfer the mixture to an ice-cream maker (follow the directions of the specific model) and churn until the mixture is of soft-serve consistency (see note). Serve or transfer to containers to freeze.

Ingredients 411: Most hazelnut butters use roasted hazelnuts, even though the label may not identify the nut butter as "roasted." You may be able to find raw hazelnut butter, but it's not necessary in this recipe.

After blending the ice-cream mixture (before churning), taste for sweetness. If you think you'd like the ice cream sweeter, now's the time to add another tablespoon or two of unrefined sugar or a touch more maple syrup. Keep in mind that the room-temperature ice-cream mixture will taste sweeter than when frozen.

Chocolate Hazelnut Ice Cream

MAKES ABOUT 3½ CUPS

wheat gluten soy **FREE**

Before becoming vegan, I loved getting Italian gelato, and chocolate hazelnut was one of my favorite flavors. This ice cream rivals the nonvegan versions, with a thick, creamy consistency with not too much chocolate to overpower the hazelnut essence.

1 (14-ounce) can coconut milk (regular, not "lite")
⅓ cup hazelnut butter (see note)
1 cup plain or vanilla nondairy milk (see chapter introduction)
⅓ cup pure maple syrup
¼ cup unsweetened cocoa powder
2 to 5 tablespoons unrefined sugar (see note)
1½ to 2 teaspoons pure vanilla extract
¼ teaspoon sea salt
¼ teaspoon (rounded) guar gum

In a blender, combine all the ingredients (starting with 2 tablespoons of sugar; see note) and blend until smooth. Transfer the mixture to an ice-cream maker (follow the directions of the specific model) and churn until the mixture is of soft-serve consistency. Serve or transfer to containers to freeze.

Ingredients 411: Most hazelnut butters use roasted hazelnuts, even though the label may not identify the nut butter as "roasted." You may be able to find raw hazelnut butter, but it's not necessary in this recipe.

After blending the ice cream mixture (before churning), taste for sweetness. If you think you'd like the ice cream sweeter, now's the time to add another tablespoon or two of unrefined sugar or a touch more maple syrup. Keep in mind that the room-temperature ice-cream mixture will taste sweeter than when frozen. I typically use 3½ to 5 tablespoons.

Make It More-ish: If you like, just before the ice cream is finished churning, throw in a handful of chocolate chunks or some chopped toasted hazelnuts (skins removed).

Chocolate Lovers Ice Cream

MAKES ABOUT 4½ CUPS

wheat gluten soy **FREE**

You'll never need to buy another creamy chocolate ice cream again, with this recipe. It is luscious, and adaptable to any extras you want to throw in there!

1 (14-ounce) can coconut milk (regular, not "lite")
3 tablespoons coconut butter (not oil, see "Plant-Powered Pantry," page xxviii)
1 cup vanilla or chocolate nondairy milk (see note)
⅓ cup unsweetened cocoa powder
⅓ cup unrefined sugar
1 to 3 tablespoons pure maple syrup
1 teaspoon pure vanilla extract
¼ teaspoon (rounded) guar gum
⅛ teaspoon sea salt
2 to 3 tablespoons vegan chocolate syrup (optional)

In a blender, puree all the ingredients (starting with 1 tablespoon of maple syrup), until smooth, stopping to scrape down the blender jar as needed. Add extra maple syrup to taste (see note). Transfer the mixture to an ice-cream maker (follow the directions of the specific machine). Once the mixture has reached a soft-serve ice-cream stage, add the chocolate syrup, if using, and stop churning very soon after—so it remains in ribbons in the ice cream. Transfer the mixture to container(s), and freeze until serving. (It will firm up more with freezing, and you may need to thaw slightly, leaving out at room temperature for 5 or more minutes, to soften before serving.)

Ingredients 411: I like to use refrigerated coconut milk (e.g., So Delicious brand) or almond milk. If using chocolate milk, you may want to add a little less sugar or maple syrup, adjusting the sweetness to taste.

After blending the ice-cream mixture (before churning), taste for sweetness. If you think you'd like the ice cream sweeter, now's the time to add another tablespoon or two of maple syrup (and consider whether you're adding any extras such as chocolate chips or cookie pieces which will make it sweeter). Keep in mind that the room-temperature ice-cream mixture will taste sweeter than when frozen.

Make It More-ish! You can add other goodies to this ice cream, including broken cookie pieces, chocolate chips, toffee pieces, toasted nuts, nondairy truffles, chocolate sauce—go on, what's Chocolate Lovers Ice Cream without some lovin' back?!

Savvy Subs and Adds: You can also try substituting raw cashew butter or macadamia butter for the coconut butter.

Strawberries 'n' Cream Ice Cream

MAKES ABOUT 3½ CUPS

wheat gluten soy **FREE**

The best strawberry ice cream can come straight from your own kitchen. With whole foods ingredients, you'll taste the difference in this dreamy dessert.

1 cup fresh strawberries, or 1 to ½ cups frozen (see note)
1 (14-ounce) can coconut milk (regular, not "lite")
½ cup raw cashews
½ cup plain or vanilla nondairy milk (see chapter introduction)
½ cup pure maple syrup or agave nectar
⅛ teaspoon sea salt
¼ teaspoon (rounded) guar gum
  Seeds from 1 vanilla bean (see "Plant-Powered Pantry," page xlii)

In a blender (I use a Blendtec), combine all the ingredients and puree until smooth, scraping down the sides of blender as needed (this may take a few minutes with a standard blender). Transfer the mixture to an ice-cream maker (follow the directions of the specific model), and churn until the mixture is of soft-serve consistency. Transfer to a container to store in the freezer.

Ingredients 411: Fresh strawberries are easier to measure. If the berries are large, cut in half or into quarters, and if smaller you can just leave them whole for measuring. Fill about 1 cup. Frozen berries are more difficult to measure and cut, so you can use anywhere between 1 and 1½ cups of the whole frozen berries. Keeping the measurement close to 1 cup will give the creamiest ice cream.

Make It More-ish! Make a pan of Berry Patch Brownies in advance. Cut into small cubes, and add to the ice cream just in the last few seconds of churning. I don't call it Dreena Dazs for nothing!

Banana Pear Soft-Serve

MAKES 2½ TO 3 CUPS

wheat gluten soy **FREE**

No ice-cream maker required for this ice cream, which is a little more like a sweet sherbet, but with the creaminess of added coconut milk and nut butter.

2½ to 2¾ cups sliced overripe banana (see "Plant-Powered Pantry," page xxv)
1 cup peeled, chopped ripe pear
¼ cup coconut milk (regular, not "lite"; use thick cream and not watery portion; see note)
2 tablespoons macadamia nut butter or raw cashew butter (see note)
1 to 2½ tablespoons pure maple syrup or agave nectar (see note)
¼ teaspoon ground cardamom
⅛ teaspoon sea salt

Place the bananas in a food processor and pulse through to break up into very bitty pieces, scraping down sides of bowl several times. Be sure the banana is quite broken down before adding the other ingredients. Add the remaining ingredients (starting with 1 or 1½ tablespoons maple syrup, and the adjusting sweetness to taste later), and process until very smooth. Taste, and add additional sweetener, if desired. Serve immediately, or store in containers and freeze.

If This Apron Could Talk: You might be able to find small cans of coconut milk (such as Earth's Choice 160 ml cans), which are very convenient for this small amount. Or, if using a larger can, save the remainder for use in curries or sauces or smoothies. Either refrigerate in a sealed container for a few days, or freeze (in ice cube trays).

If you freeze for just a few hours, the ice cream will still be easy to scoop; however, after many hours or overnight, the ice cream will become fairly hard. To serve once very hard, leave out at room temperature for 10 to 15 minutes.

Ingredients 411: Both macadamia butter and raw cashew butter have a light, creamy color, and also a more delicate flavor than other nut butters. Other nut butters will not substitute as well in this recipe.

I typically use about 2 tablespoons of sweetener, but it really depends on the sweetness of the bananas and also the ripeness of pear used, so start with a little, and add more to taste after blending. Keep in mind that the room-temperature ice-cream mixture will taste sweeter than when frozen.

Powering the Vegan Family

I became vegan in my twenties, quite a few years before having children. My husband joined me on the journey from meat eating to vegetarian and then vegan. When we started our family, the plant-powered diet fueled the way, from my first pregnancy to my third, and all the toddler years in between. Now that our children are growing a little older, we see their strength, endurance, and abundant energy as a reflection of the good food they eat daily.

It isn't an easy or obvious thing to take your family on a vegan journey. As a parent, you assume responsibility for the creation and development of another entire human. It is the ultimate accountability—every decision you make essentially affects their health and well-being. Like other vegan parents, I was questioned about whether I would continue to eat vegan through my pregnancy (at least for the first), and of course, "Would I raise our child vegan?"

Perhaps I was fortunate to have some understanding family and friends in my life at the time, as it didn't become much of an issue after I addressed the initial questions. And I understand their concerns. We are raised thinking it is not just "normal" but absolutely critical to eat meat and dairy. It is not. In fact, it is critical that we acknowledge the health pitfalls of our meat, dairy, and processed food–centric diets. But it takes time for this thinking to change, and so anyone beginning to raise a family as vegans will undoubtedly meet with resistance.

In my experience, actions speak louder than words. I didn't feel it was necessary to defend all our dietary choices, as I had researched them well, and I'd also had very positive personal experiences. I do think it is very important that new parents (and new vegans, in general) do the research they need to understand what comprises a whole-foods vegan diet—not just a vegan diet. And vegan parents need to know what might be necessary through pregnancy, early infancy, and beyond, and be armed with the resources—and ideally a supportive and informed pediatrician or naturopath—to provide guidance and assistance. With the right information, you can feel confident in your choices and prepare wholesome meals and snacks that will fuel and nourish your children. Just watch out—you might find they have such steady energy that you are wishing for a break! (I often joke with my husband that if we gave our girls some cow's milk, they'd conk out for a nice, long nap.)

Before long, your friends and family will see the vibrant health your children possess—their clear, glowing skin; shiny, bright eyes; and overall strength—and will be less inclined to challenge your decisions. My mother marvels at the variety of foods our children eat, what healthy appetites and appreciation they have for "real" food, and how excited they get when their brown rice and baked beans are topped with their favorite—guacamole! My mother told me her friends always ask, "What do they eat?" . . . "If only they could see!" she said.

Plant-Powered Beginnings

After publishing my last cookbook, *Eat, Drink & Be Vegan*, we welcomed our third daughter into our family. With every baby, I've made most of their baby food, and with our third daughter, I made virtually all of it. I'd like to share more about making your own baby food, as it becomes a critically important part of cooking for many of us, albeit for a brief period in our lives.

Making baby food is an extra job when you are already a busy mom or dad. But, homemade baby food is best for your wee one. It's most nutritious, tastes far better, and is also less expensive than buying large quantities of jarred baby food (especially the organic varieties). Fortunately, when preparing your own food, it is easy to make large batches that you can then refrigerate and freeze in smaller portions to meet your baby's mealtime needs.

It's not hard to make baby food. It does take time, though, and requires extra effort every few days. But it's worth it to know that your little one is getting freshly made, tasty, and nutritious whole foods. You don't need special culinary skills to get started, or to come up with creative food combinations to keep your baby nourished and happy. It simply requires some advance preparation, a little thinking, and a few tools to make the process simpler.

You'll need a few kitchen items to get started:

Pot to steam vegetables and fruit, or a steaming insert. This is useful for the first few months, when you are steaming most foods. Alternatively, you can cook the fruit and vegetables in just an inch or two of water and simmer until tender. Some vegetables can also be baked or roasted whole, including yellow- and orange-fleshed sweet potatoes, winter squash, beets, and white potatoes. (To do so place on a baking sheet lined with parchment paper and bake at about 400°F until tender when pierced. Let cool enough to handle, and then remove the skins or rinds to puree with some water.)

Blender or food processor to puree foods. With our first two children, I used my food processor (for larger amounts) or my immersion blender (for smaller amounts). Third time around I used my Blendtec, because it works with varying amounts easily and achieves smooth consistencies effortlessly. Sometimes you need to add a small amount of water to thin out the purees, so it's handy to have some water boiled ahead of time (let it cool down, if you want) to do so.

Glass bowls (preferably with covers) to store portions in the fridge and freezer. I have two sets of glass prep bowls with covers (twelve bowls total). When making different batches of purees, you will need many bowls. These are perfect because they are easy to store, and well suited for freezing and thawing. Any size or shape of a glass or ceramic bowl will also work well, but consider ones that have covers.

If This Apron Could Talk: I don't use a microwave, so to warm the purees, spoon out into another glass bowl the amount your baby might eat. (You won't use the full 1 cup in the early weeks/months, so spoon out just a portion to warm. This helps avoid wasting any food that your baby may not eat, as you should not save any leftovers that have made contact with your babe's hands or mouth). Place this bowl in a larger bowl and pour in enough hot/boiled water to come up to about three-quarters of the height of the inner bowl. This will quickly warm the food; you can stir it to evenly distribute the heat. Of course, make sure to test all food for the proper temperature before feeding it to your little one.

In the first weeks of introducing foods, you'll be working with single food purees, such as sweet potatoes. Later, you can start combining some of these foods. Some vegetables and fruits work better blended with others. For instance, bitter greens such as broccoli, spinach, and kale, and stronger-tasting vegetables such as beet and parsnip will be more readily accepted by your babe if blended into a puree with sweet potatoes or pears. Later, once grains and beans are introduced, more variety and flexibility comes with food preparation.

Things to consider when introducing solids:

- **Head off allergic reactions.** In my cookbook *Vive le Vegan!* I discuss baby food in depth and include a food introduction schedule that is designed to reduce possible allergenic reactions for your baby. Foods with lower allergenic potential (and better digestibility) are introduced as first foods, and foods with higher allergenic risks are delayed until your baby is more mature. This chart is unlike most baby food introduction guides, and it may seem complicated at first glance. Once you get sorted and organized, it is very easy to follow, however, and I have had very positive experiences with all three of our children, following this schedule.[*]

- **Choose organic as much as possible.** Your baby is in the biggest phase of growth and development of his or her life; organic is best to avoid exposure to harmful pesticide and chemical residues. For certain, make sure you know what the "dirty dozen" produce items are (go to www.ewg.org/foodnews), and be sure to buy those items organic.
- **Have backups.** While I advocate making your own, sometimes you'll have days when you need reinforcements! Pick up several jars of organic baby foods for your pantry.
- **What goes in must come out.** While not typical cookbook fodder, it's worth alerting you: Don't be alarmed if you see bright pink poop in your baby's diaper shortly after that meal of pureed sweet potatoes and beets! Also know that all of this food is minimally processed and fiber rich, so be prepared for two to four or more poopy diapers per day.
- **Babies will eat only pureed foods for just the first few months.** It will become easier once he or she reaches eight or nine months of age, when some finger foods (e.g., rice puff cereal, cut rice pasta, soft beans, pieces of cut fruit such as bananas, soft melon, raisins, apricots, and so on) can become part of your baby's meals. Also, food mixtures can now become somewhat chunkier and involve less preparation, such as mixing cooked quinoa or brown rice into mashed avocado or banana.

---

[*] This section is meant to give tips on making baby food specifically, rather than to detail food introduction timelines, nursing, and other nutritional specifics. For more of this detailed information, please refer to *Vive le Vegan!* Other resources you may find useful for nursing and feeding your babies and toddlers include:

Becoming Vegan: The Complete Guide to Adopting a Healthy Plant-Based Diet by Brenda Davis, RD, and Vesanto Melina, MS, RD

The Complete Idiot's Guide to Plant-Based Nutrition by Julieanna Hever, MS, RD, CPT

Dr. Jack Newman's Guide to Breastfeeding by Dr. Jack Newman and Teresa Pitman

Physician's Committee for Responsible Medicine (www.pcrm.org; see "Raising Vegan Children")

Plant-Powered Lunch Box

Just as you're in a groove and have things figured out with snacks and meals, your child starts school and things change again. Now you have to navigate snacks and lunches among party days and special events (which always involve food, and typically too much junk), and also school rules that might include allergy restrictions for nuts. Now your lunches have to work into the mold of school, and that also includes not much time for your children to eat, compared to meals at home.

Once our children entered school, the reality wasn't as scary as I had imagined (unless of course you happen to stumble upon lunch hour and get a glimpse of kids eating "lunchables," yogurt tubes, and "wagon wheels"—yep, that's disturbing)! But once you get into the swing of things, you'll find things easier than you anticipated.

For young children, you will want to let the teacher know about your diet. Most teachers are very understanding—and some, very supportive. Our first daughter's kindergarten teachers asked whether I could help them make a vegan cake for one of their classroom experiments (demonstrating the chemical reactions of baking). They would normally make a standard cake mix using eggs, but knew our daughter ate vegan, and thought it was an opportunity to be inclusive while also teaching the children about what it meant to eat vegan! I was so appreciative of their thoughtfulness (thank you, teacher Janet and teacher Glory!), and remember hearing the teacher and children still talking about yummy vegan cake at the end of the day.

Most teachers are used to allergy issues in their class, and expect to make modifications for party days and other food-related events for those allergies. So they are usually very understanding when you explain that your child doesn't eat dairy, eggs, or meat. As long as you provide the alternatives for your child for any of those food celebrations, there is rarely a hiccup. During primary grades, I left a treat bag with my daughter's teacher. When candy or cookies were being distributed for a birthday, Halloween, or Christmas, the teacher would pick out a treat from the bag for our daughter. I included such things as small dairy-free chocolate bars and small boxes or pouches of vegan cookies.

Once your children move beyond primary grades, they are capable of explaining their food choices if situations arise, and also of notifying you of any events where they might need a lunch or treat packed. There are also plenty of opportunities to share your vegan food with the classrooms if you want, for parties or bake sales. This gives your children the chance to show their friends that plant-based foods are delicious. Sure, some kids might have attitude and say something unkind about eating vegan ("Your food sucks. I'm not trying that!"). We've heard those things, but that is part of eating differently from the norm. Try to view these less-than-impressive moments as opportunities to talk to your children about why people, even kids, may say hurtful things because they are uncomfortable, defensive, or do not fully understand. These situations are the exception, as most children, parents, and teachers are open and understanding, and sometimes even interested and supportive.

On to the nuts and bolts of packing lunches. While I joked about the scary foods in some lunches, it is no joke. A lot of processed and unhealthy foods circulate through schools. Sure, these "foods" may be convenient but are devoid of nutrition, and instead deliver doses of artificial colors, flavors, high levels of sodium, saturated and hydrogenated fats, refined sugars, and refined flours. Yes, it takes some time to shop and prepare more healthful lunches and snacks, but it's worth it. I'm not saying that you have to make everything from scratch. Sure, you can have some quick fixes to pack in lunches. But there are healthier alternatives. And there are things you can do to plan ahead and put into rotation every week.

Here are some general preparation tips along with more specific lunch and snack times.

- **Make lunch when you make lunch.** My girlfriend Tanya once remarked, "I cannot stand having to pull out more food and pack lunches in the night." I said, "You're doing extra work . . . pack the lunches at lunchtime." When I get to prepping veggies, fruit, sandwiches, and so on, for lunch during the day, I get together the lunches for the next school day. That way, I'm not doing the same job two times in one day. I explained to my girlfriend that she might as well get lunches prepped for the next day while she has all the lunch fixings out for that day. It does require planning and having an extra half-hour or more to get the lunches in order and packed, but it's worth it not to dirty up your kitchen again at the end of the day. If it works better for you to prep lunches at dinner hour, then go that route. Either way, you won't have a kitchen to clean again in the evening, or worse, in the morning, when you're already squeezed to get the kids out the door.

- **Power cook.** If you have a day or two during the week or on the weekend, when you can carve out dedicated kitchen time, use it. Prepare multiple batches of your children's favorite foods (see below). And get your soup pot on! My soups are hearty and pack a punch for lunches (and dinner). Make a double batch of Kids' Cheesy Chickpea and White Bean Soup or French Lentil Soup with Smoked Paprika (see kid-friendly tips).

- **Save small leftovers.** Most of us save appreciable amounts of leftovers, but we may not keep smaller amounts to refrigerate. What's the point—*what can you do with them*, right? Well, lunch boxes are a welcome home for small amounts of foods. After all, kids love to nibble on different things, and I can often make a lunch around nibblers of roasted potatoes, bean dips, baked beans, rice, a few pieces of tofu, and more. Think about how quickly you can make a wrap with last night's leftovers of a few tablespoons of rice along with a sprinkling of beans, a drizzle of tahini sauce, and some grated or chopped veg. Voilà! A tasty, tidy wrap that made use of your "rice scraps." Or pair those roasted potatoes with some cubed

tofu or chickpeas, add some condiments, if you like, and pair with a couple of slices of whole-grain bread with fruit and/or veggies to round out the lunch. Keep handy a half-dozen or so small containers to refrigerate small portions of leftovers until it's time to pack the lunches.

- **Bake and cook in batches.** When possible, double or triple recipes that can be used in lunches. Muffins, healthy cookies, hummus, and other snacks can appear in several lunches through a week. (I triple my Tamari Roasted Chickpeas recipe from *Eat, Drink & Be Vegan* at least once a week!) So do the work once in the week rather than several times, when you can. And remember: The freezer is your friend! Dips such as hummus and baked goods such as muffins freeze very well. Store smaller portions in the freezer and then thaw later as needed for lunches.

- **You can match "hot lunches."** If your children have insecurities about eating "differently," try to find ways to have their lunches "match" the items on the hot lunch menu. This can be tricky when most of the hot lunch items are essentially junk (cheese pizza, hot dogs). Nevertheless, you can try to mirror them with healthier choices. And most kids don't mind if their lunches aren't exactly hot— they're happy to have food they enjoy to eat, cold or hot! For instance, on hot-dog days, pack up a veggie hot dog in a whole wheat bun or wrapped in a whole wheat tortilla. That cheese pizza can be shown up with a whole wheat crust version, topped with vegan cheese, veggies, and chickpeas, or even with a nut cheese. Or if you have a couple of slices of a healthy, leftover take-out pizza, send that along. Leftovers of pasta come in handy for those pasta hot lunch days. Heat frozen peas and corn in boiling water, drain off the water once warmed through, and toss with leftover whole-grain pasta along with marinara sauce or a splash of tamari and balsamic vinegar. Add protein-rich additions such as seeds, beans, or tofu or tempeh, if you like.

Here are more lunch and snack ideas:

- **Wraps.** Wraps are easy for the kids to eat, and can be filled with countless ingredients, such as baked beans, refried beans, chickpeas, lentils and other beans, corn, chopped or grated raw veggies (e.g., chopped cucumber or grated carrot), rice, quinoa, millet, or chopped leftover baked or roasted potatoes. Also, wraps are a good way to sneak in veggies they might not otherwise eat, plus other nutritional add-ins such as tahini and nutritional yeast. Sauces, mashes, and spreads can be used to help hold ingredients together (think hummus, leftover smashed sweet potatoes or Smashing Sweet Spuds, Smoky Spiked Tahini Sauce, KD Dip, or the com-

mercially available Annie's Goddess Dressing mixed with nutritional yeast [try it; it's tasty!]). If all else fails, add a squeeze of ketchup!
- **Hummus and Bean Dips.** For me, *hummus* is a catch word for any kind of tasty, smooth bean dip. I realize it might be inauthentic to make a dip out of white, black, or kidney beans and call it some variation of hummus, but for our family it works. The variety keeps lunches interesting with different colors and seasonings. Many days I simply pack up hummus along with pita bread, fruit and veggies, and another munchable, and our daughters' lunches are set. Typically I make triple (or quadruple) batches of hummus, and freeze one or more containers. Hummus thaws brilliantly (just takes a little time), so give this time-saver tip a try. Hummus can also be used in sandwiches as a spread, in wraps, as a layer on pizzas to hold veggies, or even mixed with grains such as rice or into pasta. Hummus is truly a lunch lifesaver. Make it your friend (and make it yourself; it's much cheaper and far tastier). Try Artichoke and White Bean Dip and Grilled Onion Hummus with Hemp Seeds (see kid-friendly tips). And if you are a true hummus lover and want even more recipes, check out my entire hummus chapter in *Eat, Drink & Be Vegan*!
- **Nut-and Seed-Based Dips and Spreads**. Depending on your school,

nuts may be allowed. If so, this opens up plenty of options for lunches, using not just nut butters in sandwiches, but also nut cheeses, spreads, and sauces in wraps, crackers, sandwiches, pasta, pizza, and more. For instance, pack "Vegveeta" Dip in a container along with veggies and pitas for dipping, or a wrap slathered with Truffled Cashew Cheese (see kid-friendly tips), a personal pizza with Spinach Cashew Pizza Cheese Spread, or pasta tossed with Fresh Cream Sauce and nutritional yeast (or better, Cheesy Sprinkle). If nuts are not allowed, try KD Dip for similar meals. It uses tahini as a base, and most classes allow sesame products.

- **New take on PB&J.** I doubt there is a school that allows peanut butter. But some allow nuts, and if not, seeds are usually permitted. So, circumvent the PB by making sandwiches with almond, cashew, or pecan butter. Seed butters (sunflower, sesame, pumpkin) are bitterer and less palatable for children; try adding ground cinnamon to make them naturally sweeter; I have found that the Nuts to You brand of pumpkin seed butter is a little smoother and more palatable than other brands, and substitutes pretty well for PB in a sandwich. Also, look into organic soy nut butter spreads—there are even varieties that contain cocoa, for a special treat. Then, change the J, using a drizzle of agave

nectar and sprinkle of ground cinnamon instead of jam, from time to time. You can also add raisins, or sliced dried fruit such as dates, apricots, or dried apple inside the sandwich. Next, switch the bread! Use whole-grain pita or whole wheat tortillas, instead of sliced bread. You can either roll up the fillings in the tortilla or make a quesadilla of sorts. Spread the butter over the face of the tortilla, add the dried fruit or other filling to half of the surface, fold over, and lightly toast (either under the broiler, flipping after a few minutes, or pan toast). Let cool on a cooling rack, then cut into wedges with kitchen shears. These tortilla wedges are especially fun if paired with a dip such as unsweetened applesauce or nondairy yogurt. If your children like crispbreads, you can also use those (such brands as Wasa) to create sandwiches. (Spread the nut butter on *both* crispbreads, with jam or agave in the center; that way the crispbread won't absorb the jam or agave.)

- **Soups and Stews:** As mentioned earlier, soups make a hearty, satisfying lunch for your kids. If you don't get to cooking from scratch on the weekend, there are some wholesome alternatives that are also time-savers. Amy's brand offers a number of canned, kid-friendly vegan soups such as Alphabet Soup, and No Chicken Noodle Soup. I like to add some cooked beans to these soups, just to up the nutritional ante and stretch the meal a little further, as well. So try adding kidney beans to the Alphabet Soup, for instance, or chickpeas to the No Chicken Noodle Soup. There are other vegan soups on the market, whether canned, in aseptic boxes, or sold "fresh" in-store. Pop into a thermos and combine with some whole-grain bread or crackers, along with nondairy yogurt or some fruit— lunch is served! (You might want to toss in a Cocoa Almond Jumble for "best-mom [or dad]-ever" points!)

- **Savory sandwiches.** If you have leftover grilled or baked tofu, pulse it through a mini-food processor and then mix in chopped veggies and condiments and use as a sandwich filling. Or simply use slices in sandwiches, with a tahini spread, hummus, or other condiment to hold the tofu in place. Chickpeas can be mashed or pureed and again mixed with veggies and condiments for a hearty sandwich filling, and one that looks not much different from the egg or tuna sandwiches other kids might be eating. Grilled cheese sandwiches are a favorite, and you can use any vegan cheese you prefer, or a nut or seed cheese in place of a commercial vegan cheese. Let cool before packing, and include a small container of ketchup for dipping. If your child is a true veggie lover, make simple sandwiches with chopped, sliced, or grated fresh veg-

gies or roasted veggies layered with a spread or dip, such as Truffled Cashew Cheese (see kid-friendly tips), "Almonnaise," or Creamy Carrot Miso Dip.

- **Snacks for lunches or recess.** Fresh fruit is an obvious choice, especially easy-to-eat fruit such as grapes, strawberries, and orange segments. But others such as cubed melon, plums, kiwi wedges (the kids can eat them like an orange), and half a mango (scored) are welcome changes. Also try replacing raisins with other dried fruit such as apple slices, mango, or apricots. Choose unsulfured and organic whenever possible. For snacks, our girls love to have some of these dried fruits mixed with popcorn, or added to a nut-free trail mix, or in a container with some rice crackers (the yin and yang of salty-sweet)!

- **Prepared items.** Lunches and snacks are made even easier with a few prepared items: healthier granola bars, dairy-free yogurts, whole organic fruit bars, unsweetened applesauce cups, crackers, and some treats, such as wholesome cookies. Try Cocoa Cookie Dough Balls, Monsta! Cookies, Wholesome Oat Snackles!, and Proper Healthy Granola Bars, or some of the muffin recipes (pages 3–9) to get started! If nuts are allowed, pack some raw or lightly salted cashews, pistachios, or tamari almonds for a protein-rich snack.

Let Them Eat Greens!

Now that you're whipping together nutritious lunches, it's time to talk about eating those all-important, nutrient-dense leafy greens. It's easier than you might think. I understand how intimidating bunches of kale, chard, and collards can look on those grocery shelves. Hey, I grew up eating iceberg lettuce, which I doubt qualifies as a green! So, I get it. I, too, was at first daunted by buying, cleaning, prepping, eating, and cooking greens. But I'll tell you, now I love them, and stock my fridge with bunches of kale and collards, and grow chard and kale in my garden in the summer. So I'm here to tell you—it's doable.

I must give off some vibe for my love of greens, because I'm often asked what to do with chard or kale when I'm picking it up at our local farmers' market or grocery store. Unfortunately for the person asking, I jump into a real-life version of Wikipedia tips. In case you bump into me picking out greens, I'll save you the rambling and steer you to plenty of handy tricks right here.

Admittedly, it does take some time to get used to using and working with greens, familiarizing your palate with their flavors, and making them an everyday part of your diet if you are unaccustomed to them. Children especially notice the bitter notes of dark greens, so it is more challenging for them. But, like introducing other foods to children, repetition is key to acceptance. And for the adults, before long you'll find yourself looking to eat more greens, actually loving them and wanting to have them at more than one meal. At least, I have! Are you feeling that dark-leafy-vibe yet?

Buying Greens

First, when buying greens, make sure they are very fresh. Look for vibrant dark green leafies that are crisp and full, not wilted or yellowish. In general, Swiss chard and spinach are considered milder and sweeter tasting, with beet greens and collards slightly stronger tasting, but still milder in flavor than kale. Younger, more tender leaves from these greens are also often a little sweeter than more mature, robust leaves. There are also quite a few varieties of kale (curly, lacinato or dinosaur, purple) that differ slightly in taste and bitterness. Then there are other "spicy" greens such as arugula, and mustard, and dandelion greens. I prefer to use mostly spinach, chard, collards, and kale, as they are best accepted by my whole family, but if you like those peppery greens, by all means, rotate them as much as the others. Kale and collards are also hardier greens, so I find that they are often fresher in the store, and refrigerate better. But some days the chard is the freshest at the store—or the spinach . . . so shop with freshest in mind. After buying your greens, keep them refrigerated in a plastic bag (unless already packaged). If they aren't in a plastic bag, they will dehydrate quickly and become limp. And go organic when possible. Spinach, kale, and collards have appeared on the "dirty dozen" list (www.ewg.org/foodnews). Certain vegetables are worth buying organic, and greens are one of them.

Preparing Greens

When you are ready to use your greens, give them a good bath! Get them submerged in a sinkful of cool water (unless you've bought triple-washed spinach, which just needs a quick rinse and salad-spin). Separate the leaves, and agitate a little with your hands to remove any soil and debris—and bugga-buggas! Kale especially can house little critters, so get a good wash through those leaves. Then shake off the water and transfer the greens to a salad spinner. You can use other methods to wick away the water, but I find a salad spinner most effective. Spin until mostly dry, then you're ready to use them.

For sturdy greens with tough stalks (e.g., kale, collards), you will want to remove the leaves from the fibrous stalk. You may even want to remove some of the lower portion of stalks from chard and larger spinach leaves (not from baby spinach), where it becomes thicker and more fibrous. You can do so by "stripping" the leaves. Hold the base of the leaf at the stalk in one hand, and then using your other hand, run your fingers from the base of the stalk to the tip to strip off the leafy portion. You can then discard the stalks—or use them in stock bases, if you make homemade vegetable stock. Now that you have the leafy portion, you can use them whole for smoothies or sandwiches, or chop some more to use in salads or soups, for instance. I like to julienne leafies for salads, and roughly chop them for soups or sautés. You'll get the feel once you get going, based on how you want to use the greens, how large the leaves are, how tender, how bitter, and so on (applications follow!).

Eating and Cooking Greens

There are many ways to eat greens—raw or cooked—and I'll cover many of them here. My first tip though is to start simple. Simple is best, and not intimidating. After you do simple, then you can get more creative with greens and schmancy up some recipes. But here are some simple ways to eat them daily:

- **Green Smoothie.** The almighty green smoothies—they have changed my life, and my morning routine. I swear they are the most efficient, easiest way to eat greens—and probably the most delicious way to eat them *raw*. See "'Go Green' with Smoothies," page 26, for more.

- **Salads.** I know salads seem obvious, but some tweaking might be needed here. See, some greens such as spinach and chard are milder in flavor. Many of us have had a spinach salad, for instance; no big deal. But have you ever had a kale salad? That's a different story. Some greens are bitterer than others. Kale is one of those greens, and chard to a lesser extent. So, when adding rich, dark leafy greens to a salad, chop them finely and mix with other greens or lettuces. I prefer to julienne such greens as lettuce and chard. Once you become adjusted to the flavor of bitterer greens, use them as a base for a lunch salad. Try Kale-slaw with Curried Almond Dressing, or simply toss julienned kale with a nutritious dressing that will coat the leaves but add substance and flavor, such as Raw-nch Dressing, Citrus Tahini Dressing, Creamy Cumin-Spiced Dressing, or Creamy Carrot Miso Dip. Kale is your new romaine, and these dressings your new Caesar!

- **Pestos.** Pesto is one of my very favorite recipes to make, basil pesto in particular, and usually with cashews, Brazil nuts, and/or walnuts. When basil isn't as abundant but still available in grocery stores, you can modify your pesto recipes by substituting spinach, or even Swiss chard, for some of the basil. While I'm not generally a fan of a pesto made entirely with spinach, some partial substitutions work beautifully, along with earthy nuts such as walnuts or pecans. My Spinach Herb Pistachio Pesto has become one of my favorite pesto creations.

- **Brief Cooking Methods.** Most greens benefit from only very brief cooking. Overcooking turns their vibrant green to a murky green-gray color, and also changes the flavor. I prefer the color and flavor of greens when they're cooked quickly, just to wilt and warm through the greens. Greens also lose some of their nutritional value with prolonged cooking, so brief is best, especially for more tender greens such as Swiss chard and spinach, and the leafy portions of such greens as bok choy or beet greens. Sturdier, hardier greens such as collard greens and kale usually take a little longer to become tender and pick up a brighter green color. Here are some ways to quickly warm or heat through greens—remember, cook until the color has just perked up and the leaves have softened; this is when the flavor is best:

- *Sauté.* Adding some chopped, torn, or julienned greens to a lightly oiled pan, with a touch of salt, pepper, and a little grated or minced fresh garlic, shallot, and/or ginger, if you like. Let the greens soften into the oil over medium heat for a few minutes (just a minute or two for delicate greens such as spinach, longer for tougher greens such as kale). The leaves wilt down considerably, so you may want to use far more than you think!
- *Soups and stews.* Many soups offer the perfect opportunity to get greens into your meal. Consider the stew you are having, and whether the flavors or ingredients would suit adding something like Swiss chard or collard greens. If so, add them just before serving, letting them wilt ever so slightly into the hot soup, and then serve immediately. Try Beans 'n' Greens Soup and also the other soup and stew recipes in Chapters 4 and 6.
- *Pasta.* Much like soups, pasta can be even more delicious with the addition of some greens—especially if the pasta has a generous sauce just looking for something to cling to! Again, add close to serving, tossing the greens through the finished pasta and sauce to warm through. Try the wilted greens option in Tomato Artichoke Pasta, for instance, or with other pasta sauces (see Chapter 8).
- *Steam.* Greens can be steamed in just a matter of minutes, and then are particularly delicious topped with some kind of sauce, such as Peanut Tahini Sauce, Moroccan Carrot Dip, or Creamy Curried Almond Dressing.

Keep Trying

You may have tried some of these ideas, or others, but are still not convinced. Try again. I know it took a little time for me to get used to working with greens and eating them daily. So, keep at it, and try another technique or another recipe. You will get the green-vibe, sooner or later!

Guide to Cooking Grains (Stovetop)

Grain (per 1 cup dry measure)	Water Needed to Cook	Cooking Time (minutes)
Amaranth	2½–3 cups	20–25
Barley (hulled)	3 cups	70–80
Barley (pearl)	3 cups	40–50
Barley (pot)	3 cups	55–65
Buckwheat	2 cups	15–20
Bulgur (see note)	2 cups	15–20
Cracked wheat (see note)	2 cups	20–30
Kamut	4 cups	70–90
Millet (see note)	2½–3 cups	18–25
Oat groats	3 cups	50–60
Oats (rolled)	2 cups	10–20
Oats (steel-cut)	3 cups	20–30
Quinoa (see note)	2 cups	12–15
Rice (short-grain brown)	2 cups	35–45
Rice (long-grain brown)	2 cups	40–50
Rice (brown basmati)	2 cups	35–45
Rye berries	3–3½ cups	60
Spelt berries	3 cups	55–70
Wheat berries	3 cups	55–70
Wild rice	3 cups	45–60

For all grains, rinse before cooking to remove any dust or other particles (amaranth and quinoa will need to be rinsed in a very fine strainer). To cook, simply combine the grain and cooking water, bring to a boil, then lower the heat to low, cover, and simmer for the specified time (per the chart). About 5 minutes before the cooking time is complete, check for doneness—the water should be almost totally absorbed and the grains tender. It is okay for a smidgen of extra water to remain, as it will absorb with standing time. Once the grains are cooked, remove from the heat and let stand covered for 4 to 5 minutes.

You can add a pinch or two of salt to grains while they cook, or choose not to season if you don't want the added salt. Other seasonings and aromatics can be added to grains during cooking.

Cooking times are meant as a guide, and can vary slightly. In general, if you shorten the cooking time, the grains will be firmer and chewier. If you increase the cooking time (adding a little more water), the grains will be softer.

Some grains (e.g., amaranth and amaranth) take on a nuttier flavor and are more separate and less sticky if toasted before cooking: simply add the dry grains to a dry skillet on medium heat and toast for 2 to 3 minutes, stirring occasionally, until there is a nutty aroma. You can also sauté them with a little olive oil before adding water.

Ingredients 411: Bulgur differs from cracked wheat in that cracked wheat is the raw wheat kernel that is cracked, whereas bulgur is the wheat kernel cracked after first steaming and then drying. The steaming precooks the bulgur, so it requires less cooking time and can also be eaten after merely soaking (until tender). You can cover bulgur with water and let soak for about an hour until tender; then it's ready to eat or use in recipes.

For millet, more water (3 cups or more) and a longer cooking time (25 minutes or more) will yield a softer, creamier texture; do not stir millet while simmering. For a fluffier texture similar to that of rice, use less water and a shorter cooking time.

Rinse quinoa before using to remove its natural bitter coating. Certain brands are prerinsed, but some bitterness may still remain. To be sure, rinse for several minutes.

Guide to Cooking Beans (Stovetop)

Legume	Cooking Time
Adzuki beans	45–60 minutes
Black beans	60 minutes
Black-eyed peas	45–60 minutes
Cannellini beans (white kidney)	60–90 minutes
Chickpeas (garbanzos)	1½–2 hours
Kidney beans (red) (see note)	1½–2 hours
Lentils (brown/green) (see note)	30–40 minutes
Lentils (Le Puy/French) (see note)	35–45 minutes
Lentils (red) (see note)	15–25 minutes
Mung beans (see note)	40–50 minutes
Navy beans	70–90 minutes
Peas, split (see note)	40–60 minutes
Pinto beans	60–90 minutes
Soybeans	3 hours

With the exception of lentils, mung beans, and split peas, dried beans should be soaked before cooking—it shortens the cooking time and helps improve the digestibility of the beans. You can either soak the beans overnight or do a "quick soak" (method follows). To soak overnight, first rinse the dried beans and remove any dirt, stones, particles, or beans that are split or shriveled. Combine three to four parts water with one part beans and soak for at least 6 hours. Then drain, rinse again, and proceed to cook (method follows).

To "quick soak" beans, first rinse the dried beans and remove any dirt, stones, particles, or beans that are split or shriveled. Combine three to four parts water with one part beans in a large pot. Bring to a boil on high heat, and let boil for 5 to 7 minutes. Turn off the heat, cover, and let sit for 1½ to 2 hours. Drain the beans and rinse again. Also, rinse out the cooking pot and wipe clean to remove any cooking residues. Then proceed to cook (method follows).

To cook beans, combine three to four parts water with one part presoaked beans (see note for exceptions to soaking) in a large pot. Bring to a boil on high heat, then lower the heat to low and simmer partially covered until tender, using the chart as reference. Ensure that the beans simmer, not boil, throughout the cooking time to prevent their skins from splitting. In general, 1 cup of dried beans will yield 2 to 2½ cups of cooked beans. Do not add salt or acidic ingredients such as lemon, vinegar, or tomatoes to the cooking water, as they will lengthen the cooking time; add them when the beans are tender. Aromatics such as onion and garlic can be added at the beginning of the cooking process, however.

Once the beans are cooked, they can be frozen for later use. (Be sure to cook the beans in large enough batches that you can freeze extra portions.) I usually freeze 2- or 3-cup portions in resealable plastic bags or other containers, as these are the amounts needed for most recipes. Ensure they have an airtight seal and are labeled to identify the type of bean and quantity.

To use frozen beans, simply thaw. To hasten the process, hold the container under hot running water for a few seconds to loosen. Alternatively, add a whole chunk of frozen beans to soups or stews, letting them thaw as the dish cooks. If you plan to puree them, you can place the frozen beans in a bowl and cover with some boiled water. Let sit until thawed, then drain before using.

Of course, canned beans can be used, but your own cooked beans (particularly organic) usually taste better. If using canned, always drain and rinse before using.

Ingredients 411: A note about digestibility: In general, beans that are classified as softer are easier to digest than are those classified as hard. Softer beans include lentils, adzukis, and black-eyed peas. Harder beans include cannellini, kidney beans, and chickpeas. Soybeans are the hardest bean to digest, but soy products such as tempeh and tofu are more digestible.

Red kidney beans contain a high concentration of a toxin called phytohaemagglutnin (don't ask me to pronounce it; just know if it looks this nasty, it probably is that nasty!). This toxin is also found in other bean varieties, but in much lower levels. Red kidney beans must therefore be thoroughly cooked at a high temperature, requiring boiling and not just simmering. With all dried beans, but especially red kidney beans, be sure to cook in fresh water (after soaking or quick-soaking through boiling), and then boil for at least 10 minutes, or longer, before simmering to continue cooking. Undercooked red kidney beans can induce nausea. Cooking from dried form in a slow cooker is not recommended because the low cooking temperature does not destroy the toxin, and undercooked beans are actually more toxic than when in their raw form. Canned red kidney beans are perfectly fine, as they have been precooked at high temperatures.

Lentils, mung beans, and split peas do not need to be presoaked. Just sort to remove any dirt, stones, or particles, rinse, and cook.

Metric
Coversions

The recipes in this book have not been tested with metric measurements, so some variations might occur.

Remember that the weight of dry ingredients varies according to the volume or density factor: 1 cup of flour weighs far less than 1 cup of sugar, and 1 tablespoon doesn't necessarily hold 3 teaspoons.

General Formula for Metric Conversion

Ounces to grams	multiply ounces by 28.35
Grams to ounces	multiply ounces by 0.035
Pounds to grams	multiply pounds by 453.5
Pounds to kilograms	multiply pounds by 0.45
Cups to liters	multiply cups by 0.24
Fahrenheit to Celsius	subtract 32 from Fahrenheit temperature, multiply by 5, divide by 9
Celsius to Fahrenheit	multiply Celsius temperature by 9, divide by 5, add 32

Volume (Liquid) Measurements

1 teaspoon	=	1/6 fluid ounce	=	5 milliliters
1 tablespoon	=	½ fluid ounce	=	15 milliliters
2 tablespoons	=	1 fluid ounce	=	30 milliliters
¼ cup	=	2 fluid ounces	=	60 milliliters
⅓ cup	=	2⅔ fluid ounces	=	79 milliliters
½ cup	=	4 fluid ounces	=	118 milliliters
1 cup or ½ pint	=	8 fluid ounces	=	250 milliliters
2 cups or 1 pint	=	16 fluid ounces	=	500 milliliters
4 cups or 1 quart	=	32 fluid ounces	=	1,000 milliliters
1 gallon	=	128 fluid ounces	=	4 liters

Volume (Dry) Measurements

¼ teaspoon	=	1 milliliter
½ teaspoon	=	2 milliliters
¾ teaspoon	=	4 milliliters
1 teaspoon	=	5 milliliters
1 tablespoon	=	15 milliliters
¼ cup	=	59 milliliters
⅓ cup	=	79 milliliters
½ cup	=	118 milliliters
⅔ cup	=	158 milliliters
¾ cup	=	177 milliliters
1 cup	=	225 milliliters
4 cups or 1 quart	=	1 liter
½ gallon	=	2 liters
1 gallon	=	4 liters

Weight (Mass) Measurements

1 ounce	=	30 grams		
2 ounces	=	55 grams		
3 ounces	=	85 grams		
4 ounces	=	¼ pound	=	125 grams
8 ounces	=	½ pound	=	240 grams
12 ounces	=	¾ pound	=	375 grams
16 ounces	=	1 pound	=	454 grams

Linear Measurements

½ in	=	1½ cm
1 inch	=	2½ cm
6 inches	=	15 cm
8 inches	=	20 cm
10 inches	=	25 cm
12 inches	=	30 cm
20 inches	=	50 cm

Oven Temperature Equivalents, Fahrenheit (F) and Celsius (C)

100°F	=	38°C
200°F	=	95°C
250°F	=	120°C
300°F	=	150°C
350°F	=	180°C
400°F	=	205°C
450°F	=	230° C

Acknowledgments

To my readers: I started this book because I felt such excitement and support after *Eat, Drink & Be Vegan*. You e-mailed and commented on my blog to thank me, and I am always grateful for this feedback. Your good spirits and support fueled my passion to keep on and to challenge myself even further with my recipes. I think I've brought my "A-game" in this book—I hope you do too!

To my testing squad: You ladies really strengthened my confidence in these recipes, and helped me fine tune those that needed it. I very much appreciate the time you put in to test recipes and give feedback, and also the genuine interest you have for my work. My sincere thanks to: Julie Tegg, Michelle Bishop, Jenni Mischel, Stefania Moffatt (and daughter Giorgia for some recipe-naming assistance!), Aimee Kluiber, Christina Marquis, Rebekah Youngers, Carrie Bagnell Horsburgh, Nora Kuby, Donna Forbes, Michelle Sorensen, Jenny Howard, Heather Davis, Sara Rob-

son Francoeur, Judy Panke, and Angie Ramsay.

To the talented cookbook author and photographer Hannah Kaminsky. You brought life to my recipes through your gorgeous photos. I am continually impressed by your skill and professionalism, and am grateful that you agreed to work on this project. It was lovely to develop a friendship with you, and I hope to work with you again.

To Julieanna Hever and Mark Reinfeld. Thank you for taking the time to review my book and for contributing your generous endorsement quotes.

To the group at Da Capo, and to Cisca Schreefel, Iris Bass, Timm Bryson, and Renée Sedliar in particular. Cisca: my gratitude for your organization and attention to detail with this book, and your understanding with my changes—as I can have many. Iris: for tackling those long hours of copyediting which eventually brought harmony to this book. Timm: For the impressive clean layout (in spite of how wordy my recipes are)! And finally to Renée . . . thank you for seeing my vision with me, for understanding my place in this cookery world, and for valuing the sweat and tears I put into my creations. I also greatly appreciate how you helped to shape my work better than I had imagined, all while injecting humor along the way; I've greatly enjoyed working with you.

To my sisters for not just supporting my projects, but also actually using and enjoying my recipes (Dayle, hit the Creamed Cheese Brownies with Salted Dark Chocolate Topping first)! And, to my friends—Tanya and Vicki especially—for being my sounding boards for ideas and my personal cheering squad. Tanya, one day we'll work out that tofu thing.

To my mother, who cooked many meals from scratch for six children. While I might not pass down your signature dishes to my family, I will pass the memories and love.

To my father. Though I only knew you in life for eleven years, I know you are with our family and our girls every day in spirit. I think you influenced my journey into this lifestyle with some of your own unconventional ways of thinking and living.

To my family. With utmost gratitude and love to my husband, Paul. Most importantly, I thank you for your selfless love and support as a husband and father (we are blessed). Next, for always showing appreciation for my hard work in the kitchen, whether it's a special dinner or burger night—*and* for your honesty with my edits and recipe trials. It must be tough to tell me if something needs improving! Finally, to our three strong, beautiful daughters—Hope, Bridget, and Charlotte. You give me the three best reasons to make nutritious, delicious foods from scratch every day. I love you so.

Index